Knowledge and Pain

At the Interface

Volume 84
A volume in the *Making Sense of* series
'Pain'

Probing the Boundaries

Knowledge and Pain

Edited by
Esther Cohen, Leona Toker, Manuela Consonni
and Otniel E. Dror

Rodopi

Amsterdam - New York, NY 2012

In Cooperation with the Mandel-Scholion Library
Scholion – Interdisciplinary Research Center in the Humanities and Jewish Studies
The Hebrew University of Jerusalem

The paper on which this book is printed meets the requirements of "ISO 9706:1994, Information and documentation - Paper for documents - Requirements for permanence".

ISBN: 978-90-420-3582-9
E-Book ISBN: 978-94-012-0857-4

Printed in the Netherlands

Table of Contents

Introduction: In Despite

Leona Toker and Esther Cohen

humani nihil a me alienum puto
- Terentius

Reasoning by analogy never gives more than a probability; yet there are numerous cases in which that probability is so high that it amounts to practical certainty.
- Henri Bergson

The Biblical statement that 'he that increaseth knowledge increaseth sorrow' (Ecclesiastes 1:18) may be read as a tragic view of the human condition: the more we learn of human history and life the clearer they emerge as histories of pain, and the stronger the tension between the hurt of knowledge and the anaesthetic effects of its enhancement.[1] Would the Solomonic proportionate relationship work if the terms were reversed? Does pain increase knowledge, does it expand, or, on the contrary, contract one's awareness and understanding of what is outside the self? Part of the reason for the notorious unavailability of pain to linguistic expression is that people with a direct knowledge of pain do not necessarily want to *give* their pain to others; what they want is for the other to *know that* there is pain, and possibly to act on this knowledge.

This volume reflects the work of a three-year long collaborative research sponsored by the Scholion Interdisciplinary Centre for Jewish Studies of the Hebrew University of Jerusalem and culminating in an international conference. The editors are grateful to the Scholion Centre for having granted generous support to this research even though its relationship to Jewish Studies is somewhat tangential. Indeed, the project deals with a common human predicament, some aspects of which can be usefully highlighted by a specifically Jewish historical experience. The findings of the project confirm the philosophically grounded intuition[2] that there is at least one way in which pain is conducive to the enhancement of knowledge: one's own pain, its *knowledge* in the sense of having experienced it, is a basis for recognition of the pain of the other. But one ought to see this possibility as contingent on the sort of humility that rejects the barriers between the self and the other, barriers that are all too often based on class, race, gender, level of education, ethnicity, religion or ideas of retributive and distributive justice. Empathetic recognition is usually analogic ('What she is going through I have also experienced'), but it may be enhanced by semiotic proficiency ('I think I know what this particular mannerism may stand for'). The empathetic knowledge thus largely depends, like all scientific or scholarly knowledge, on repetition, aggregation and replicability. One may never achieve the full understanding of the pain of another - we are prepared to grant that much. But we also say that given empathy, humility and repetition, one may, for all practical purposes, come close enough. 'Reasoning by analogy,' notes Henri Bergson, 'never gives more than a probability; yet there are numerous cases in which that probability is so high that it amounts to practical certainty.'[3] If the analogy involved is with our own suffering, then, in the words of Bernard Harrison, 'instead of thought contriving somehow to make sense of suffering, it may be that suffering makes sense of thought.'[4]

The connection between one's own pain and knowledge of the pain of others is brought into high relief by literary representations. Solzhenitsyn's *Gulag Archipelago*, for example, forcefully conveys the suffering of millions through the analogies between autobiographical episodes and numerous cases of experience of other prisoners as variants, often much harsher ones, of the author's own. Marguerite Duras's *The War: A Memoir* (*La Douleur*) situates the autobiographical persona's tormenting anxiety for her husband while his fate in the German concentration camps is unknown against a similar agony of others; she does not take any credit for uniqueness of her own suffering. In the same book by Duras, however, retributive justice becomes a pretext for the author's avatar to turn into a torturer under the delusion of a search for truth: a transformation that is likewise not unique.

If most survivors of concentration camps find it difficult to convey their memories to others, this is largely because of the radical difference between their experience and any past suffering that their audiences can recall for the sake of analogy. In the words of the writer Ka-Tzetnik, Auschwitz is 'another planet' - those who have been there need no explanation, while those who have not, must accept the limited scope of what it is in their power to imagine, despite the massive amount of data at their disposal. What we do know, however, is that withholding attention increases the sufferer's pain.

The International Association for the Study of Pain (IASP) has defined pain as 'an unpleasant sensory and emotional experience associated with actual or potential tissue damage, or described in terms of such damage.'[5] Emotional suffering that is not triggered by a sensory component evades this definition, as if it were a separate category. By contrast, in our attempt to map paths to the understanding of what is involved in the experience of pain, we suspend the distinction between the physical and the emotional pain or at least register the porousness of the dividing line between them.

The study of pain has a medical/neurobiological component and a cultural one; the present volume is devoted to the latter. The very distinction between pain and 'other unpleasant experiences, for example sadness, guilt or nausea,'[6] is culture-bound. The content of the semantic field of *pain* and the responses it elicits vary also with time and place. Indeed, the 'intricate experience' of pain and its treatments are 'culturally embedded. Moreover, the symbolic processes that interrelate body and self with meanings and relationships change as part of wider societal and cultural transformations.'[7] The chapters in this collection deal with the cultural embedding of pain and the socio-historical transformations in its perception and treatment. While the essays do not touch on the vast subject of Oriental perspectives on pain, the communities studied in the different chapters reflect the multiplicity of attitudes even in the one conceptual framework of 'Western culture.'

In the humanities, attitudes to pain in its relationship to knowledge fall into roughly two groups. One is the belief that pain, especially physical, is a totally negative experience, except when perceived as a warning symptom: pain reduces the sufferer's world, obliterating language, consciousness, and interaction. This position is represented by Elaine Scarry's *The Body in Pain* (1985). The other view, rooted in older concepts and partly refracted in David Morris's *The Culture of Pain* (1991), is that pain can lead to intellectual growth, moral benefit, soul-fashioning. This idea is often associated with varieties of religious practices[8] and is a subject of numerous literary explorations. Between these two diametrically opposite attitudes, discussed in more detail in the concluding part of Shlomith Rimmon-Kenan's chapter in this collection, one can situate a number of secular positions, as well as the religious born-again experience or, on the contrary, the experience of a religious crisis caused by suffering, the loss of faith - liberating for some yet tragic for others. Though the experience of physical pain is *ex tempore* perceived as 'tissue damage,' emotional suffering is more readily and more often associated with the opposite phenomenon, spiritual growth.

To put the question of the impact of pain on knowledge in another way, is our knowledge of the practical world (as well as the accumulated scholarship and science) a matter of delusion, a distraction from the 'real thing,' which *is* pain? Conversely, do pain and sorrow interfere with 'the real thing,' which is personhood, culture, knowledge, communication and understanding? The attitudes of chronic-pain patients and the doctors and anthropologists who treat them teeter on both sides of this divide; any generalising answer is vulnerable to counter-examples. One can, however, isolate a number of tendencies in the effects of suffering, responses to suffering and epiphenomena of these responses. A particularly vexed aspect of this issue, and likewise analysable only as a matter of tendencies, is, as noted above, the extent of one's knowledge of the pain of others, the roles of sympathy and empathy in achieving or responding to such introspection-based knowledge, the function of re-enactment, replicability or analogy in isolating the intersubjective area in a specific kind of suffering, the ethical obligations imposed by whatever limited awareness is attained. On the other side of the gap between the sufferer and the witness is the problem of the social capital: change in social status resulting from noticeable pain can be a partial compensation for pain, or its deplorable aftermath, or its epiphenomenon, positive or negative, as the case might be.

This volume examines the cultural and intellectual responses to physical and/or emotional pain from the perspective of analytic philosophy, phenomenology, history, oral history, history of science and literary criticism. The methodological common denominator of the chapters coming from these varied disciplines is the analogy in human experience (recorded in different disciplinary languages) that provides a critical mass for a discernment of widespread tendencies. What is shared delineates the contours of the intersubjective domains that can reduce (or partly make up for) what is essentially unknowable in the pain of another. Belief in some form of intersubjectivity is the root of all attempts to connect with the pain of the 'other.' Compassion, pity, sympathy, empathetic attention, attempts to help - all these are based upon our acknowledgement that others suffer and that we know that they do. The volume's emphasis on the replicability of the data is the rationale for the sequence of its materials: with the exception of the philosophical inquiry following this introduction, chapters are arranged not by artificially watertight disciplinary frameworks but by historical periods as marking intellectual and cultural contexts for intersecting views. In terms of methodological orientation and subject repertoire, the chapters about specific historical periods fall under the following rubrics: Antecedents, Reconceptualisations, Decodings, Epiphenomena, Narratives, and Images.

The first chapter in the volume is a philosophical examination of the issues of the knowledge of pain, another's and one's own. S. Benjamin Fink's 'Knowing Pain' discusses what can be meant by *knowing pain* and by *knowing that* there is pain in a specific given case. The former is based on having had a similar experience, but extrapolation from this experience, our knowledge of the presence of pain, especially in another person, is not reliable. Moreover, as Fink's deconstruction of the above-quoted IASP definition shows, pain is not a single concept but a plethora of concepts. Orientation among ideas of pain calls for a study not just of pain as a mental state but also of the contexts and relationships in which it is experienced. The collection pursues this agenda, maintaining awareness of mutually explanatory as well as potentially mutually obfuscating relationship between the general and the cultural/particular, as well as between the past and the present features of the human interactions in response to suffering.

The study starts with late medieval discourse formations as *antecedents* of modern views. Esther Cohen's chapter surveys medieval attitudes to the pain of others - the pain of religious martyrdom, the pain of illness and the pain of torture - in terms of the possibility of empathy with the sufferer on the part of the observer or of the person inflicting the pain. She demonstrates that emotional recognition of the pain of the other depended on the status of that other, in social, racial, moral/religious, or gender terms - no sympathy, for example, was to be accorded to the sinners in hell or criminals under torture. The dependence of participative emotion on the status of the sufferer is a comment that medieval history makes on modern times: 'The pain of the other may be intellectually apprehended, but empathy varies according to the manner in which we see the sufferer.' Conversely, distancing the sufferer morally or racially from oneself is an apt way of (and a justification for) pre-empting the interference of sympathetic response with the efficiency of the perpetrator's or even a bystander's agenda.

R. F. Yeager's chapter moves from the general feature of medieval attitudes to suffering towards a specific episode in the early modern artistic representation of pain. It deals with a case of the literary processing of the emotional pain of another - the handling of the Biblical story of Jephtah and his daughter in the work of Middle English poets Geoffrey Chaucer and John Gower. The exploration of the tragically clashing commitments in the literature and visual art of the period and of their codes for signalling pain demonstrates an empathic awareness of emotion; this constituted a new development in fourteenth-century culture. The chapter lends indirect support to Cohen's observation that empathy depended on the status of the sufferer, in this case, a kingly military leader and a proto-martyrial virgin.

The general and the individual tend to be conflated when it comes to prescribing treatment. Two late medieval healing professions addressed the pain of ordinary people: the medical establishment and the clergy. Na'ama Cohen-Hanegbi's chapter focuses on the notion of pain (*dolor*) as an emotion, the pain of the soul (*dolor animi*), and the pain of remorse (*contritio*), within both contexts. These types of pain are on the periphery of the established definition of pain yet they were perceived as legitimate objects of medical and spiritual succour. Nevertheless, the discourse around these kinds of suffering suggests not so much the healer's empathy with the sufferer as the imperative need to assert the healer's professional authority.

Whereas the vocabulary of the semantic field of pain in medieval texts points to limitations in the response to the pain of others, early modern *reconceptualisations* of pain suggest a broader spectrum of attitudes, a more complex awareness of different kinds of pain and a further subversion of the conceptual boundary between physical and emotional pain. One example of this expanded awareness is discussed in Michal Altbauer-Rudnik's chapter on the illness of love. The chapter follows the permutations of the medical diagnoses and definitions of lovesickness, concentrating upon the transition from its early modern varieties to modern erotomania and showing that the changes in the description and recommended treatment of the disease have been grounded in each specific socio-historical and scientific context. The social problems of unequal attachments in the seventeenth century are, for instance, a considerably weaker factor for twentieth-century troubled lovers; and, indeed, the aetiology of the disease has metamorphosed from frustrated love to delusional attachments.

The credibility of the accounts of suffering and the effectiveness of the calls for help likewise depended on the manner they were presented to their intended audience. Emotional rhetoric, it seems, is often a trope rather than proof of genuine sympathy towards sufferers. Michèle Bokobza Kahan's chapter deals with an extraordinary early eighteenth-century event: a series of miraculous cures at the grave of the noted Jansenist Deacon Pâris. The chapter discusses the manner in which the miracles are presented in the written account, concentrating upon the visualising rhetoric of the narrative and evaluating the impact of the detailed and frightful descriptions of female bodies in pain. The analysis shows that empathy with the sufferers is here not a goal in itself; it is placed in the service of a proselytising rhetoric, as is the repetitiveness of the aggregated material, which helps to simulate the results of empirical research. The effect of the collection of Jansenist testimonies is thus based both on the Enlightenment agenda of systematising knowledge and on the widespread cultural agenda of the expansion of sympathies, which made the empathetic appeal of the narratives serve its counter-rational goals. Once empathy with others became a norm, it could be transposed into a more disingenuous discourse.

The history of science shows that empathy eventually comes to embrace the other who is all too distinct from the self. Yet empathy does not become a dominant value. Nathaniel Wolloch's chapter investigates the attitudes of Enlightenment *savants* to the pain of animals: late eighteenth-century thinkers deplored the infliction of unnecessary pain on animals yet maintained the hierarchical view that prioritised human interests over those of animals. Whenever the comfort or needs of humanity required hurting animals and the cause of human progress was at stake, animal rights were seen as ethically sacrificed to this cause - pointing to the inescapable dialectics between the progressive refinement of humanitarian sensibilities on the one hand and the material conditions of human life along with its social structuring on the other.

With humanitarian sensibilities radically expanded, nineteenth-century literature and culture could afford to turn from continuing calls for sympathy to ways of *decoding* the presence and the nature of pain. In this collection the research into nineteenth-century approaches to understanding and registering pain is represented by two issues which may be seen as the bookends of a virtual library. Otniel E. Dror's chapter deals with what in nineteenth-century science was seen as a direct connection between affect and visceral-physiological processes. It is at this point in the history of science, when the visceral basis for emotions attracted sustained attention of the medical community, that the borderline between physical and emotional pain practically collapsed. The discourse on the physiology of emotions contributed to the expansion of the field of emotions beyond the existing vocabulary but also transformed the concept of the viscera: numerous processes on the visceral level were henceforth re-interpreted in terms of emotions. One of the consequences of this development was the physiologists' marginalisation of the spoken word, the overt gesture, and other exteriorisations of the psychologically felt.

Nineteenth-century scepticism concerning the expressibility of pain through verbal and body language (largely compensated for by the possibility of registering it through the data on visceral processes) provides a context for Natalia Pervukhina's chapter, which discusses the indirect, muted, coded literary expressions of pain in Anton Chekhov's stories and plays. The humdrum coding, which characterises Chekhov's treatment of pain foregrounds the possibility of miscommunication, of the readers' and characters' failure or reluctance to acknowledge suffering; this, in its turn, is associated with Chekhov's staging of miscommunications that express or lead up to a callous neglect of the pain of helpless old people among Chekhov's personages.

Twentieth-century literary audiences may be trusted to develop a semiotic proficiency to register and decipher the signals of a character's pain. Yet when the experience of pain transcends the normal expectancies, decoding can break down. Manuela Consonni's chapter shows that the suffering of another may be inaccessible to the imagination when ordinary language is found to be incommensurable with prolonged acute suffering, such as the pain of concentration-camp experience as described, in particular, by Charlotte Delbo and Primo Levi. Within concentration-camp realities, words such as 'hunger,' 'cold,' 'thirst,' 'shoes,' are endowed with meanings that are unthinkable under ordinary conditions of life in society. Literary memoir-narratives, the chapter shows, help the reader build up the worlds in which such words make sense in a different way, with death taking precedence over their denotative meanings and over ordinary habitual complexes of nuance and connotation. The experience of reading such narratives may still fail to create the imaginative leap from the world of the readers to that of the camp-inmate authorial personae, but it can, at least, enhance our intellectual awareness of semantic shifts in the wake of camp experience, as well as awareness of the limits of our capability for imaginative reconstruction of camp existence.[9]

The breakdown of culturally determined codes leads to individual explorations of the meaning of pain. Records of such explorations likewise reveal repeating patterns. Leona Toker's chapter deals with an *epiphenomenon* of the unbearable suffering within concentration camps: literary accounts of concentration-camp experience (the experience of the prisoners of the Gulag indirectly commenting on that of the Nazi camps, and vice versa) repeatedly present the breakdown of what the chapter calls 'folk theodicy.' Faith-based beliefs that under normal circumstances facilitate ethical orientation turn out to be inadequate for attempts to justify or come to terms with prolonged acute suffering.[10] In so far as knowledge is antithetical to faith-based certainties, pain may thus be said to enhance knowledge, but the mechanisms of the loss of faith and some of the fantasies that replace it are shown to have an affective rather than an intellectual base.

Moving back to pain as an ordinary part of the human condition, Paula Michaels's chapter deals with another epiphenomenon of pain - the rise and fall of the Lamaze method of controlling birth-pangs. Advocates of the psycho-prophylactic methods used to view any birth accompanied by pain as a failure of the parturient's mental strength to withstand what they considered psychogenic pain. The chapter goes on to trace the developments following the disenchantment with the promises of the Lamaze method in the late 1970s: the view of childbirth pain as normal was restored; links between it and weakness of character (or the original sin) were largely abandoned. By the end of the century, a growing percentage of parturient women on both sides of the Atlantic started to demanded pharmacological aid for pain.

The relationship of physical suffering and emotional distress is a pervasive motif of Anna Leimumäki's research into narratives of Finnish cardio-vascular patients. The common narrative patterns isolated in this bio-ethical oral-history research is further evidence of the replicability of human experience beyond the cultural stencils of its formatting and conceptualisation. The chapter demonstrates, among other things, how concepts developed in analyses of literary works can help a researcher construct the meanings inherent in non-literary illness narratives.

Shlomith Rimmon-Kenan's chapter discusses a specific autobiographically-based *literary* illness narrative, Christine Brooke-Rose's *Life, End of*, as a strikingly articulated expression of one way in which individual creativity transcends the experiential confines imposed by a cardio-vascular and neurological disease. Making use of Michel de Certeau's distinction between physical 'place' and the subjectively perceived and constructed 'space,' Rimmon-Kenan outlines the ways in which the spiritual life traced in Brooke-Rose's book transforms the narrowing down of the protagonist-narrator's physical location (place) into expanding spaces of her linguistic and philosophical inner freedom.

Rebecca Bitenc's chapter is devoted to literary narratives dealing with demented patients. Literary works present the intense suffering of the sick as subsiding in the progress of the illness; they also probe the possibility of compensatory stages. The chapter argues for seeing dementia patients as subjects in their own right, subjects of intrinsically interesting experience, rather than merely as factors in the lives of others. It also shows that though their painful experience remains essentially unknowable, the techniques of narrative fiction may have the power of simulating it and of giving the reader the sense of what this experience may be like.

Study of the dialectics of the individual and the common-human experience is continued in Nourit Melcer-Padon's chapter on David Grossman's novel *To the End of the Land* (*Ishah Borachat miBesorah*), a narrative in which individual experience is represented as reaching the boundary with the idiosyncratic. The chapter deals with improvisations in attempts to escape sorrow or pre-empt uncontrollable fatalities. In the novel these improvisations recurrently take the shape of lexical innovation which eventually turns out to be based on the intersubjective regularities that bind all the speakers of the language. The blending of the voices of the protagonists and the authorial narrator of the novel further suggests a resonance in the personal narratives of trauma and sorrow: for all the irreplaceable individual differences, there is a common path where individual life-stories meet.

Beyond the narratives of pain lie *images* of pain, and the ethics of their production, observation and recording. Rebecca Adelman's chapter critiques academic responses to the pictures of torture and humiliation that emerged from the Abu Ghraib military prison camp; she gazes back at the academic gaze and finds it ethically wanting. Adelman problematises the issue of empathy vs. distribution of blame and guilt as responses that either appropriate the suffering of another or obtund it, losing sight of the connections between the observer's emotional response (or lack thereof) and its intellectual processing. Indirectly the chapter also suggests that the absolutely blameless inner response to the images of another's suffering is a matter of ethical utopia, but this does not deny the possibility of humanitarian legislation and ethical codes.

The volume closes with another chapter on images - Ariela Freedman's exploration of the possibility to convey pain through the techniques of graphic narrative. As all the chapters on the literary representations of pain and its consequences show, the potential of the literary narrative in impressing the intensity of human pain on the reader (who is not invited to re-enact it) is sometimes a matter of hermeneutic perplexity. It is a challenge to normalize the extraordinary in human conduct or thought, only to discover that causality is not identical to norm. Yet a more direct (perhaps even psychedelic) transmission of the awareness of pain is likewise often a matter of techniques and devices specific to different art forms and unavailable to scientific and scholarly discourse. The subject of graphic narrative is particularly challenging in view of the tradition of representing sanitised painless violence in the genre of comics (Spiegelman's *MAUS* is a notable exception). The case for the availability of the genre for empathy and for evocation of genuine suffering is made on the material of

David Small's *Stitches: A Memoir.* That memoir, and the chapter about it, end on a note of hope, as does, in relation to the public sphere, Rebecca Adelman's chapter. Despite recidivistic replications of pain in human experience, the accumulating knowledge about it may help to keep it within bounds.

Thus the present collection of research-records partly sides with Elaine Scarry's negative estimation of the impact of pain on the sufferer's experience, yet it sees the positive influence of individual experience of pain in the growth of compassion as a social force. It traces the shifts of empathy from the suffering God, through the tragic pain of kings and heroes, to the pain of sufferers who are closer to oneself and to the ethics of response to remoter pain brought to our doorstep by narrative and image. It also points to the potential abuses of compassion when it becomes normative.

Though the research represented in this volume accepts the ultimate unavailability of full knowledge of the pain of another, it testifies to the success, albeit partial, of scholarly attention to the replicability of experience in improving our understanding of the suffering of others. It also shows some of the ways in which literary evocations of suffering can help lay the ground for unstructurable insights even into the ineffable facets of human pain. The horizon of this inter-disciplinary inquiry includes an attempt to translate pain as an epistemological problem into an ethical, social, and political challenge.

The editors are grateful to Israel Yuval, the founding director of Scholion Interdisciplinary Center of the Mandel Institute for Jewish Studies, for his unflagging attention, kind and demanding, to the work of the 'Knowledge and Pain' research group. We wish to acknowledge the advice of the peer reviewers, whose uncompromising standards have enhanced the value of the collection. We thank the current director of the Center, Daniel Schwartz, for timely input at the final stages of the work on the collection. The organisational and administrative support of Zohar Marcovich, and, at the final stages, Maya Sherman, facilitated the research for and the composition of this volume, as did the dedicated help of research assistants Adam Farkash and Michal Margalioth, and the technical support provided by Eti Mizrahi and by Scholion's computer wizard, Boris Patkin. Special thanks go to Hannah Landes for her thoughtful stylistic editing.

Notes

[1] Cf. Geoffrey Galt Harpham: 'To be human is to think, and thinking of suffering is the beginning of converting it into nonsuffering' ('Trading Pain for Knowledge, or, How the West Was Won,' *Social Research* 75 [2008]: 509). Yet Harpham is well aware that some forms of pain, one's own or

another's, are too overwhelming to be converted into knowledge even by the most dedicated volition (Ibid., 508).

[2] See, for instance, Bernard Harrison, 'Wittgenstein and Scepticism,' in *Meaning Scepticism*, ed. Klaus Puhl (Berlin: Walter de Gruyter, 1991), 34-69.

[3] Henri Bergson, *Mind-Energy* (Basingstoke: Palgrave Macmillan, 2007), 6.

[4] Bernard Harrison, *Inconvenient Fictions: Literature and the Limits of Theory* (New Haven: Yale University Press, 1991), 184.

[5] U. Lindblom et al. 'Pain Terms: A Current List with Definitions and Notes on Usage,' *Pain* 24 (1986): supplement 1, S217.

[6] Horacio Fabrega and Stephen Tyma, 'Culture, Language, and the Shaping of Illness: An Illustration Based on Pain,' *Journal of Psychosomatic Research* 20 (1976): 324.

[7] Arthur Kleinman et al., 'Pain as Human Experience: An Introduction,' in *Pain as Human Experience: An Anthropological Perspective*, ed. Arthur Kleinman et al. (Berkeley: University of California Press, 1992), 1-28.

[8] Ariel Glucklich's *Sacred Pain: Hurting the Body for the Sake of the Soul* (Oxford: Oxford University Press, 2001) is devoted to the latter connection. For an earlier attempt to deal with this problem, see Talal Asad, 'Notes on Body Pain and Truth in Medieval Christian Ritual,' *Economy and Society* 12 (1983): 288-98; reprinted in *Genealogies of Religion: Discipline and Reasons of Power in Christianity and Islam* (Baltimore: Johns Hopkins University Press, 1993), 83-124.

[9] Cf. Sara Liu's argument about the need of accepting one's own 'illiteracy' in respect to the Holocaust, 'The Illiterate Reader: Aphasia after Auschwitz,' *Partial Answers* 7 (2009): 319-42.

[10] The adverse effect of prolonged acute moral suffering on religious faith is also discussed in Yael Feldman's forthcoming article '"When my flesh decays . . . my lips cannot sing the praise of God": Agnon's Holocaust Critique of "Holy" Pain.'

Bibliography

Asad, Talal. 'Notes on Body Pain and Truth in Medieval Christian Ritual.' *Economy and Society* 12 (1983): 288-98; reprinted in *Genealogies of Religion: Discipline and Reasons of Power in Christianity and Islam*, 83-124. Baltimore: Johns Hopkins University Press, 1993.

Bergson, Henri. *Mind-Energy*. Translated by H. Wildon Carr. Edited by Keith Ansell Pearson and Michael Kolkman. Basingstoke: Palgrave Macmillan, 2007.

Fabrega, Horacio, Jr., and Stephen Tyma. 'Culture, Language and the Shaping of Illness: An Illustration Based on Pain.' *Journal of Psychosomatic Research* 20 (1976): 323-37.

Glucklich, Ariel. *Sacred Pain: Hurting the Body for the Sake of the Soul.* Oxford: Oxford University Press, 2001.

Harpham, Geoffrey Galt. 'Trading Pain for Knowledge, or, How the West Was Won.' *Social Research* 75 (2008): 485-510.

Harrison, Bernard. *Inconvenient Fictions: Literature and the Limits of Theory*. New Haven: Yale University Press, 1991.

———. 'Wittgenstein and Scepticism.' In *Meaning Scepticism*, edited by Klaus Puhl, 34-69. Berlin: Walter de Gruyter, 1991.

Kleinman, Arthur, Paul E. Brodwin, Byron J. Good, and Mary-Jo DelVecchio Good, editors. *Pain as Human Experience: An Anthropological Perspective*. Berkeley: University of California Press, 1992.

Lindblom, U., H. Merskey, J. M. Mumford, P. W. Nathan, W. Noordenbos, and S. Sunderland. 'Pain Terms: A Current List with Definitions and Notes on Usage.' *Pain* 24 (1986): supplement 1, S215-S221.

Liu, Sarah. 'The Illiterate Reader: Aphasia after Auschwitz.' *Partial Answers* 7 (2009): 319-42.

Morris, David. *The Culture of Pain*. Berkeley: University of California Press, 1991.

Scarry, Elaine. *The Body in Pain: The Making and Unmaking of the World*. Oxford: Oxford University Press, 1985.

Knowing Pain

S. Benjamin Fink

Abstract
We might have different projects in mind when we ask whether we know pain. Can I know what someone else is going through when they say they are feeling pain? Do you and I always know that we are in pain when we are in pain? Can we know something about pain in general, about its essence, what makes it a pain? In nursing, McCaffery's Principle states that pain is whatever a patient says it is whenever the patient says it is. But this principle, while being morally cautious, is no guideline for knowledge. This article queries the epistemic strength of knowledge-claims about pain from different perspectives, such as the definition of the International Association for the Study of Pain. I assess how accurate we may be given such existing pain phenomena as pain asymbolia, emotional pain, or Weltschmerz. One of the conclusions derived is that the phenomena grouped under the label 'pain' are not homogeneous, which challenges a mono-disciplinary pain science and undermines the strength of most of our knowledge claims concerning pain. I close with an outlook on the limits of our knowledge about pain and suggest that currently marginalised methods in pain science may help to improve our knowledge about pain in general in the light of the heterogeneity of phenomena labelled 'pain'.

Key Words: Epistemology of pain, homogeneity of pain, pain asymbolia, pain ascription, self-ascription of pain, IASP definition of pain.

*****

1. Introduction

Do you know what I feel when I tell you I am in pain? I hope so, especially if you are my doctor or nurse. But hope is a poor guide to knowledge: I hope that I will not die, but we all know that death is inevitable. So, do I know that you and I agree on what pain is?

Much depends on whether we know what pain is or is not, but, depending on our roles, we have different goals in mind. Pain scientists want to know the nature of pain and its connection to our body's activity, anatomy and chemistry. Caregivers want to know what you are going through so they can treat you accordingly: is it an intense and burning pain? Can you localise it? Does it spread? Are you confusing a pressure experience with pain? Might you even be a hypochondriac? All this matters for providing the right treatment. Lastly, your friends and family want to relate to your suffering. Sometimes, they may excuse your misbehaviour because you are in intense pain: think of a wife swearing at her husband while she is in labour, or a father cursing in front of his kids after hitting his thumb with a hammer. In some sense, even adequate empathy for pain is connected to knowledge about pain since it requires a similarity between your experience and my idea of that experience. If my idea of your pain is one of a little tingle while you are suffering immensely, my empathy is likely to seem shallow or even sarcastic to you.

So, do we know pain? Let me offer three interpretations of the question: (1) Can we know what someone is experiencing when they use the expression 'pain' or its synonyms? (2) Do I know when I myself am in pain? (3) What can we know about pain in general and what may be the limits of our knowledge?[1]

Nothing seems to be clearer to ourselves than the feeling of pain. There is, some philosophers claim, such a self-intimating moment in experiencing pain that we immediately know that we are in pain: there is no feeling pain without knowing that you are in pain.[2] Pain is epistemically luminous: it 'shines' so brightly that we are automatically informed when we have it.[3] Conversely, our beliefs about pain can be seen as transparent: whenever I believe that I am in pain, I am in pain. That at least is a standard assumption in healthcare: '[p]ain is whatever the experiencing person says it is, existing whenever he says it does,' writes Margo McCaffery.[4] We immediately see through the belief to the referent that the belief pertains to. Being in pain and believing to be in pain suggests knowledge that we are in pain.

A belief about one's pain is, thus, self-warranting: if one has this belief, it is true and justified.[5] So the answer to (2) would be positive. If we ask somebody whether she is in pain and, if she answers without wanting to deceive, we know that she is in pain. Yet, we do not know what kind of pain she is in or what this pain is like. This may be revealed by further description. Or my belief that her pain is like that may be warranted by her present and my past pain experiences being identical in quality. If people answer truthfully or if qualities are shared, the answer to (1) is also positive. If pain truly is such a self-intimating phenomenon, then—concerning (3)—there seem to be very few boundaries to what we might know about it.

Unfortunately, the story is more complicated. In a slightly different context, Fred Dretske provides strong reasons for doubting the connection of the self-intimating aspect of pain and knowledge about pain: we must distinguish between awareness of things and awareness of facts.[6] Things are linguistically expressed in nominal phrases, like 'ball' or 'the woman my father married.' Facts, on the other hand, are linguistically expressed in sentences, like 'My father married a woman.' The knowledge demanded by the three questions posed above is knowledge that or propositional knowledge: when you have knowledge that, then you have (at least in the classical picture of knowledge) a justified true belief.[7] Beliefs are stances or attitudes a person has towards a proposition: you think that a proposition p is true. In the case of knowledge, p is actually true. As an example, consider me knowing that I am short-sighted. For the sentence to be knowledge, it actually has to be true—I really have to be short-sighted to know that I am short-sighted. That is why knowledge can be called a factive mental state.[8]

Knowledge of things is not propositional; it is not knowing that. Consider the sentences 'I know Bob,' 'I know Paris,' or 'I know karate.' These sentences seem to express a kind of knowing how: that we know how Bob acts, we know how to get around in Paris, and we know how to chop boards in half with bare hands. Compare this with a different kind of knowledge, knowing what-it-is-like, which is knowledge of the qualitative feeling of mental states: knowing what it is like to eat cheesecake or knowing what it is like to dream of flying.[9] Regarding the knowledge of pain, it seems obvious that the knowing subject has to have had the experience. An analgesic, somebody who is unable to feel pain, cannot know what it is like to have pain, even though she may have complete propositional knowledge. She may understand the phrase and have an idea about it due to others telling her, but in a way her understanding of pain resembles the understanding of colour by a blind person.[10]

Strictly speaking, one cannot know what another's pain is like because nobody can have another person's pain: the subject being in pain is an inextricable part of the pain experience. This does not exclude the possibility that there are resemblances, shared structures or properties, between different people's pain experiences. We can state that our pains share properties, but this transcends knowing-what-it-is-like: stating identities between properties two objects are having is propositional, not phenomenal knowledge. We are back at knowing that.

Therefore, our three questions aim at knowing that. Thus, even if awareness entails knowledge, awareness of pain must be awareness of a fact to entail this kind of knowledge. When we ask the last question—what can we know about pain?—we ask also for general facts about pain, e.g. the fact that pain is a mental state or that pain is unpleasant. However, when we stand in such an intimate relation to the state of pain, we relate to an object, namely the mental state of hurting. We do not stand in the same relation to a general fact: in the moment you feel pain, you do not experience pain as a mental state, that is, you do not experience that pain belongs to a larger class of objects such as thoughts, emotions and desires. The arguments from self-intimacy do not bring us any closer to answering the three questions above: our awareness of pain is the awareness of a thing; and even if awareness necessarily leads to knowledge, it does not lead to the propositional knowledge needed for understanding somebody else's pain or knowing something scientifically about pain.

We must therefore focus on propositional knowledge. (1) partly rests on whether everyone assents to the same analysis of 'pain.' Any accepted analysis of 'pain,' e.g. the definition by the International Association for the Study of Pain (IASP), can be the starting point of this inquiry. But that two people must assent to a similar analysis has been questioned on pragmatic grounds in nursing—for example, by Margo McCaffery's statement that pain is whatever the patient says it is. If this is the way pain scientists and healing professionals approach their target phenomenon, we also ought to consider use-conditions of the term 'pain.'[11] Wittgenstein mentions use conditions of 'pain' in the Philosophical Investigations numerous times, specifically concerning what makes sense to say and what does not.[12] I am not in a position to add a meaningful exegesis of my own; therefore I follow a different methodology: I contrast documented usages of the phrase with one of the most successful analyses of 'pain', the IASP definition.

2. What Is This Thing Called Pain?

The definition of the International Association for the Study of Pain (IASP) has determined our scientific understanding of pain since 1986. No textbook on pain does without it. It reads:

> Pain: an unpleasant sensory and emotional experience associated with actual or potential tissue damage or described in terms of such damage.[13]

There are four good reasons to accept this as a fitting analysis of our concept of pain. First, it is intuitive: most of us assent to this analysis without further theoretical reflection or scientific training—it simply mirrors our usage as laypersons. This makes it a *real* definition that reflects our way of speaking in contrast to a *nominal* definition, where we define arbitrarily, e.g. 'justice' as 'every prime number larger than 13.'[14] Second, the definition is scientifically useful. By stating the parts of pain, the definition suggests which sciences contribute to our understanding of pain, e.g. sensory neuroscience, affective psychology, etc. If a phenomenon is complex, it has been a successful strategy in the past to 'divide and conquer.'[15] Third, the definition clearly covers our most paradigmatic pain experiences: broken bones, headaches, stomach aches, muscle cramps, labour pains, toothaches, and so on. Lastly, as a real definition, it is fallible. The IASP recognizes this. In a footnote to the definition we find:

> Many people report pain in the absence of tissue damage or any likely pathophysiological cause. … If they regard their experience as pain and if they report it in the same ways as

> pain caused by tissue damage, it should be accepted as pain.[16]

The generality of the IASP definition is thus under threat from non-standard usage of the term. If we hold on to the thesis that 'pain' picks out a homogeneous group of phenomena, we have to change the definition in light of such usage: if a sufficiently large portion of our community of speakers use the expression 'pain' without assenting to specific parts of the definiendum, such as actual or potential tissue damage, we could conclude that this is not a necessary part of our idea of pain. This encourages us to test the applicability of the IASP definition in fringe cases. Influential as the IASP definition is, it does not pass this test.

A class of fringe cases leads to the rejection of parts of the IASP definition as necessary. To refute a connection to hedonic valence (pleasantness or unpleasantness) in general, we may refer to pain asymbolia.[17] Patients with this pathology do feel pain: they can report about their pain threshold, their pain's location and its intensity.[18] What is lacking in pain asymbolia is pain's motivational impetus, its emotional force. A telling example comes from a surgeon working in India, whose patient suffered under extreme vaginal cramps, so painful that she turned to brain surgery for relief. After the surgery was performed with a simple wire (!), she stopped complaining about pain. Years later, the surgeon visited her again and asked about her pain-free life. She answered:

> 'Oh, yes, it's still there [the pain]. I just don't worry about it anymore.' She smiled sweetly and chuckled to herself. 'In fact, it's still agonizing. But I don't mind.'[19]

This account is coherent with other reports by pain asymbolics, who show no sign of rational or linguistic impairment as well. Apparently, something in their experience is sufficiently pain-like to be worthy of the label 'pain.' This dissociation of pain affect and evaluation from pain sensation is not limited to neural pathologies: pain felt while in a hypnotic trance (e.g. during dentistry), can be experienced as such while lacking any motivation for action;[20] sitting pains during meditation can be calmly attended to without emotional evaluation or distress. An experience has to be neither unpleasant nor emotional to be considered pain.

Let me then focus on association with tissue damage, which bears a conceptual problem. Association is an arbitrary cognitive act: anything can be associated with anything else. There is nothing wrong with associating Freud with mothers, Donald Duck with Nixon, or triangles with tissue damage. Still, we rightly hesitate to call images of triangles 'pain,' even when they are associated with tissue damage. The association with tissue damage is therefore not sufficient for pain, but is it necessary?[21] If it were necessary, pain illusion, like the thermal-grid illusion (the Thunberg illusion), ought to be impossible: placing your hand on a grid of alternating cool and warm bars results in a strong pain sensation, yet the grid does not even potentially provoke tissue damage.[22]

Perhaps it is the feeling as if one's tissue is damaged that ought to count. This, however, still does not cover emotional, social and cognitive pains. Such expressions are part of our everyday language (which is used by scientists as well).[23] Consider emotional pain due to the loss of a loved one, either by death or divorce. This feeling of grief is not associated with tissue damage—yet it still seems natural to talk of pain. Association with tissue damage is therefore not amongst the necessary use conditions.

Nor does pain present itself as a language-like mental state analogous to a belief or thought. A feeling of pain does not need description to become a pain. That we ascribe pains to beings deemed incapable of language-like mental states supports this. Otherwise no baby, animal, or mentally disabled human could be said to have pains. Apart from our intuitions, there is also no scientific support for language being a component of pain: significant overlap between those areas in the brain associated with language and those correlating with pain has not been shown. The activity of nociceptor activation spreads over the thalamus to the insular cortex, the anterior cingulate cortex, as well as the primary and secondary somatosensory cortex.[24] The most prominent neural substrates of language are Broca's area, Wernicke's area, the supramarginal gyrus, the angular gyrus and the primary auditory cortex.[25] Although there might be some overlap in the supramarginal gyrus, the neural evidence that pain and language are tightly connected is slim at best. Furthermore, description of pain usually *follows* pain. To make description a necessary condition of one's pain experience therefore matches neither the neuroscientific data nor phenomenology.

But what if the description of pain need not come from the person in pain herself? Some researchers, especially those with sociological, relativist or constructivist tendencies, argue that it is the acknowledgement of pain *by others* that brings pain into existence.[26] Only if someone else can or does describe a pain, it exists. Pain, in this picture, is socially constructed. Obviously, some cultural influences have been recorded. In the O-Kee-Pa hanging ritual, for instance, a person is suspended by hooks through the skin of the chest, resulting in an extremely intense pain. This ritual pain, part of the Mandan culture, is desired for spiritual reasons.[27] Yet, even here we find a core which is not culturally but biologically determined. Claiming an exclusively social construction of pain by acknowledgement would be tantamount to thinking that there has not been any pain throughout evolution until socialisation of higher primates—a stark contrast to our idea of pain being an alarm system with evolutionary advantage. A strong social constructivist view also ignores evidence that parts of the pain matrix can be traced back to simple life forms such as ringworms.[28] Therefore, description by others should not count as a necessary component for pain any more than description by the sufferer herself.

The IASP definition has thus shrunk to a sensory experience—which pain is in paradigmatic cases. But consider such literary usages as Jean Paul's *Weltschmerz.*[29] It describes a painful emotion due to the world's balefulness and one's incapability to change it. This mental state, which incorporates a complex set of beliefs about oneself and the state of the world, does have accompanying sensations, but these vary and need not be of any specific sensory modality such as sound, sight or nociception. The term *Weltschmerz* has caught on since the 19th century, which suggests that it is meaningful to many people. If *Weltschmerz* is 'pain,' as the etymology suggests, then pain is not necessarily limited to sensory experience. And if the tie to sensory modalities breaks down, we are left with pain as an experience—which is too unspecific to be helpful.

Is the IASP definition of pain at least sufficient? Imagine the following scenario: Gertrude, an analgesic, insensitive to pain from birth, cannot feel and has never felt any pain in her life. One morning, she wakes up in a hotel, and scrapes her hand on the rough plaster of the wall. Seeing the fresh blood on her knuckle right after waking up angers her. The anger and the sight of blood are unpleasant to her, and both are associated with tissue damage on her hand. Even though Gertrud fulfils all conditions for the IASP definition, she still feels no pain.

If the IASP's use-conditions for 'pain' are neither necessary nor sufficient, we are forced to give up the assumption of homogeneity: we are dealing with a varied field of phenomena grouped together only by loose resemblance. Pain is not one but a family of phenomena. How does this affect our knowledge of pain in ourselves and others?

3. Knowing Pain?

We have now seen how much difference there is in the usages of pain expressions and mental states associated with them, from sensational pain asymbolia to cognitive-affective Weltschmerz. The first conclusion has been that pain is not a homogeneous type. How does this affect our knowledge about pain? Clearly, we might confuse knowledge about one subtype of pain with knowledge about another. This raises the question: how justified are we in our knowledge claims about pain? How safe is our propositional knowledge about pain?

Safety has become a technical term in modern epistemology. To determine the safety of a knowledge claim, we consider closely resembling alternate scenarios and see with how little change knowledge turns into false belief. Under safety, if someone knows that p, then she believes that p when p is true in (nearly) all alternate scenarios in which she forms her belief in the same manner as she forms her belief in the actual scenario.[30] Consider the Chicken Sexer Case: it is notoriously difficult to determine the sex of a freshly hatched chicken, therefore experts in sexing chicks are highly valued in factory farms.[31] One of these professionals, Gladys, thinks she reliably tells the sex by smell, while her colleague Dorothy thinks she does it by weight. Let us assume that there is only one way to reliably tell the sex of a chick, and that is by smell. An *internalist* in matters of justification does not ascribe knowledge about the sex of a specific chick to Dorothy, as she is internally unjustified—she believes the wrong justification, namely that she sexes by weight, while *externalists* do claim knowledge for Dorothy: even if she is not aware of it, she still has the sense of smell that allows for proper sexing. How much do we need to change to see if Gladys's and Dorothy's knowledge about the sex of a specific chick is safe? Not much: a runny nose is a minor change in the scenario, yet it might make all the difference.

Considering such alternate scenarios is a powerful philosophical tool: besides asking whether we can know something about pain—and obviously, we sometimes know something about pain—we add the question whether our possible knowledge is safe. We are able to distinguish knowledge from believing truly simply because we are lucky, by asking whether our claimed justification is sensitive to the changing situation. If it is, then we know; if it is not, then we do not know.

4. Can We Know What Someone Is Experiencing when They Say 'Pain'?

What may be the inner procedure we use to form a belief about the experience that another person is having when she is talking about pain? We might consider an analysis or theory of pain. The IASP definition covers at least paradigmatic cases—statistics is on its side—but it cannot claim *safe* knowledge, especially not when we are facing a pain asymbolic, a person in grief, or someone feeling *Weltschmerz*. They all use the expression 'pain,' but this usage does not convey enough to know safely what the experience is like, whether it is more sensational, cognitive, or affective. Even if I bracket a theory-based account and simply pose my own pain as a pseudo-referent of her utterance, I cannot claim safe knowledge: there might only be minimal resemblance between her and my pain. The usage of 'pain' alone neither suggests nor rejects this possibility: our knowledge of the pain of others based on the usage of the linguistic expression is unsafe. Yet, the probability that our belief is accurate may be heightened by further independent sources such as non-verbal and contextual constraints: observing body language and attending to the social and psychological context of a subject in pain do much more work than hearing the word 'pain.'[32] Pain asymbolics, for example, show less facial grimacing when in pain even as they report pain verbally.[33]

5. Do I Know when I Myself Am in Pain?

The question about propositional self-knowledge concerning pain (knowing that I am in pain) is complicated by a lack of research about the connection of an experience and the conceptualisation of this experience. There may be no method at all. Instead, there may be immediate processes, like mental pointing, attention or inner perception. If so, are our abilities to conceptualise our experience as reliable as we might think?

Ned Block has introduced a distinction between phenomenal consciousness ('phenomenal' being the property by which something has experiential character) and access consciousness ('access' being the property by which a mental state can influence other mental states such as beliefs, emotions or behavioural dispositions). According to Block, this distinction is supported by empirical findings as well as by conceptual analysis.[34] Consider, for example, change blindness: a subject is presented with a complex stimulus, e.g. a scene at the market. After a short switch to grey, the same picture is flashed again but with a detail changed, e.g. the colour of the trousers of one of the vendors. It takes most people quite some time to realise what specifically has changed (therefore: change blindness). Though you sense that a change in your experience has occurred, this experiential change is inaccessible to belief formation at the time of its occurrence.[35] If there is a difference between attending and experiencing, it seems at least possible that you will have an experience of pain to which you are not attending, and therefore may not conceptualise it. If someone has a headache while watching a thriller that person may at first be preoccupied with this pain, but as the suspense rises in the movie, she is increasingly drawn into the story—until she forgets about her headache. Does she still have a headache if she is not attending to it? There is at least the conceivable possibility that pain is still present. Some minor pains may be below the threshold and are not conceptualised at all. If so, there might be a pain that one does not know that one is having it. Therefore, that pain is not *luminous*.[36]

This means that when one is in pain, one is not necessarily aware that one is in pain. But how about wrongly believing that one is in pain? How about transparency? Our intuitions deny this possibility: if I believe I am in pain, I am in pain. Nursing manuals promote this view: the subjects are always right about their pain—remember Margo McCaffery. In the practice of nursing, giving the subject such an authority may well be justified for pragmatic and moral reasons: we do not want a person to remain in pain even if we might have to nurse a few hypochondriacs from time to time. But this pragmatic stance does not apply to self-ascription. One reason to doubt transparency of pain beliefs—being in pain whenever I believe that I am in pain—is misconceptualisation. Consider the spiciness of hot food, produced by capsaicin, which occurs naturally in chilli peppers. Most consider this experience a taste—it tastes hot or spicy—but this chemical compound docks to the nociceptors of the tongue, the dedicated pain receptors: on the transducer level the experience of chilli ought to count as pain. Amongst tastes, spicy hotness is unique: imagine the sugariness of candy in the corner of your eye. This is hard for most people. Now imagine the spicy hotness of a chilli in your eye. This comes easy to most. You would not hesitate to call this imagined experience pain. By parity, the 'taste' of spicy hotness of food should also be considered as pain on the introspective level. If it is possible to mislabel the taste of spiciness as pain, why should it not be possible that the concept 'pain' is misapplied in other cases as well? Allow me another example: at the dentist's, my friend Jonas' jaw was sedated, and the dentist asked him whether a certain procedure was painful. Jonas winced in reply. 'That is not pain,' said the dentist, and suddenly pushed his instrument under the teeth-ridge: '*That* is pain.' What is remarkable is not the sadism of a licensed dentist, but Jonas' comment: 'The dentist was right; I did not feel pain before, only pressure.' The misattribution of the concept of pain is therefore plausible. Since such cases exist, our own self-ascriptions of pain—believing that I am in pain now—might be neither transparent nor (even if true) as safe as intuitively expected. Pain's privacy (only I myself can be the proper judge of whether I am in pain) makes it hard to evaluate the degree of safety of our knowledge about it. Intuitively, these cases seem marginal, yet how marginal they are is still an open question.

6. What Can We Know about Pain?

Our insight into the non-homogeneous diversity of the phenomena commonly subsumed under 'pain' and our limited understanding of the pain of others as well as our own pain affects our knowledge of the nature of pain in general. 'Nature' may be understood in two ways. As a metaphysical notion, 'nature' refers to the essential properties that make an entity what it is, in this case: pain. But pain experience also relates to our biological nature, in the sense of our evolutionary history and neural make-up.

The metaphysical notion has already been subverted by the failure of the IASP definition: necessary conditions for something to be subsumed under 'pain' (other than it being a mental state) cannot be found. If there are no identity criteria for pain, it may follow that pain does not exist—'no entity without identity.'[37] We meet this challenge by giving up the homogeneity assumption, that is, by regarding pain as not one but many different kinds of experience, grasped by a plethora of concepts grouped together by family resemblance where no single feature is universally shared under one term at the surface: 'pain.'

There are still facts that we can know about this group as a whole even if they do not suffice for a definition, e.g. that every pain is a mental state. Knowing that more than one kind of phenomena fall under 'pain,' we lean toward sub-categorisation. That is, we may know the nature of pain (a), pain (b), pain (c), etc. At the moment, we are far from grasping all of these sub-phenomena. Progress towards such knowledge must involve expanding our awareness of the different contexts of pain phenomena and of the subtle differences between them in different cultures and periods. Historical, ethnological and anthropological studies will further our ability to distinguish sub-phenomena of pain. On the other hand, literature, oral history and visual representations may further broaden our horizon of what is possible in pain. This inquiry may never be exhausted, especially since some possible categories of pains may have not yet been felt or conceptualised by humans.[38] Using only one's own pain as a study object, as in auto-phenomenological enquiry, sacrifices statistical significance and may even enforce stereotypes, since a single person is not likely to experience all subtypes of pain.

Our inquiry into the biological nature of pain faces similarly grave problems: if we cannot know in which sub-type of pain a person is, we cannot yet determine what the specific neural correlate of that specific type of pain is. Scanning 230 patients may reveal certain regularities in neural activation, yet we might overlook subtle difference in this averaging process: 42 of them might have pain-type (a), while 37 are in pain (b), with the rest being in pain (c), except 3 being in a rare pain (d). Examining each group separately could reveal different correlates, but our proven weak categorisation skills might hide a vast diversity, e.g. under the label 'pain (a)', which now will all be correlated with only one shared type of neural activation pattern. This is not a problem of neuroscience per se, but of our impaired classificatory access to our own mind—we have not yet provided the concepts that neuroscience can reduce.[39] The best strategy may be to use multiple and independent methods and triangulate the findings.[40]

Revealing minimally sufficient neural correlates is one of the most central goals in the quest for the neural substrates of pain experiences—experiences without description, conceptualisation or belief. Without minimal sufficiency, our results do not reflect what we are looking for, namely the neural correlates of pain experience, not (pain experience + x). If we were to mistake the correlate of (pain + conceptualisation) as the correlate for pain, we might ignore the pain of non-lingual beings like babies, animals or the comatose. Focusing on (pain + x) instead of just pain may side-track us in our search for the phylogeny of pain. There must have been a break-off point in our ancestry: somewhere between single-cell organisms and higher primates like homo sapiens there was a mental quantum leap after which animals could feel pain. Searching for this dividing line is crucial for animal ethics as well as for animal experiments in pain research. Emphasis on (pain

+ x) may exclude animals from the group of pain-feelers. A prominent example is the discussion of the pain of fish: James D. Rose argues that in humans pain experience has its basis in thalamo-cortical loops of activation; as fish have no cortex, they cannot have thalamo-cortical loops, and they therefore cannot feel pain.[41] This is wrong: the same capacity may be instantiated in two different ways, e.g. in two different brain areas (e.g. after a stroke, other brain areas take over, to some extent, the duties of injured areas), in different brains (e.g. your and my brain both instantiate the ability to understand language), or in a brain and a silicon chip (e.g. calculating). Philosophers call this feature of the mind *multiple realisability*.[42] It does not follow directly from the lack of a certain brain anatomy that a type of experience is impossible for this brain: pain may be differently instantiated in fish than in humans. Rose is conflating a sufficient condition—having a cortex—with a necessary condition. A multi-facetted approach in contrast to a solely neural one in assessing pain in non-humans may minimise such mistakes. Dale Langford and his colleagues, for instance, have established a facial coding system for mice to determine the severity of their pain on the basis of facial expressions like whisker or ear position.[43] Again, the multi-facetted nature of pain seems to favour methodological pluralism and epistemic triangulation over single-method-approaches, including neural or auto-phenomenological ones. Any scientific approach is merely a honing in to truth and knowledge, if one believes Popper.[44] The main issue for philosophers in this multi-disciplinary and multi-methodological quest is how to structure this discourse and distinguish valid from invalid trans-disciplinary critique.

7. Our Limits and Our Prospects

So far, my assessment of our ability to gain knowledge about pain has been grim. Even our most intuitive, paradigmatic and scientific take on the phenomenon, the IASP definition, fails in a broad range of cases, from eating spicy food to pain asymbolia, from Weltschmerz to the anger of an analgesic about her scratch. Even if we are sometimes right in our diagnosis of what others feel when they say that they feel pain, our knowledge of another's pain is not strictly safe. The same applies to knowing our own pains, as pain is not luminous and our beliefs about our pains are not necessarily transparent. This limits our prospect of knowing pain with the help of science, auto-phenomenology, introspection or empathy alone.

I therefore recommend that we give up the assumption of homogeneity. To know more about different pains means also learning a more fine-grained vocabulary to describe and distinguish them from each other and from other experiences in general. We should not see pain as having only an internal structure (as the IASP definition suggests), but be open to the idea that what makes pain a pain is reliant on other concurrent mental states. Further research questions should pertain to contexts: When and why does a person use a pain expression? When are they only metaphorical? When is some pain welcomed and desired? When is pain despised? Studies of extra-phenomenal contexts, those that stand outside the experience of the subject in pain—linguistic, social, ethnological and cultural ones—can complement other extra-mental approaches such as neurology or pharmacology, as well as the study of intra-phenomenal contexts which may reveal which phenomena co-occur 'in' the subject. The study of pain should not be confined to the mental state of pain and its inner structure; it should take into account ways in which this state is embedded in our situation and our mind when feeling pain. Triangulation of conceptual, contextual and neuroscientific tools may lead to the breakthroughs we hope for.

Notes

[1] These questions relate to three central debates in philosophy: (1) our knowledge of other minds, (2) self-knowledge and the epistemic status of self-ascriptions, and (3) our knowledge of the metaphysical nature of specific mental states. These three questions also have a highly practical impact on nursing, pain treatment and bedside dialogues. That talking to a patient may actually inform a diagnosis is an indicator that at least (1) can be answered affirmatively; there is at least *something* that we can know about *that specific individual pain* when the person who experiences it talks about it. It also suggests that there is at least some answer for (3). Quite probably, answers on the philosophical side will influence recommendations for field work in health care. Conversely, if success is an indicator for truth, successful therapies might warrant certain philosophical positions as more plausible than others. In this article, however, the main focus is not on practices or treatment but on the relationship between pain and knowledge.

[2] See René Descartes, *Principia philosophiae* (Amsterdam: Elzevier, 1641) and Saul A. Kripke, *Naming and Necessity* (Cambridge, MA: Harvard University Press, 1980), 152-153.

[3] See Timothy Williamson, *Knowledge and Its Limits* (Oxford: Oxford University Press, 2002). It is quite another question whether pain may also be *absent*-luminous: whether we always know when we are *not* in pain. We often are aware of pain's onset, yet seldom can we say when a pain has ceased. When you take a pill against headache, you will realise after a while that the pain is gone, but you will not be able to determine the exact moment when it has stopped. Hence, there must have been a period when you were not aware whether you were in pain or not.

[4] Margo McCaffery, *Nursing Practice: Theories Related to Cognition, Bodily Pain, and Man-Environment Interactions* (Los Angeles: UCLA Student

Store, 1968). Quoted in Caroline Bunker Rosdahl and Mary T. Kowalski, *Textbook of Basic Nursing* (Philadelphia: Lippincott Williams & Wilkins, 2007), 704.

[5] William Alston, 'Varieties of Privileged Access,' *American Philosophical Quarterly* 8 (1971): 235.

[6] F. Dretske, 'The Epistemology of Pain,' in *Pain: New Essays on Its Nature and the Methodology of Its Study*, ed. M. Aydede (Cambridge, MA: MIT Press, 2006), 59-73.

[7] Doubts about this classical picture of knowledge being justified true belief have been raised most prominently by Timothy Williamson (*Knowledge and its Limits*, 2002). Williamson states that knowledge is a *distinct* mental state (21-48).

[8] Williamson, *Knowledge and Its Limits*, 21-48.

[9] Frank Jackson, 'Epiphenomenal Qualia,' *Philosophical Quarterly* 32 (1982): 127-136.

[10] This may be a temporary state. If our ability to manipulate the human brain progresses further, it is not impossible that we may induce colour experiences in the blind, or pain experiences in the analgesic. Furthermore, it is not yet certain that an identity statement of conscious states with brain states is false, even though strong arguments for this have been put forward. In this case, even an analgesic may know what it is like to have a pain state under the guise of knowledge of neural activity. At the moment, both cases are utopian. For an overview see P. Ludlow, Y. Nagasawa and D. Stoljar, eds., *There's Something about Mary: Essays on Phenomenal Consciousness and Frank Jackson's Knowledge Argument* (Cambridge, MA: MIT Press, 2005).

[11] There is a danger in making use of a single determinant of whether something is in pain or not, however practical and ethical this approach might be. If we say that pain science is determined by what people call pain, and there are no restrictions on what people can call pain, as McCaffery seems to imply, then pain science is in danger of losing its homogeneity. Furthermore, pain would emerge not as a natural phenomenon, but as a constructed one: everything that is called a pain is pain. This marginalises fruitful evolutionary and neuroscientific approaches.

[12] See, for instance, Wittgenstein's *Philosophische Untersuchungen: Kritisch-genetische Edition* (Frankfurt: Wissenschaftliche Buchgesellschaft, 2001 [1953]), §248ff. See also Bernard Harrison, 'Wittgenstein and Scepticism,' in *Meaning Scepticism*, ed. Klaus Puhl (Berlin: de Gruyter, 1991), 34-69.

[13] U. Lindblom et al. 'Pain Terms: A Current List with Definitions and Notes on Usage,' *Pain* 24 (1986): supplement 1, S217.

[14] Albert Menne, 'Definition,' in *Handbuch philosophischer Grundbegriffe,* ed. H. Baumgarten and C. Wild (München: Kösel, 1973); H. M. Nobis and G.

Gabriel, 'Definition,' in *Historisches Wörterbuch der Philosophie,* ed. J. Ritter and K. Gründer (Basel: Schwabe, 1980); Frederick Suppe, 'Definition,' in *A Companion to the Philosophy of Science,* ed. W. Newton-Smith (Oxford: Blackwell, 2002). In cases of real definitions, it is permissible to use analysis and definition interchangeably, as I do in this article.

[15] A good example has been the study of life, seen as an irreducible *élan vital,* until a specific level of understanding reproduction, metabolism and homeostasis was achieved (cf. Churchland, 2002). With the IASP definition, pain might receive a similar treatment.

[16] See n. 13 above.

[17] Grahek distinguishes the phenomenology of normal pain, pain asymbolia and analgesia (loss of pain affect) with the distinction between *feeling pain* and *being in pain,* a distinction which points toward the involvement of the self. Normal pain experiences have both, while pain asymbolics only feel pain, but are not in pain; analgesics lack both features. N. Grahek, *Feeling Pain and Being in Pain* (Cambridge, MA: MIT Press, 2007 [2001]).

[18] J. L. Rubins and E. D. Friedman, 'Pain Asymbolia,' *Archives of Neurology and Psychiatry* 60 (1948): 554-573; M. Berthier, et al., 'Pain Asymbolia: A Sensory-Limbic Disconnection Syndrome,' *Annals of Neurology* 24 (1988): 41-49; V. S. Ramachandran, 'Consciousness and Body Image: Lessons from Phantom Limbs, Capgras Syndrome, and Pain Asymbolia,' *Philosophical Transactions of the Royal Society* (1998): 1851-1859.

[19] P. Brand and P. Yancey, *The Gift of Pain* (Michigan: Zondervan Publishing, 1997), 220ff.

[20] Theodore X. Barber, 'Toward a Theory of Pain: Relief of Chronic Pain by Prefrontal Leucotomy, Opiates, Placebos, and Hypnosis,' *Psychological Bulletin* 56 (1959): 430-460; Ernest Hilgard and Josephine Hilgard, *Hypnosis in the Relief of Pain* (London: Routledge, 1994), 190.

[21] In the case of *allodynia,* pain is elicited by non-noxious stimuli and associated not with tissue damage but with an effect on the nociceptors themselves. One might argue that this is still damage. Then again, certain types of neuropathic pain—pain due to lesions in the central nervous system—produce pain which is not felt at the location where the actual tissue damage is. Phantom-limb pain is another example: a patient feeling a pain in a hand she no longer has is mis-associating the felt location with the actual tissue damage. We could compromise by saying that the association must not be subjective. It may be sufficient for an outside observer to associate correctly the felt pain with a tissue damage of the subject in pain. This, however, would entail that the subject herself cannot know whether she is in pain or not, as pain is now dependent on an objective association not available to the subject.

[22] This illusion is known since 1896; for a newer discussion see Bouhassira, et al., 'Investigation of the Paradoxical Painful Sensation ('Illusion of Pain') Produced by a Thermal Grill,' *Pain* 114 (2005): 160-167.
[23] Randolph Nesse, 'What Good Is Feeling Bad? The Evolutionary Benefits of Psychic Pain,' *The Sciences* (1991): 30-37; Jaak Panksepp, 'Feeling the Pain of Social Loss,' *Science* 302 (2003): 237-239.
[24] See A. Craig, 'Pain Mechanisms: Labelled Lines versus Convergence in Central Processing,' *Annual Review of Neuroscience* 26 (2003): 1-30; A. Craig, et al., 'Quantitative Response Characteristics of Thermoreceptive and Nociceptive Lamina I Spinothalamic Neurons in the Cat,' *Journal of Neurophysiology* 86 (2001): 1459-1480; P. Romanelli and V. Esposito, 'The Functional Anatomy of Neuropathic Pain,' *Neurosurgery Clinics of North America* 15 (2004): 257-268.
[25] See N. Dronkers et al., 'The Neural Architecture of Language Disorders,' in *The New Cognitive Neurosciences*, ed. Michael S. Gazzaniga (Cambridge, MA: MIT Press, 2000), 949-958; P. Lieberman, 'On the Nature and Evolution of the Neural Bases of Human Language,' *Yearbook of Physical Anthropology* 45 (2002): 36-62.
[26] See Hildur Kalman and Naomi Scheman, 'Inflicting Pain,' in *Making Sense of Pain: Critical and Interdisciplinary Perspectives*, ed. Jane Fernandez (Oxford: Inter-Disciplinary Press, 2010), 100-107.
[27] See George Catlin and John Ewers, *O-kee-pa, A Religious Ceremony, and Other Customs of the Mandans* (Lincoln: University of Nebraska Press, 1976).
[28] See D. M. Tobin and C. I. Bargmann, 'Invertebrate Nociception: Behaviors, Neurons and Molecules,' *Journal of Neurobiology* 6 (2004): 161-174.
[29] 'Nur sein Auge sah alle die tausend Qualen der Menschen bei ihren Untergängen. Diesen Weltschmerz kann er, so zu sagen, nur aushalten durch den Anblick der Seligkeit, die nachher vergütet.' ['Only his eyes saw all the torment of humanity in its decline. This *Weltschmerz* he can only bear, so to say, by contemplating the bliss that compensates afterwards.'] Jean Paul, *Selina oder über die Unsterblichkeit* (Stuttgart: J. G. Cotta'sche, 1827), 132, my translation.
[30] See Duncan Pritchard, *Epistemic Luck* (Oxford: Oxford University Press, 2005), 163.
[31] See R. B. Brandom, *Articulating Reasons: An Introduction to Inferentialism* (Cambridge, MA: Harvard University Press, 2000), 100ff.
[32] See M. L. Hill and K. D. Craig, 'Detecting Deception in Pain Expressions: The Structure of Genuine and Deceptive Facial Displays,' *Pain* 98 (2002): 135-144; K. D. Craig, et al., 'Perceiving Pain on Others: Automatic and Controlled Mechanisms,' *The Journal of Pain* 11 (2010): 101-108.

[33] See Berthier et al., 'Pain Asymbolia: A Sensory-Limbic Disconnection Syndrome,' *Annals of Neurology* 24 (1988): 41-49.
[34] See Ned Block, 'On a Confusion about the Function of Consciousness,' *Behavioral and Brain Sciences* 18 (1995): 227-247; 'Consciousness, Accessibility, and the Mesh between Psychology and Neuroscience,' *Behavioral and Brain Sciences* 30 (2007): 481-548.
[35] For a list of related phenomena see Victor A. F. Lamme, 'Towards a True Neural Stance on Consciousness,' *Trends in Cognitive Sciences* 10 (2006): 496.
[36] Further support can be drawn from the work of Eric Schwitzgebel, who raises doubts about knowing our own current conscious states, indicated by our hesitation and insecurity. A person can have many emotions at a given moment, but still find it hard to give them a definitive label. Eric Schwitzgebel, 'How Well Do We Know Our Own Conscious Experience? The Case of Visual Imagery,' *Journal of Consciousness Studies* 9 (2002): 35-53; 'Introspective Training Apprehensively Defended: Reflections on Titchener's Lab Manual,' *Journal of Consciousness Studies* 11(2004): 58-76; 'No Unchallengeable Epistemic Authority, of Any Sort, Regarding our own Conscious Experience contra Dennett?' *Phenomenology and the Cognitive Sciences* 6 (2007): 107-113; 'The Unreliability of Naive Introspection,' *Philosophical Review* 117 (2008): 245-273.
[37] W. Quine, 'Speaking of Objects,' *Proceedings and Addresses of the American Philosophical Association* 31 (1957-1958), 20.
[38] I believe that pain metaphors, i.e. metaphors used to describe the specificity of a pain, are a valuable tool in gaining further insight into pain difference because they rely on structural similarities between different sections of reality. The use of specific metaphors to describe a specific pain suggests structural parameters that lay the basis for classification.
[39] One may hope for a mutual influence: a careful neuroscientific study might reveal subtleties that we may then explore from the first-person perspective.
[40] Even in careful studies we may misidentify the neural correlates of pain *per se* due to the difference between phenomenal and access consciousness. If these are different processes, they must have different implementations in the brain. It is, however, only our belief that we are in pain that counts as an indicator that we are experiencing pain now. Measuring in this instances will give us, even in the best of circumstances, only a measurement of a state being phenomenal *and* accessible; Ned Block has called this 'Epistemic Correlationism' or 'Phenomenal Consciousness → Reportable Principle' ('Consciousness, Accessibility, and the Mesh between Psychology and Neuroscience,' *Behavioral and Brain Sciences* 30 [2007], 483-485). As phenomenal consciousness is different from access consciousness, we need to subtract the activation of access consciousness from the whole measured

activation. This raises a problem: as long as we do not know the neural correlate of access, we cannot know the minimally sufficient correlates of pain experience. Unfortunately, access consciousness needs something to access, and that is phenomenal consciousness. Therefore, Block states, we face a hurdle in getting to the neural correlates of pure phenomenal consciousness due to our methodology.

[41] See James D. Rose, 'The Neurobehavioral Nature of Fishes and the Question of Awareness and Pain,' *Reviews in Fisheries Science* 10 (2002): 1-38.

[42] See Hilary Putnam, 'Psychological Predicates,' in *Art, Mind, and Religion*, ed. W. H. Capitan and D. D. Merrill (Pittsburgh: University of Pittsburgh Press, 1967), 37-48; Jerry Fodor, 'Special Sciences: Or the Disunity of Science as a Working Hypothesis,' *Synthese* 28 (1974): 97-115; 'Special Sciences: Still Autonomous After All These Years,' *Philosophical Perspectives* 11(1997): 149-163.

[43] Dale Langford, et al., 'Coding of Facial Expressions of Pain in the Laboratory Mouse,' *Nature Methods* 7 (2010): 447-449.

[44] Karl Popper, 'A Note on Verisimilitude,' *The British Journal for the Philosophy of Science* 27 (1976): 147-159.

Bibliography

Alston, William. 'Varieties of Privileged Access.' *American Philosophical Quarterly* 8 (1971): 223-241.

Barber, Theodore X. 'Toward a Theory of Pain: Relief of Chronic Pain by Prefrontal Leucotomy, Opiates, Placebos, and Hypnosis.' *Psychological Bulletin* 56 (1959): 430-460.

Berthier, M., S. Starkstein, and R. Leiguarda. 'Pain Asymbolia: A Sensory-Limbic Disconnection Syndrome.' *Annals of Neurology* 24 (1988): 41-49.

Block, Ned. 'On a Confusion about the Function of Consciousness.' *Behavioral and Brain Sciences* 18 (1995): 227-247.

———. 'Consciousness, Accessibility, and the Mesh between Psychology and Neuroscience.' *Behavioral and Brain Sciences* 30 (2007): 481-548.

Bouhassira, D., D. Kern, J. Rouaud, E. Pelle-Lancien, and F. Morain. 'Investigation of the Paradoxical Painful Sensation ("Illusion of Pain") Produced by a Thermal Grill.' *Pain* 114 (2005): 160-167.

Brand, P., and P. Yancey. *The Gift of Pain.* Michigan: Zondervan, 1997.

Brandom, R. B. *Articulating Reasons: An Introduction to Inferentialism.* Cambridge, MA: Harvard University Press, 2000.

Catlin, George, and John Ewers. *O-kee-pa, A Religious Ceremony, and Other Customs of the Mandans.* Lincoln: University of Nebraska Press, 1976.

Churchland, Patricia Smith. *Brain-Wise: Studies in Neurophilosophy.* Cambridge, MA: MIT Press, 2002.

Craig, A. 'Pain Mechanisms: Labelled Lines versus Convergence in Central Processing.' *Annual Review of Neuroscience* 26 (2003): 1-30.

Craig, A., K. Krout, and D. Andrew. 'Quantitative Response Characteristics of Thermoreceptive and Nociceptive Lamina I Spinothalamic Neurons in the Cat.' *Journal of Neurophysiology* 86 (2001): 1459-1480.

Craig, K. D., J. Versloot, L. Goubert, T. Vervoort, and G. Crombez. 'Perceiving Pain on Others: Automatic and Controlled Mechanisms.' *The Journal of Pain* 11 (2010): 101-108.

Descartes, René. *Principia philosophiae*, Amsterdam: Elzevier, 1641.

Dretske, F. 'The Epistemology of Pain.' In *Pain: New Essays on Its Nature and the Methodology of Its Study.* Edited by M. Aydede, 59-73. Cambridge, MA: MIT Press, 2006.

Dronkers, N., B. B. Redfern, and R. T. Knight. 'The Neural Architecture of Language Disorders.' In *The New Cognitive Neurosciences.* Edited by Michael S. Gazzaniga, 949-58. Cambridge, MA: MIT Press, 2000.

Fodor, Jerry. 'Special Sciences: Or the Disunity of Science as a Working Hypothesis.' *Synthese* 28 (1974): 97-115.

———. 'Special Sciences: Still Autonomous after All These Years.' *Philosophical Perspectives* 11(1997): 149-163.

Grahek, N. *Feeling Pain and Being in Pain.* Cambridge, MA: MIT Press, 2007 [2001].

Harrison, Bernard. 'Wittgenstein and Scepticism.' In *Meaning Scepticism.* Edited by Klaus Puhl, 34-69. Berlin: de Gruyter, 1991.

Hilgard, Ernest, and Josephine Hilgard. *Hypnosis in the Relief of Pain*. London: Routledge, 1994.

Hill, M. L., and K. D. Craig. 'Detecting Deception in Pain Expressions: The Structure of Genuine and Deceptive Facial Displays.' *Pain* 98 (2002): 135-144.

Lindblom, U., H. Merskey, J. M. Mumford, P. W. Nathan, W. Noordenbos, and S. Sunderland. 'Pain Terms: A Current List with Definitions and Notes on Usage.' *Pain* 24 (1986): supplement 1, S215-S221.

Jackson, Frank. 'Epiphenomenal Qualia.' *Philosophical Quarterly* 32 (1982): 127-136.

Kalman, Hildur, and Naomi Scheman. 'Inflicting Pain.' In *Making Sense of Pain: Critical and Interdisciplinary Perspectives*. Edited by Jane Fernandez, 100-107. Oxford: Inter-Disciplinary Press, 2010.

Kripke, Saul A. *Naming and Necessity*. Cambridge, MA: Harvard University Press, 1980.

Lamme, Victor A. F. 'Towards a True Neural Stance on Consciousness.' *Trends in Cognitive Sciences* 10 (2006): 494-501.

Langford, Dale, et al. 'Coding of Facial Expressions of Pain in the Laboratory Mouse.' *Nature Methods* 7 (2010): 447-449.

Lieberman, P. 'On the Nature and Evolution of the Neural Bases of Human Language.' *Yearbook of Physical Anthropology* 45 (2002): 36-62.

Ludlow, P., Y. Nagasawa, and D. Stoljar, editors. *There's Something about Mary: Essays on Phenomenal Consciousness and Frank Jackson's Knowledge Argument*. Cambridge, MA: MIT Press, 2005.

McCaffery, Margo. *Nursing Practice: Theories Related to Cognition, Bodily Pain, and Man-Environment Interactions*. Los Angeles: UCLA Student Store, 1968.

Menne, Albert. 'Definition.' In *Handbuch philosophischer Grundbegriffe*. Edited by H. Baumgarten and C. Wild. München: Kösel, 1973.

Nesse, Randolph. 'What Good Is Feeling Bad? The Evolutionary Benefits of Psychic Pain.' *The Sciences* (November/December 1991): 30-37.

Nobis, H. M., and G. Gabriel. 'Definition.' In *Historisches Wörterbuch der Philosophie*. Edited by J. Ritter and K. Gründer. Basel: Schwabe, 1980.

Panksepp, Jaak. 'Feeling the Pain of Social Loss.' *Science* 302 (2003): 237-239.

Paul, Jean. *Selina oder über die Unsterblichkeit*. Stuttgart: J. G. Cotta'sche Buchhandlung, 1827.

Popper, Karl. 'A Note on Verisimilitude.' *The British Journal for the Philosophy of Science* 27 (1976): 147-159.

Pritchard, Duncan. *Epistemic Luck*. Oxford: Oxford University Press, 2005.

Putnam, Hilary. 'Psychological Predicates.' In *Art, Mind, and Religion*. Edited by W. H. Capitan and D. D. Mer, 37-48. Pittsburgh: University of Pittsburgh Press, 1967.

———. *Representation and Reality*. Cambridge, MA: MIT Press, 1988.

Quine, W. 'Speaking of Objects.' *Proceedings and Addresses of the American Philosophical Association* 31 (1957-1958): 5-22.

Ramachandran, V. S. 'Consciousness and Body Image: Lessons from Phantom Limbs, Capgras Syndrome and Pain Asymbolia.' *Philosophical Transactions of the Royal Society* (1998): 1851-1859.

Romanelli, P., and V. Esposito. 'The Functional Anatomy of Neuropathic Pain.' *Neurosurgery Clinics of North America* 15 (2004): 257-268.

Rosdahl, Caroline Bunker, and Mary T. Kowalski. *Textbook of Basic Nursing*. Philadelphia: Lippincott Williams & Wilkins, 2007.

Rose, James. D. 'The Neurobehavioral Nature of Fishes and the Question of Awareness and Pain.' *Reviews in Fisheries Science* 10 (2002): 1-38.

Rubins, J. L., and E. D. Friedman. 'Pain Asymbolia.' *Archives of Neurology and Psychiatry* 60 (1948): 554-573.

Schwitzgebel, Eric. 'How Well Do We Know Our Own Conscious Experience? The Case of Visual Imagery.' *Journal of Consciousness Studies* 9 (2002): 35-53.

———. 'Introspective Training Apprehensively Defended: Reflections on Titchener's Lab Manual.' *Journal of Consciousness Studies* 11 (2004): 58-76.

———. 'No Unchallengeable Epistemic Authority, of Any Sort, Regarding our own Conscious Experience: Contra Dennett?' *Phenomenology and the Cognitive Sciences* 6 (2007): 107-113.

———. 'The Unreliability of Naive Introspection.' *Philosophical Review* 117 (2008): 245-273.

Suppe, Frederick. 'Definition.' In *A Companion to the Philosophy of Science.* Edited by W. Newton-Smith. Oxford: Blackwell, 2002.

Tobin, D. M., and C. I. Bargmann. 'Invertebrate Nociception: Behaviours, Neurons and Molecules.' *Journal of Neurobiology* 6 (2004): 161-174.

Williamson, Timothy. *Knowledge and Its Limits*. Oxford: Oxford University Press, 2002.

Wittgenstein, Ludwig. *Philosophische Untersuchungen. Kritisch-genetische Edition.* Frankfurt: Wissenschaftliche Buchgesellschaft, 2001 [1953].

Part I

ANTECEDENTS

'If You Prick Us, Do We Not Bleed?' Reflections on the Diminishing of the Other's Pain

Esther Cohen

Abstract
The article surveys medieval attitudes to the pain of others—the pain of religious martyrdom, of illness, and of torture—in terms of the possibility of empathy with the sufferer on the part of the observer or the person inflicting the pain. It demonstrates that emotional recognition of the pain of the other depended on the status of that other, in social, racial, moral/religious, or gender terms—no sympathy, for example, was to be accorded to the sinners in hell or suspected criminals under torture. Within the medical sphere, a healer's over-identification with the patient was regarded as conducive to an unscientific bias in the healer's mind and to distorting his judgment. The dependence of participative emotion on the status of the sufferer is a comment that medieval history makes on modern times: The pain of the other may be intellectually apprehended, but empathy varies according to the manner in which we see the sufferer. Conversely, distancing the sufferer morally or racially from oneself is an apt way of (and a justification for) pre-empting the interference of sympathetic response with the efficiency of the perpetrator's or a bystander's agenda. The key to efficient (albeit emotionally neutral) treatment resided in respect for the patient's status, not in an emotional response to his/her suffering.

Key Words: Middle Ages, empathy, martyrdom, crucifixion, hell, illness, torture, criminals, interrogation, physicians.

*****

> If you prick us, do we not bleed? If you tickle us, do we not laugh? If you poison us, do we not die? And if you wrong us, shall we not revenge?[1]
> -William Shakespeare

Thus Shylock asserts in *The Merchant of Venice* the universal vulnerability to pain which, he claims, affects also Jews. What he is saying, in other words, is that Jews are human, something his opponents very much doubt. The ability to suffer pain and, even more importantly, to communicate to others this sensation, has been a yardstick of humanity since the expulsion from Eden. Furthermore, in Christianity it became the hallmark of divinity. A Jew like Shylock who claims to bleed and suffer in a Christian context was therefore claiming, quite incredibly, to be akin to Christ in his human sensibilities.

In Western culture, subjective sensitivity to pain is clearly scripted and consistent. One finds in medieval texts that in hell the same fire affects different people to differing degrees. Thus, great sinners suffer much more than lesser ones from the same fire.[2] Women are more vulnerable than men, virgins more sensitive than sexually experienced women, higher-class people susceptible to pain more keenly than peasants.[3]

The scientific tradition of subjective pain sensitivity goes back to seventeenth-century philosophy, when some philosophers (not Descartes) denied the sensitivity of animals to pain, given their lowly place in the hierarchy of life. Victorian anthropologists often claimed that women were more resistant to pain than men,[4] savages more insensitive than civilised people, and white Caucasians more prone to pain than Africans, Native Americans, or any other kind of 'native.'[5]

The modern version of this theory surfaces in the first serious work of pain anthropology, Mark Zborowski's *People in Pain*, which demonstrates that Jews and Italians are far more vociferous in hospitals than what he termed 'old Yankees.'[6] In the wake of the criticism aroused by Zborowski's simplistic division,[7] other anthropologists have noted that indeed, communicating pain in hospital situations is worthwhile, especially for those groups who are still somehow considered less sensitive to pain.[8] It is obvious, therefore, that—while there is still no quantitative manner of measuring pain —there are at least two different yardsticks. One is the entirely subjective sensation of the sufferer, faced with what others consider her or his pain. The other measurement, from the opposite side, is no more objective: beings of higher status are credited with more sensitivity and suffering. There is not one 'other' that suffers. There are several.

This chapter examines attitudes towards different sufferers in the later middle Ages through the prism of identification and sympathy. Who ought to receive most sympathy and closeness in suffering, and whose pain should be ignored with a shrug? Note that the question is not based upon the injury received, for the same injury affects different people differently, like the fires of hell. I examine three fields: popular devotion to the Crucifixion of Christ, the professional attitude of physicians towards their suffering patients, and the theories of pain underlying the infamous practise of judicial torture by civil law courts.

The identification of pain with a higher position in any social or intellectual hierarchy also took place within the body. Galen, following Alexandrian Hellenistic medicine, distinguished noble organs from non-noble ones in the human body. Noble organs were mostly the internal ones (brain, heart, liver, etc.), but included the eyes too. Notably, Hellenistic physicians agreed that noble organs were more sensitive to pain than plebeian ones, such as hands or feet. This tradition was summarised and re-enforced in Galen's writings, and came to permeate medieval medicine.[9] In the fifteenth century, the jurist Bartholomé Chassenée still recommended punishing a criminal's eyes rather than his ears (ear-cropping being far more common than blinding), for eyes were nobler and hence, more sensitive.[10]

The trend of identifying pain with 'us' and not with 'the other' is consistent in medieval culture. When, beginning in the late eleventh century, the cult of Christ was metamorphosed from awe before a superhuman universal ruler to an emphasis upon empathy with the sufferer Christ became humanised and sensitive to pain. Long scholastic discussions and preachers' manuals detail his human ancestry from a virgin woman and discuss his medically perfect complexion. Typically, this perfection allows not invulnerability, but its opposite—the greatest possible sensitivity to pain. Christ's pain was greater than any other human pain precisely because of his superior, noble and pure physical nature.[11]

Though the term 'empathy' did not exist at the time, meditational practises and writings insisted upon every detail of Christ's suffering, adding much to the rather terse description of the Gospels. Here is one example from a vernacular fourteenth-century treatise:

> Alas, then the suffering began. … And they took him by the hair and threw him on the cross—he could have broken apart completely. … They took his right hand and pulled it to the hole in the arm of the cross and drove a nail through it. The nail was blunt and triangular and the edges were sharp as a knife, and they carried the skin of the hand and quite a lot of the flesh through the hole of the cross. … They took his other hand and pulled it over the arm of the cross. The hand was so far from the hole that they could not reach it. Then they took rope and put a line on his hand and pulled it so powerfully that the veins and limbs pulled apart so that the hand reached the hole. … Then it happened that his feet were not able to reach the hole by quite a few handspans. Then they took a rope and fastened a line to both of his feet and pulled it … until his feet reached the hole.[12]

The recurring theme in all of these meditations and prayers is that each and every believer ought to try and sense in her or his body the same pains. Indeed, the height of religious experience, as recorded by late medieval mystics, was feeling and having the *stigmata*—the wounds of Christ. St Francis is traditionally credited with being the first to receive this sign of grace in 1224 and was therefore acclaimed by his followers as 'the other

Christ.' Several other mystics followed in the ensuing centuries.[13] The constant prayer of these mystics to receive the stigmata was, in a way, a request for proof that they had joined the very select club of people who could imitate Christ to the utmost and therefore set a standard for empathy with him.

This empathetic trend, it must be noted, was limited to the cult of the Passion (both of Christ and his mother). Late antique Christian literature is a rich field of martyrology tales, each one detailing more atrocious tortures than the previous. Nevertheless, the telling is quite different from the narratives of the Passion. The stories extol the martyrs' courage and endurance—often claiming that they were miraculously immune to what was inflicted upon them—but they never exhort audiences to follow in their path and seek pain in martyrdom. Examples of martyrial suffering ran throughout medieval Christianity in sermons and liturgy as a testimony of courage. The intended audience was not meant to pity martyrs for two reasons: for one, they were often immune to pain, and for another, they were imitating Christ of their own free will, as every Christian ought to do. There is a rich literature of imitation of Christ, but none concerning the imitation of martyrs as a practise recommended to the laity. When a group of Christians under Muslim rule tried to become martyrs in ninth-century Cordoba, the movement got short shrift from the papacy.[14]

The stress laid upon a practical imitation of Christ with an almost total prohibition of imitating martyrs seems to run counter to my original position. Martyrs were unquestionably human and admirable but Christ was both divine and human. True, the late medieval Christ was almost completely humanised, but martyrs were never supra-humanised. I believe that the devotional difference between Christ and the martyrs was meant to clarify beyond all doubt the essential distinction between god-become-human and humans-born-human. Of the two, Christ—the nobler—naturally suffered far worse than the martyrs. Mostly, this was not due to the ferocity of his torture, but to his own subjective nature. And it was with this subjectivity that people were called to identify.

Who, then, were the sufferers who merited no empathy or even sympathy? If we remain in the realm of religion, sinners in hell were beyond any participatory feelings of the living. Scholasticism, preaching manuals and sermons all relied upon the detailed visions of hell produced by various visionaries (especially Cistercians monks) to describe its horrors. These, too, of course, were subjectively assigned: the greater sinners suffered more than the lesser ones, but for the most part, despite Dante's unusual and original divisions, mainstream narratives of hell made little quantitative difference among the various circles. Boiling lakes of pitch and freezing swamps stood next to each other, and souls were constantly tossed from one to the other. Nevertheless, these descriptions made it clear that the sufferers were beyond the pale. They had forfeited any possible redemption, and all that one could feel for them was regret. In fact, preachers were far more interested in eliciting their audiences' fear of such a terrible future than pity for the lost souls. The iconography of hell from the twelfth century onwards consistently shows the writhing, screaming figures of the lost souls. They often look only half-human in their contortions, and they are designed to inspire fear, not empathy.[15]

In contrast, sinners in purgatory were to be pitied, heard and seen in dreams of their living relatives. They could not be spared from pain, but they could certainly be helped. Preachers usually suggested the commonplace means of subventions to the church in order to shorten their period of suffering, but a few holy women found far more original ways of doing so. They willingly undertook to endure on earth the pains of purgatory for others.[16] Nevertheless, these 'gifts' to suffering souls formed no more than a footnote in the lives of holy women who spent their entire existence in self-inflicted pains. Catherine of Siena, for example, undertook to suffer for her father, who was in purgatory, but this pain was minor compared to that of her stigmata, hidden from sight but felt nonetheless. There is a distinct difference between the intense emotional range of identifying with Christ and the matter-of-fact way in which measures to shorten purgatorial suffering are described. To the reader, it almost seems as though the pain was the saint's main aim, with redemption of souls from purgatory as an excuse.

But the most familiar segment of humanity, that of the living, merited very little pity or empathy. True, living saints washed the sores of lepers and fed the hungry, but these were expressions of humility and self-mortification rather than of empathy. Francis, who associated with lepers, and Catherine of Siena, who drank the pus of their wounds, considered these actions as, first and foremost, an exercise in self-discipline. They did not imitate the lepers or seek leprosy, rather they identified with the lowest outcasts of society. When it came to charity, all Christians were enjoined to practise it, but within reasonable limits. Adopting total poverty, as identification with Christ, earned Spiritual Franciscans the label of heretics and, in the fourteenth century, the pyre.[17] Poverty was admirable, but not imitable. The multitudes of beggars were to be helped mainly so that one might practise the virtue of charity, not so that the beggars might be freed of their poverty. Thus the pain of living others was considered at best as useful, at worst a nuisance.

The pain of poverty was also useful since it allowed the wealthy to collect credits in the heavenly ledger of their lives. The usefulness of the other's pain is most obvious in the writings of physicians and jurists. Both professions dealt with pain: jurists by ordering torture during their investigations of crime and physicians by treating diseases. In both cases, the literature they produced is clear evidence of the total distancing of the observer (and manipulator) of pain from the suffering subject.

In the case of medicine, Galen had laid the groundwork for using different types of pain as diagnostic tools. His view, however, was that simply classifying types of pain was a useless exercise, as words failed to convey genuine sensations, especially words used by lay patients. In his opinion, only somebody who had suffered all possible types of pain, and was (incredibly enough) immune to their emotional impact, could analyse the pain of the other in an accurate manner. In order to decode pain, claimed Galen, one needed to know not only the type but also the location of the pain and the circumstances leading to its formation. In short, total identification and yet total distance was required for diagnosing pain. This caveat, however, did not stop Galen and his followers from using pains as a diagnostic tool.

Medieval followers of Galen's writings nevertheless stuck to a taxonomy of pain types, each of which carried some diagnostic meaning. Pains could indicate an illness, or be an illness in themselves (as in the case of ear- or tooth-ache), or even cause another illness. In each case the discussion is dispassionate, revealing neither sympathy for nor empathy with the patient. Witness the words of Bernard de Gordon (ca. 1258-1320):

> There are many types of pain according to Avicenna. According to Galen, they can be reduced to three or four, as he says in the commentary [on the Hippocratic] aphorism *Spontaneous lassitude indicates disease* and in his book *Regimen of Health.* There is a pain called sharp [*acutus*], stabbing [*pungitivus*], and ulcerative pain; there is another [called] stretching [*extensivus*] pain; another is *inflativus* and another *gravativus* or apostemous. If there are other kinds, they can be reduced to these.[18]

These words are taken from a classroom text. In texts referring to the practise of medicine and clinical treatment, medieval physicians modified their dispassionate tone. They insisted upon the importance of maintaining the patient's trust in his physician as an essential component of healing. This trust, however, is to be gained by an exhibition of knowledge and authority, not through sympathy.[19] Occasionally physicians did recommend pain alleviation, but only when the intensity of pain might endanger the patient's life, especially in the case of wounds.[20] Surgery was performed without anaesthesia, since anaesthetics were extremely dangerous and liable to cause death rather than painlessness. Even in cases of individual advice, or *consilia*, there is no particular sympathy towards the patients, merely prescriptions for restoring their health.[21]

Intriguingly, while medical literature failed to demand any emotional response from physicians and surgeons, there was another category of healers whose sympathy, though not empathy did come through the interstices of the texts. Many ill people in the middle Ages, unable to afford medical care, turned to saints' shrines in hope of a cure. Given that miraculous cures were recorded by clerics at the saint's shrine and subsequently used as propaganda in miracle collections, the descriptions of the sufferers, before and after their cure, were far more stirring and emotional, deliberately so. Ill and crippled pilgrims seeking cure are often described in a manner reminiscent of the souls in hell: thrashing uncontrollably, screaming and moaning, gesticulating, rolling on the ground like mad people, all because of the intensity of the pain. Following their cure, naturally, they recovered the proper respectful norms of behaviour towards the saint and his or her servants.[22] These texts, geared towards clergy and literate laity, are not manuals for healing; they are descriptions of thaumaturgic miracles. The suffering pilgrim may have been an 'other,' but the nature of the text generated a hyperbolic style that would create at least sympathy with that other.

The idea of the other's insensitivity to pain took a further turn when the other was not a patient but a suspect. When inquisitors began questioning witchcraft and heresy suspects, they resorted to torture in order to extract confessions.[23] Much to the perplexity of the inquisitors, on occasion the suspects proved immune to the pain of torture or punishment. Had the phenomenon taken place in the second century, the sufferer would unquestionably have been pronounced a martyr. Thirteen hundred years later, the *Malleus maleficarum* (1485), the most notorious witch-hunting manual, posited immunity to pain as one of the conclusively incriminating characteristics of a witch. She could therefore not be efficiently tortured unless the devil abandoned her to her fate.[24] Thus, the ordeal of red-hot iron was practised in the early modern era in order to see whether the witch could recite the creed while holding it, cry, or react to the pain.[25] In practise, on the Continent people suspected of witchcraft were also tortured, for even witches could sometimes be sensitive to pain. Furthermore, many broke down under torture and confessed to their illicit relationship with the devil, thus paving the way for their execution by burning.

English legal procedures were somewhat different, but the methods used to elicit a confession across the English Channel were also predicated upon pain and painlessness. The assumption in sixteenth- and seventeenth-century England was that witches had marks of teats all over their bodies (from which the devil sucked), and these spots were insensitive to pain. The office of a self-appointed witchfinder, who specialised in finding those spots and pricking them, so that they could be proven immune to pain, was familiar in early modern England.[26]

Witches were probably the ultimate other. As historians have shown, they were often women of dubious social position, but their theological stance was clear.[27] They were traitors to God, allies of the ultimate enemy of God and of humanity. They had lost all claims to compassion or sympathy. But even more importantly, their status as human beings was near the bottom of the scale—so low, that they sensed no pain. If empathy and sympathy were born out of awareness and identification with the other, total repudiation cancelled such feelings.

A step above the witch stood the heretic and the criminal. Both categories were human and (theoretically, at least), redeemable. On the road to redemption, however, they underwent torture as a matter of course. From the early thirteenth to the eighteenth century, torture, as a method of interrogation, was standard practise in European courts. A great many treatises on torture were written during the later Middle Ages and the early modern era. The tractates mention grounds for investigative torture, types of torture, limitations and degrees of severity. There is seldom any reference to pain. Only on occasion do they even mention the lasting damage done to the human frame by torture. Pain does appear in the standard definition of torture (*quaestio*), taken verbatim from Roman law: 'pain of the body for the purpose of eliciting the truth.'[28] The only other place where pain does appear is when jurists discuss the unusual phenomenon of the recalcitrant suspect who, immune to pain, will not confess under torture. As in the case of witches, a suspected criminal's refusal to confess was no proof of innocence. On the contrary, it merely implied that he possessed either unusual natural fortitude or supernatural means to combat pain. Curiously, not a single jurist assumed that such people had had recourse to standard analgesics. Combating pain with medical painkillers would have promoted the subject's status to that of a normal human being, very much like an ill person aided by analgesics. The criminals' means had to be either superhuman or supernatural.

Jurists were not the only ones to write about the silent suspect. Trial protocols also show that some people survived various forms of torture without confessing, and were eventually freed for lack of proof, but banished for their stubbornness (*duritia, dureté*).[29] Nevertheless, protocols do not investigate the phenomenon or ascribe any special meaning to it. It remained for jurists to interpret hardihood as tricks or effects of incantations.

On one point all jurists agreed. These powers were not available to an innocent person who had fallen foul of the judicial system. They were part of the imaginary culture of the underworld (for which we have only the jurists' evidence), and only professional criminals possessed them. Odofredus (d. 1265) from Bologna mentioned some who were so hardened that they slept throughout torture. Franciscus Brunus (fl. 1493) corroborated this observation, testifying that some professional criminals merely presented the aspect of sleep or death while tortured, opening their eyes when the session was over. A third jurist even described a man willing to undergo strappado for a few coins, replacing more sensitive colleagues. The stories jurists told include myths concerning criminals who trained secretly by torturing each other, so that they might resist a real situation; of others who, like Houdini, knew the trick of keeping their shoulder joints so flexible that the strappado did not dislocate them; and those who knew the system well enough to realise that one session was all they would suffer unless new evidence was forthcoming, which gave them the necessary endurance. The explanation, therefore, lay in the physical capabilities of hardened criminals and their familiarity with criminal law of torture:

> There are some who are so terrible and robust that they fear neither pain nor torture, as though somebody else was feeling it in his body. ... Some of them [survive] by the strength of their body and arms, others by their lightness, for they lift a light weight; some, who can turn their arms from the back forwards and over their heads through suppleness, so that it seems they feel only a light pain, or none. And I have seen others too.[30]

In all of these stories, there was no suggestion of the supernatural.[31] This changed in the sixteenth century. Sixteenth-century jurists borrowed the alleged insensibility of the witch as an explanation for the criminal who, presumably, also dabbled in witchcraft.[32]

Unlike earlier jurists, who could view hardened criminals in a detached, somewhat admiring manner, sixteenth-century jurists were concerned with witchcraft and its cosmic dangers. The ability of witches to withstand torture was not a sports competition or a matter for anecdotes. These men and women possessed the gift of insensibility without any professional criminal training. The resistance of some witchcraft suspects, as well as criminals using supernatural means, supported this belief. A series of potions, scrolls and incantations could help the tortured suspect remain silent without feeling any pain, a fact that jurists found most disturbing. Most of the stories about supernatural resistance derive from sixteenth-century jurists. Paulus Grillandus had gained most of his fame for his demonological work. In his view, a silent 'patient' was automatically guilty, either as a professional criminal or as a witch. Like all his predecessors, Grillandus claimed to have encountered the phenomenon himself. As we have seen above, he begins by describing the naturally hardened. Subsequently, however, the same author provides the new interpretation:

> I found some others who, with the aid of sorcery and incantations of the evil art, are so strengthened physically, or levitate, or fall into a deep sleep after being lifted, so that they suffer absolutely no pain in their body. And this is called the witchcraft of silence or insensibility (*maleficium taciturnitatis sive insensibilitatis*).[33]

At this point, Grillandus enumerates specific means of resisting torture. First, he mentions an analgesic known from antiquity, the Egyptian *Mesites* stone; next, a number of incantations. One charm wishes that just as Mary's milk was sweet to Christ, so should the upcoming torture (obviously strappado) be sweet to the victim's arms. The theme of Christ hanging from the cross, his arms wrenched backwards, recurs in the incantations of men or women about to be put in a somewhat similar, and equally painful, physical position. The same theme recurs in the recommendation to recite all the words Christ said from his capture until his death. All this Grillandus knew from experience.

Grillandus actually managed to capture such a charm, a small piece of parchment embedded in the recalcitrant suspect's hair, with the following text upon it: '†Iesus auem [*sic*] transiens† per medium illorum ibat.† os non comminuetis ex eo.†' The mangled Latin defies translation, but the warning not to open one's mouth is explicit. All the same, upon being raised again, the suspect resorted to another charm, a recited one this time and once more remained silent. Apparently, it did not occur to Grillandus that the man might be displaying hardihood. Once caught with a charm, he was classified as a witchcraft-user. The judge tried torture methods other than the strappado (the *taxillum*, small dice put between the toes), with no result, 'always impudent, he was strengthened in his denial' (*sed in sua negativa semper audacius convaluit*). Could he simply have been a professional? The frustrated magistrate was forced to close the case, and he had encountered similar ones in which other judges were baulked by the silent suspect.[34]

What have early modern horror stories to do with present-day attitudes towards the pain of others? I believe that they illustrate in a nutshell the subconscious rules governing human attitudes towards un-sensed but known pain. The pain of the other may be intellectually apprehended, but empathy varies according to the manner in which we see the sufferer. If empathising with her is expected to bring us salvation, we will induce ourselves and our senses to feel, to the best of our ability, *with* the subject. If, however, the acknowledgment of pain in the sufferer forces us to recognise her humanity, we are likely to try and alter—in the sense of making the subject into 'the other'—the subject, distance him so far from us that his pain would in no manner elicit a sympathetic or empathic response.

Notes

[1] William Shakespeare, *The Merchant of Venice*, act 3, scene 1.
[2] Gregory the Great, *Dialogi*, ed. A. de Vogüé. Sources Chrétiennes 265 (Paris: Éditions du Cerf, 1980): 158-160.
[3] Esther Cohen, 'The Animated Pain of the Body,' *American Historical Review* 105 (2000): 91.
[4] This claim goes back to antiquity, when barbarian women were supposed to give birth painlessly; see Augustine, *Contra Iulianum opus imperfectum*, book 6: 'Hunc parturitionum dolorem compertum est pro parientium corporibus viribusque variari. Barbarorum certe feminae, et pastorum, quae exercitatione indurescunt, in mediis itineribus tanta facilitate pariunt, ut non intermisso uiandi labore fetus suos procurent, et statim uehant, quae nihil pariendi difficultate marcentes, onera uentris ad humeros suos transferunt.' PL 45: col. 1577 ('The pain of childbirth is found to vary according to the body and strength of the parturient. Indeed, barbarian women and shepherdesses, hardened by [constant] efforts, give birth in the middle of the road with such facility that they do not interrupt the trip, because they notice no difficulty, transferring the weight of the belly to their shoulders.')
[5] Cynthia E. Russett, *Sexual Science: The Victorian Construction of Womanhood* (Cambridge, MA: Harvard University Press, 1989), 56; Diane E. Hoffman and Anita J. Tarzian, 'The Girl who Cried Pain,' *Journal of Law, Medicine and Ethics* 29 (2001): 13-27.
[6] Mark Zborowski, *People in Pain* (San Francisco: Jossey-Bass, 1969).
[7] See articles in Alan E. Radley, ed., *Worlds of Illness: Biographical and Cultural Perspectives on Health and Disease* (London: Routledge, 1995).
[8] John Blacking, ed., *The Anthropology of the Body* (London: Academic Press, 1977), 93.
[9] Rosa María Moreno Rodríguez and Luis García-Ballester, 'El dolor en la teoría y práctica médicas de Galeno,' *Dynamis* 2 (1982): 3-24.
[10] Bartholomé Chassenée, *In consuetudines ducatus Burgundiae, fereque totae Galliae, commentarii amplissimi* (Paris: Apud Antonium Vincentium, 1552), Vols. 43a, 46b.
[11] Bonaventura, 'Commentaria in quatuor libros sententiarum magistri Petri Lombardi,' in *Doctoris seraphici S. Bonaventurae Opera Omnia* 2-5 (Quaracchi: Collegium Sancti Bonaventurae, 1885): 348-51; Durand de St Pourçain, *Petri Lombardi sententias theologicas commentariorum libri IIII* (Venice: Guerrea, 1571), fol. 240v; John Duns Scotus, 'Quaestiones in tertium librum sententiarum,' in *Opera Omnia* 14 (Paris: Vivès, 1894): 591.

[12] Translated and quoted in Thomas H. Bestul, *Texts of the Passion: Latin Devotional Literature and Medieval Society*, Middle Ages Series (Philadelphia: University of Pennsylvania Press, 1996), 145-146.
[13] A survey of the vast literature on stigmata and stigmatization is beyond the scope of this chapter. Two of the most important works are Arnold I. Davidson, 'Miracles of Bodily Transformation, or How St. Francis Received the Stigmata,' *Critical Inquiry* 35 (2009): 451-480, and Alain Boureau, 'Miracle, volonté et imagination: La mutation scolastique (1270-1320),' in *Miracles, prodiges et merveilles au moyen âge* (Paris: Société des historiens médiévistes de l'Enseignement supérieur public, 1995), 159-172.
[14] Jessica A. Coope, *The Martyrs of Cordoba: Community and Family Conflict in an Age of Mass Conversion* (Lincoln: University of Nebraska, 1995).
[15] See articles in *The Iconography of Hell*, ed. Clifford Davidson and Thomas H. Seiler (Kalamazoo: Medieval Institute Publications, 1992).
[16] Jo Ann McNamara, 'The Need to Give: Suffering and Female Sanctity in the Middle Ages,' in *Images of Sainthood in Medieval Europe*, ed. R. Blumenfeld-Kosinski and T. Szell (Ithaca: Cornell University Press, 1991), 199-221.
[17] Bernard McGinn, 'Angel Pope and Papal Antichrist,' *Church History* 47 (1987): 155-173.
[18] Bernard de Gordon, *Lilio de Medicina*, ed. B. Dutton and M. Nieves Sánchez (Madrid: Arco/Libros, 1993), 186; Esther Cohen, *The Modulated Scream: Pain in Late Medieval Society* (Chicago: University of Chicago Press, 2010), 155.
[19] Henry E. Sigerist, trans., *Bedside Manners in the Middle Ages: The Treatise* De cautelis medicorum *Attributed to Arnald of Villanova* (Durham, NC: Duke Medical Center Library, 1946); Michael R. McVaugh, 'Bedside Manners in the Middle Ages,' *Bulletin of the History of Medicine* 71 (1997): 201-223.
[20] See for example, Guy de Chauliac, 'Guigonis de Caulhiaco Inventarium sive Chirurgia Magna,' ed. M. R. McVaugh, *Studies in Ancient Medicine* 14 (Leiden: Brill, 1997); Two centuries after Guy de Chauliac, Ambroise Paré, a field surgeon, prescribed sedation for all wounds—not in order to ease the patient, but because pain was a source of inflammation. See Ambroise Paré, *Oeuvres Complètes* (Geneva: Slatkine, 1970 [1840-1841]), 1: 442.
[21] There is an open question concerning the validity of *consilia* as individual documents. Nancy G. Siraisi, *Taddeo Alderotti and his Pupils: Two Generations of Italian Medical Learning* (Princeton: Princeton University Press, 1981), 270-282, among others, argues that some cases might well be

theoretical rather than real. However, in some cases the author mentions a patient's specific name, thus authenticating the case.
[22] Cohen, *The Modulated Scream*, 133-135.
[23] It must be noted that the church did not invent questioning under torture; the practise was present and known by the end of the eleventh century. See Ibid., 59-60.
[24] Heinrich Kramer [Institoris], *Malleus maleficarum*, trans. and ed. C. S. Mackay (Cambridge: Cambridge University Press, 2006), 1: 616-619.
[25] Stuart Clark, *Thinking with Demons: The Idea of Witchcraft in Early Modern Europe* (Oxford: Oxford University Press, 1997), 591.
[26] Craig Cabell, *Witchfinder General: The Biography of Matthew Hopkins* (Stroud: Sutton Publishing, 2006).
[27] Keith Thomas, *Religion and the Decline of Magic: Studies in Popular Beliefs in 16th- and 17th-Century England* (London: Penguin, 1988); John Demos, *Entertaining Satan: Witchcraft and the Culture of Early New England* (Oxford: Oxford University Press, 1982).
[28] There are several variations of this sentence: See Piero Fiorelli, *La tortura giudiziaria nel diritto comune*, 2 vols. (Milan: Giuffré, 1953-1954), 1: 186-187.
[29] *Registre criminel du Châtelet de Paris du 6 septembre 1389 au 18 mai 1392*, edited by H. Duplès-Agier, 2 vols. (Paris: Techener, 1861-1864), 1: 502-508, 2: 137-147.
[30] 'Nonnulla tamen reperiuntur adeo terribili set robusti qui nullum timent dolorem necque cruciatum aliquem sentire videntur in corpore etiam si mille tractibus quassarentur; quod pluribus modis contingere solet; quidam enim robustitate corporis et brachiorum alii vere levitate qui levi pondere comprimuntur, quidam alii membrorum abilitate quorum brachia ex modica elevatione ex retro antea resolvuntur supra caput directo rendunt adeo quod levem aut nullum cruciatum sentire videntur et ego alias in facto habui.' Paulus Grillandus, *Tractatus de hereticis: et Sortilegijs omnifariam coitu eorumque penis. Item de questionibus et torturae ac de relaxatione carceratorum Domini Pauli Grillandi Castilionei ultima hac impressione summa cura castigatus: adaitis ubilibet Summariijs: prepositosque perutili: Repertorio speciales sententias aptissime continente*, (Lyon: Apud Jacobum Giuncti, 1545), fol. 97a.
[31] Fiorelli, *La tortura*, 1: 215-16; Franciscus Brunus, *Tractatus de indicijs et tortura* (Siena, 148…), fol. 231v; Jodocus Damhouder, *Praxis rerum criminalium* (Antwerpen: J. Beller, 1562), 38: 19; Grillandus, 'De questionibus & tortura tractatus,' in *Tractatus diversi super maleficiis, nempe Do. Alberti de Gandino, Do. Bonifacii de Vitalini, do. Pauli Grillandi, do.*

Baldi de Periglis, Do. Jacobi de Arena (Lyon: Apud Haeredes Iacobï Iunta 1555), 672-74; Grillandus, *Tractatus de hereticis*, fols. 97a-99b.
[32] Kramer [Institoris], *Malleus maleficarum*, 1: 623-624.
[33] Grillandus, 'De questionibus et tortura,' 672.
[34] Ibid., 672-673.

Bibliography

Augustine. *Contra Iulianum opus imperfectum*. PL 45: cols. 1049-1608.

Bernard de Gordon. *Lilio de Medicina*. Edited by B. Dutton and M. Nieves Sánchez. Madrid: Arco/Libros, 1993.

Bestul, Thomas H. *Texts of the Passion: Latin Devotional Literature and Medieval Society*. Middle Ages Series. Philadelphia: University of Pennsylvania Press, 1996.

Blacking, John, ed. *The Anthropology of the Body*. London: Academic Press, 1977.

Bonaventura. 'Commentaria in quatuor libros sententiarum magistri Petri Lombardi.' In *Doctoris seraphici S. Bonaventurae opera omnia* 2-5. Quaracchi: Collegium Sancti Bonaventurae, 1885.

Boureau, Alain. 'Miracle, volonté et imagination: La mutation scolastique (1270-1320).' In *Miracles, prodiges et merveilles au moyen âge*, 1591-1572. Paris: Société des historiens médiévistes de l'Enseignement supérieur public, 1995.

Brunus, Franciscus. *Tractatus de indicijs et tortura*. Siena, 1483.

Cabell, Craig. *Witchfinder General: The Biography of Matthew Hopkins*. Stroud: Sutton Publishing, 2006.

Chassenée, Bartholomé. *In consuetudines ducatus Burgundiae, fereque totae Galliae, commentarii amplissimi*. Paris: Apud Antonium Vincentium, 1552.

Clark, Stuart. *Thinking with Demons: The Idea of Witchcraft in Early Modern Europe*. Oxford: Oxford University Press, 1997.

Cohen, Esther. 'The Animated Pain of the Body.' *American Historical Review* 105 (2000): 36-68.

———. *The Modulated Scream: Pain in Late Medieval Society*. Chicago: The University of Chicago Press, 2010.

Coope, Jessica A. *The Martyrs of Cordoba: Community and Family Conflict in an Age of Mass Conversion*. Lincoln: University of Nebraska, 1995.

Damhouder, Jodocus. *Praxis rerum criminalium*. Antwerpen: J. Beller, 1562.

Davidson, Arnold I. 'Miracles of Bodily Transformation, or How St. Francis Received the Stigmata.' *Critical Inquiry* 35 (2009): 451-480.

Demos, John. *Entertaining Satan: Witchcraft and the Culture of Early New England*. Oxford: Oxford University Press, 1982.

Durand de St. Pourçain. *Petri Lombardi sententias theologicas commentariorum libri IIII*. 2 vols. Venice: Guerrea, 1571.

Fiorelli, Piero. *La tortura giudiziaria nel diritto comune*. 2 vols. Milan: Giuffré, 1953-1954.

Gregory the Great. *Dialogi*. Edited by A. de Vogüé. 3 vols. Sources Chrétiennes 265. Paris: Editions du Cerf, 1980.

Grillandus, Paulus. *Tractatus de hereticis: et Sortilegijs omnifariam coitu eorumque penis. Item de questionibus et torturae ac de relaxatione carceratorum Domini Pauli Grillandi Castilionei ultima hac impressione summa cura castigatus: adaitis ubilibet Summariijs: prepositosque perutili: Repertorio speciales sententias aptissime continente*. Lyon: Apud Jacobum Giuncti, 1545.

———. 'De questionibus & tortura tractatus.' In *Tractatus diversi super maleficiis, nempe Do. Alberti de Gandino, Do. Bonifacii de Vitalini, do. Pauli Grillandi, do. Baldi de Periglis, Do. Jacobi de Arena*. Lyon: Apud Haeredes Iacobï Iuntae, 1555.

Guy de Chauliac. *Guigonis de Caulhiaco Inventarium sive Chirurgia Magna*. Edited by M. R. McVaugh. 2 vols, Studies in Ancient Medicine 14. Leiden: Brill, 1997.

Hoffman, Diane E. and Anita J. Tarzian. 'The Girl who Cried Pain.' *Journal of Law, Medicine and Ethics* 29 (2001): 13-27.

The Iconography of Hell. Edited by Clifford Davidson and Thomas H. Seiler, Kalamazoo: Medieval Institute Publications, 1992.

John Duns Scotus. *Quaestiones in tertium librum sententiarum.* In Opera Omnia 14. Paris: Vivès, 1894.

Kramer [Institoris], Heinrich. *Malleus maleficarum.* Translated and edited by C. S. Mackay. 2 vols. Cambridge: Cambridge University Press, 2006.

McGinn, Bernard. 'Angel Pope and Papal Antichrist.' *Church History* 47 (1987): 155-173.

McNamara, Jo Ann. 'The Need to Give: Suffering and Female Sanctity in the Middle Ages.' In *Images of Sainthood in Medieval Europe.* Edited by R. Blumenfeld-Kosinski and T. Szell, 199-221. Ithaca: Cornell University Press, 1991.

McVaugh, Michael R. 'Bedside Manners in the Middle Ages.' *Bulletin of the History of Medicine* 71 (1997): 201-223.

Moreno Rodríguez, Rosa María and Luis García-Ballester. 'El dolor en la teoría y práctica médicas de Galeno.' *Dynamis* 2 (1982): 3-24.

Paré, Ambroise. *Oeuvres Complètes.* 6 vols. Geneva: Slatkine, 1970 [1840-1841].

Radley, Alan E., ed. *Worlds of Illness: Biographical and Cultural Perspectives on Health and Disease.* London: Routledge, 1995.

Registre criminel du Châtelet de Paris du 6 septembre 1389 au 18 mai 1392. Edited by H. Duplès-Agier. 2 vols. Paris: Techener, 1861-1864.

Russett, Cynthia E. *Sexual Science: The Victorian Construction of Womanhood.* Cambridge, MA: Harvard University Press, 1989.

Sigerist, Henry E., trans. *Bedside Manners in the Middle Ages: The Treatise* De cautelis medicorum *Attributed to Arnald of Villanova.* Durham, NC: Duke Medical Center Library, 1946.

Siraisi, Nancy G. *Taddeo Alderotti and his Pupils: Two Generations of Italian Medical Learning*. Princeton: Princeton University Press, 1981.

Thomas, Keith. *Religion and the Decline of Magic: Studies in Popular Beliefs in 16th- and 17th-Century England.* London: Penguin, 1988.

Zborowski, Mark. *People in Pain*. San Francisco: Jossey-Bass, 1969.

Gower and Chaucer on Pain and Suffering: Jephte's Daughter in the Bible, the 'Physician's Tale' and the *Confessio Amantis*

R. F. Yeager

Abstract
Recent scholarship has effectively traced the intellectual framework of bodily pain—what it was, whether and whence it emanated in life and death, the nature and degree of Christ's suffering—to scholastic debate beginning in the twelfth century. Little attention, however, has been paid to how pain and suffering beyond the bodily kind were experienced at the close of the Middle Ages. Literature, more than the visual arts, is our best evidence of how people felt: clearly, fourteenth- and fifteenth-century writers and readers recognised emotional registers of pain at least equivalent to corporeal forms, such as torture, that dominated the concerns of the scholastics. This essay takes the case of a familiar biblical story, Jephte and his daughter, from Judges 11:30-39, as used by two of the foremost poets of late medieval England—Geoffrey Chaucer and John Gower—to examine and vivify the emotional and psychological components of pain and suffering. Beginning with a presentation and discussion of the biblical account itself, the essay proceeds to examine in detail the treatment Chaucer gives 'Jephte' in the 'Physician's Tale' (*Canterbury Tales*), and Gower in Book IV of his *Confessio Amantis*. It shows that both poets recognised the nature, extent and significance of emotional suffering—and by reference to an illustration of Jephte beheading his daughter found in the mid-fifteenth century Morgan manuscript (New York, Pierpont Morgan Library, MS M.126, fol. 76 recto) that one reader—the illuminator—understood Gower's text accordingly. The essay concludes that the work of Chaucer and Gower provides us with tangible evidence of the degree of thoughtful laymen's sensitivity to suffering of the heart and mind, not merely of the body.

Key Words: Affective suffering, empathy, father-daughter relations, Jephte, emotional pain, human sacrifice, rape, virginity, MS Morgan 126, visualisation.

*****

Consider three narratives of the same event, all versions of Judges 11:30-39, the story of Jephte the Galaadite, who vowed to offer to the Lord as a 'burnt offering' the first living thing to emerge from the doors of his house if he defeated the Ammonites. He is victorious, but his joyful homecoming is disastrous. First the Biblical account:

> 34: And when Jephte returned into Maspha to his house, his only daughter met him with timbrels and with dances: for he had no other children.
>
> 35: And when he saw her, he rent his garments, and said: 'Alas! my daughter, thou has deceived me, and thou thyself art deceived: for I have opened my mouth to the Lord, and I can do no other thing.'
>
> 36: And she answered him: 'My father, if thou hast opened thy mouth to the Lord, do unto me whatsoever thou hast promised, since the victory hath been granted to thee, and revenge of thy enemies.'
>
> 37: And she said to her father: 'Grant me only this, which I desire: Let me go, that I may go about the mountains for two months, and may lament my virginity with my companions.'
>
> 38: And he answered her: 'Go.' And he sent her away for two months. And when she was gone with her comrades and her companions, she mourned her virginity in the mountains.
>
> 39: And the two months being expired, she returned to her father, and he did to her as he had vowed, and she knew no man.[1]

Next, Geoffrey Chaucer's version, found in the tale of the Physician, from the *Canterbury Tales*:

> And whan this worthy knyght Virginius, [when]
> Thurgh sentence of this justice Apius [Because of]
> Moste by force his deere doghter yiven [Must; give]
> Unto the juge, in lecherie to lyven, [lechery; live]
> He gooth hym hoom, and sette him in his halle, [goes; home]
> And leet anon his doghter calle, [had...called]
> And with a face deed as asshen colde, [dead; cold ashes]
> Upon hir humble face he gan beholde, [began to look]
> With fadres pitee stikynge thurgh his herte,

Al wolde he from his purpos nat converte. [But would not]
'Doghter,' quod he, 'Virginia by thy name,
Ther been two weyes, outher deeth or shame, [either]
That thou most suffre; allas, that I was bore! [born]
For nevere thou deservedest wherefore [for any reason]
To dyen with a swerd or with a knyf.
O deere doghter, endere of my lyf, [ender]
Which I have fostred up with swich plesaunce [such pleasure]
That thou were nevere out of my remembraunce!
O doghter, which that art my laste wo, [final sorrow]
And in my lyf my laste joye also,
O gemme of chastitee, in pacience [gem]
Take thou thy deeth, for this is my sentence, [order]
For love, and nat for hate, thou most be deed;
My pitous hand moot smyten of thyn heed. [smite off]
Allas, that evere Apius the say! [saw you]
Thus hath he falsly jugged the today' [judged you]
And tolde hire al the cas, as ye before [how it all was]
Han herd; nat nedeth for to telle it moore. [no need]
'O mercy, deere fader!' quod this mayde, [said]
And with that word she bothe hir armes layde
About his nekke, as she was wont to do.
The teeris bruste out of hir eyen two, [burst]
And seyde, 'Goode fader, shal I dye?
Is there no grace, no remedeye?'
'No, certes, deere doghter myn,' quod he.
'Thanne yif me leyser, fader myn,' quod she, [give]
'My deeth for to compleyne a litel space;
For, pardee, Jepte yaf his doghter grace [by God]
For to compleyne, er he hir slow, allas! [killed]
And, God it woot, no thyng was hir trespas, [knows]
But for she ran hir fader first to see, [Except that]
To welcome hym with greet solempnitee.'
And with that word she fil aswowne anon, [fainted]
And after, whan hir swownyng is agon,
She riseth up, and to hir fader sayde,
'Blissed be God, that I shal dye a mayde!
Yif me my deeth, er that I have a shame; [before]
Dooth with youre child your wyl, a Goddes name!' [in]
And with that word she preyed hym ful ofte [many times]
That with his swerd he sholde smyte softe; [sword; strike]
And with that word aswowne doun she fil.
Hir fader, with ful sorweful herte and wil, [will]

Hir heed of smoot, and by the top it hente, [struck; seized]
And to the juge he gan it to presente,
As he sat yet in doom in consistorie.[2] [judgment; court]
CT VI.204-50

And then John Gower's, from the *Confessio Amantis*, Book IV:

The Maiden, whan sche wiste of this, [knew]
And sih the sorwe hir fader made, [saw; sorrow]
So as sche mai with wordes glade [might]
Conforteth him, and bad him holde [bade]
The covenant which he is holde [had made]
Towardes god, as he behihte. [promised]
Bot natheles hire herte aflihte [nonetheless; feared]
Of that sche sih hire deth comende; [Because; saw; coming]
And thanne unto the ground knelende
Tofore hir fader sche is falle, [Before]
And seith, so as it is befalle [as it happened]
Upon this point that sche schal deie, [About]
Of o thing ferst sche wolde him preie, [one; would]
That fourty daies of respite
He wolde hir grante upon this plit, [cause]
That sche the whyle mai bewepe
Hir maidenhood, which sche to kepe
So longe hath had and noght beset; [never compromised]
Wherof hir lusti youthe is let, [Therefore; lost]
That sche no children hath forthdrawe [produced]
In Mariage after the lawe, [according to]
So that the poeple is noght encressed.
Bot that it mihte be relessed, [Unless; rescinded]
That sche hir time hath lore so, [lost]
Sche wolde be his leve go [wished his leave to go]
With othre Maidens to compleigne, [bewail]
And afterward unto the peine [pain]
Of deth sche wolde come ayein. [again]
The fader herde his doughter sein, [daughter's words]
And thereupon of on assent [by agreement]
The Maidens were anon asent, [instantly sent for]
That scholden with this Maiden wende. [go]
So forto speke unto this ende, [to bewail in this way]
Thei gon the dounes and the dales [hills and dales]
With wepinge and with wofull tales,
Compleigneth upon thilke nede, [this cause]

That sche no children hadde bore,
Wherof sche hath hir youthe lore,
Which nevere sche recovere mai:
For so fell that hir laste dai [Until it happened]
Was come, in which sche scholde take
Hir deth, which sche may noght forsake.
Lo, thus sche deide a wofull Maide [died]
For thilke cause which I saide [this]
And thou hast understonde above.[3]

CA IV.1550-95

While these three accounts share an outline and result—the father's rash vow yields victory but at the unexpected cost of his daughter's life—in their final form they diverge significantly. Such divergence is instructive. Through a close examination, a good deal can be learned about what constituted pain and suffering for Chaucer and Gower, and through their examples, as premier poets of their time and place, also about the attitudes of their late medieval English readership.[4] This is the task of the following pages: to observe and draw conclusions from Chaucer's and Gower's narratives, involving (or *not* involving) descriptions of suffering and/or pain.

Striking, especially in comparison with Chaucer's and Gower's treatments, is the spareness of the original story as it appears in the Book of Judges. The events unfold matter-of-factly, and despite the appalling nature of the circumstances—Jephte must kill his only child - there is no register of emotion on anyone's part, save the single gesture, in 11:35, when Jephte 'rent his garments, and said: 'Alas! my daughter, thou hast deceived me, and thyself art deceived: for I have opened my mouth to the Lord, and I can do no other thing.' That Jephte feels helpless before the irrevocability of his vow is clear, but the passage is rendered ambiguous by his framing of the circumstances as initiated by deceptions—of himself by his daughter, and of her by something unnamed. One wonders what deceived her, and how she deceived him? The result, however, is to render indeterminate the source of such understated feeling as Jephte shows when he rends his garments and says 'Alas!' Is it horror or grief that he expresses—either or both of which under the circumstances one could expect—or a kind of anger difficult to comprehend because the introduced deception is mysterious? In any case, there is no ambiguity about the placidity of his unnamed daughter. Her father's promise is her death-warrant, and neither its inevitability nor the justice of her becoming 'a burnt offering' for greeting him joyously seems to her subject to question. Her only request is for two months' grace to 'bewail [her] virginity' in the mountains amongst her friends. Granted this, she returns at the allotted time, and Jephte kills his only child. Notably, neither the actual moment, nor the method is described in Judges. In fact, the violent culmination of the narrative is euphemistically occluded there: 'she returned to her father, and he did to her as he had vowed.'

In Chaucer's hands, the story of Jephte and his daughter is put to a different purpose, and consequently resonates quite differently. The story is introduced at an emotional high-point in the larger narrative of 'Apius and Virginia,' which Chaucer reworked for the Physician from Livy's *History* by way of the *Roman de la Rose*.[5] Despite its brevity, as seen above (the actual Jephte narrative occupies just seven lines in the 'Physician's Tale' (*CT* VI.237-44), the story's placement lends it a power out of proportion to its size. Virginia, the maiden daughter of the upright Roman knight Virginius, has just been told by her father that he must kill her to save her from the corrupt jurist Apius, who has rigged court testimony to secure her sexual enslavement. It is at this point that Virginia brings up the story of Jephte and his daughter, apparently to obtain from Virginius the same 'grace/ For to compleyne, er he hir slow' granted by Jephte—that is, two months' respite before she must die. But of course for her no such alternative is possible. Where the Lord in the Judges account was, for once, agreeably patient, the lustful Apius will not be, and Virginius does not have Jephte's power to control the clock. Perhaps Virginia realises this, which causes her to swoon (a Chaucerian addition) for the first of two times. Psychologically, there is truth in that sequence, even if we as readers cannot know for certain how Chaucer imagined his character's mind. What we *do* know from Chaucer's inclusion of the Jephte story into his version of 'Apius and Virginia' (and include it he did, since in none of his sources or analogues do these two narratives appear together) is that by claiming Jephte's daughter as a spiritual sister to Virginia, Chaucer opens a door for himself to envision the emotional agonies of his characters so humanly understandable yet so notably underplayed and/or ignored not only in the biblical account but, importantly enough, in Livy's *History* and by Jean de Meun as well.

That exploring the suffering of fathers and daughters in exigency is at the core of Chaucer's interest in both the stories of 'Apius and Virginia' and of Jephte is seldom suggested amongst readings of the 'Physician's Tale,' a narrative that continues to unsettle many.[6] Yet the intimacy and charged, emotional accuracy of the details that Chaucer adds to the interaction of Virginius and Virginia in the 'Physician's Tale' are demonstrably spun from his own imagination, and stand out. Both of his sources are essentially pedestrian narratives. Upon reflection, it is difficult to locate the attraction of any other aspect of these narratives for him. Indeed, Chaucer's delving into his characters' suffering recalls Ovid's in its empathy, and in its elevation of that suffering as a poetic subject.[7]

Let us look closely at what Chaucer does in these 'Physician's Tale' passages. It is as if he deliberately sought out a malleable analogue to the spare account of Jephte, in order to breathe 'life' into it by adding exactly those affective elements that, in the Book of Judges, are so strikingly withheld. These are the 'normal' elements, we might say: the sensory details by which experience is classified and memorial artefacts are made. In this case, they are registers of overwhelming pain. What does a father look like, staring into the 'humble face' of his 'deere doghter' with news such as Virginius has to impart? 'Deed as asshen colde': an extraordinarily layered and economical four words that simultaneously summon the visual (Virginius' bloodless grey face), the tactile ('colde'), the emotional (every spark of living feeling extinguished), while also foreshadowing Virginia's tragic end. How does he feel, steeling himself ('Al wolde he from his purpos nat converte') to tell his only child that she shall die by his hand? 'With fadres pitee stikynge thurgh his herte'—a grief so powerful that even pity itself impales. How does his shocked daughter react when told that she must 'in pacience' take her death? She cries out, 'O mercy, deere fader!'

> And with that word she bothe hir armes layde
> About his nekke, as she was wont to do. [often did]
> The teeris bruste out of hir eyen two,
> And seyde, 'Goode fader, shal I dye?
> Is there no grace, no remedeye?'

These are images that quicken emotions with the clear intent to capture and mould the reader's empathetic response. The simplicity and familiarity ('as she was wont to do') of Virginia's embrace is excruciatingly perceptive in all it conveys, her tears and her questions being precisely what such circumstances would invoke. Pointedly, they are lacking from the Judges account—and just as pointedly, it is precisely here that Chaucer introduces the Jephte story:

> 'No, certes, deere doghter myn,' quod he.
> 'Thanne yif me leyser, fader myn,' quod she, [leisure]
> 'My deeth for to compleyne a litel space;
> For, pardee, Jepte yaf his doghter grace
> For to compleyne, er he hir slow, allas!
> And, God it woot, no thyng was hir trespas, [crime]
> But for she ran hir fader first to see,
> To welcome hym with greet solempnitee.' [ceremony]

Through Virginia's agony and plaintive appeal, in Chaucer's richer context, the stifled suffering of daughter and father in Judges is vividly unpacked, and powerfully thrust home. For those who knew the bible as well as Chaucer did, the tandem innocence of both young women, and the undeserved nature of their deaths juxtaposed in this fashion would have been a pathetic engine that must have worked on his readers, as it does on us, in an irresistible way.

Nevertheless, there is a certain danger in acceding too fully to this pathos. While legitimate in its causes and capacity to move, perhaps in the scheme of the *Canterbury Tales* as a larger, purposeful work it should be credited at its most bathetic expression to the named narrator of the tale, the shallow (and likely corrupt) character called the Physician, rather than to that far more complicated author, Chaucer himself. For the value of chastity in the 'Physician's Tale' differs radically from what is at stake in the Book of Judges' account of Jephte. Indeed, the focus of the suffering is inverted. In Judges, the tragedy pointedly bypasses the daughter of Jephte herself. Her significance, first to society (and to God, we must also assume), next even to her father, is centred in her potential capacity to bear children. Brought onstage in Judges neither as a young girl and nor as a daughter, but essentially as a vessel, her death there is less mourned than the squelching of her unrealised fertility is regretted. Hence, her namelessness; hence the reiteration of her virginity ('and she knew no man') as the final detail of the narrative, a location that underscores its importance. Hence too the author's purpose, surely, in telling us that Jephte 'had no other children.' We as readers are not expected to find pathos in this. Her loss is the loss of seed, and dooms her father's line—both are reasons of grief and pain, but, importantly, of a social, even (one might say) of a more cerebral kind that fully justifies the anaemic emotionality of the Judges account.

Chaucer, however, and his fictive narrator, take aim in different directions, although they 'both' weave the tale of Jephte into the larger story of 'Apius and Virginia.' It is not my intention here to offer a full reading of the 'Physician's Tale.' Like all the Canterbury narratives, it has been the subject of numerous, and quite varied, interpretations, most of which are not germane to the way Chaucer renders suffering and pain. It is important, however, in illuminating the latter to emphasise the distinction between the simpler lesson the fictive narrator claims for his story, and beyond that what Chaucer the author perhaps had in mind. For the Physician the point is, apparently (his fuzziness about this has generated controversy), 'Of alle tresons sovereyn pestilence/ Is whan a wight bitrayseth innocence' (*CT* VI.91-92). In 'his' portrayal of Virginia (beginning, one should note, with her name) he goes to some length to establish the girl's probity, her rectitude, her habits free of any vice (e.g., *CT* VI.40-66); and it seems to be offered as another way of emphasizing her guiltlessness that the Physician plucks the case of Jephte's equally guiltless daughter out of the bible to incorporate it into the Roman Virginia's plea to her only-too-Roman father to spare her life. Without question, it is the Physician's extended representation of Virginia's moral spotlessness as an achievement of a self-aware girl-child that makes plausible in any degree whatsoever her remarkable statement, upon regaining consciousness from her first swoon, 'Blissed be God, that I shal dye a mayde!/ Yif me my deeth, er that I have a shame.'

Virginia's request is remarkable for two reasons. It is, first, a full reversal of her plea for life uttered just prior to fainting—and since whatever thought processes led her to this new resolve are beclouded within her 'swownyng,' it comes upon the reader as a complete surprise. Possibly one might accept that the Physician is a fully independent narrator, as some Chaucerians do, and so argue his lack of competence to move seamlessly from source to source, and his consequent failure to notice, or care about, narrative disjuncture. Yet do we know enough about the fictive Physician to weigh his awareness that Virginia's request to die rather than be deflowered inverts (and this is the second remarkable thing about it) the state of 'knowing no man' from *cost*, in the Judges account of Jephte, to *value*? In any case, because this transformation of attitude toward virginity defines, in one very real sense, the chasmic division of Judaism and Christianity, it might be too much to expect such nice consciousness in a narrator whose 'studie was but litel on the Bible,' as Chaucer describes him in the General Prologue (*CT* I.438).

What we can expect of Chaucer the *author*, however, is another thing entirely. If there are contradictions and reversals brought to light by the juncture *sui generis* of the stories of Jephte's daughter and Virginia, it seems most unlikely that Chaucer, who studied the bible in depth, did not have them in mind as part of his purpose when writing the 'Physician's Tale.' Again, my intent here is not to unpack the entire tale, but rather to establish that, *inter pares* at least, if not in fact *primus* among his various motives, Chaucer carefully constructed the 'Physician's Tale' in order to foreground pain and suffering, in general, as human conditions worthy of exploration *in situ*, and also—more immediately—of a particular kind, i.e., of father and daughter *in extremis*. To do this, he began at the beginning, essentially by defining the condition. That he offset 'Apius and Virginia' with an invocation of the Jephte story is evidence of this, I think; but to clarify Chaucer's endeavour further, it is helpful to consider a third case, the parallel effort of Chaucer's friend and contemporary, John Gower, to confront the Jephte story. We shall return to Chaucer later.

In one important sense, Gower's approach to the Jephte story is closer to the Judges account than is Chaucer's. As in Judges, Gower focuses on the social loss of Jephte's daughter dying a virgin: 'the poeple is noght encressed.'[8] He mentions 'wepinge' and 'wofull tales' by the daughter and her friends during the forty days granted her to mourn—but, significantly, the grieving is not described in detail. This is not the young girl's *cri de coeur* of Chaucer's account, the utterance of a victim dramatically and visibly expressing pain at a death so undeserved and cruel. Rather, its expressed focus is the as-yet intact 'maidenhiede':

That sche no children hadde bore,
Wherof sche hath hir youthe lore,
Which nevere sche recovere mai

Indeed, Gower affords the daughter's feelings but a single line ('Bot natheles hire herte aflihte/ Of that sche sih hire deth comende') which, while one more than in Judges, is not much. Context, and narratorial viewpoint in particular, however, play a determining part in the *Confessio Amantis*—as, of course, is true of Chaucer's poem and in the Bible. Just as Chaucer nominally presents the Jephte story through the mouth of the Physician, while simultaneously pursuing other purposes with the story in the larger body of the *Canterbury Tales*, so too Gower proffers his version of the tale via an invented narrator with his 'own' fictive intent while Gower himself harbours weightier, authorial ones for its place in the *Confessio* as a whole. It is Genius, the priest of Venus and the confessor of Amans, the lover supplicant to the goddess for her help, who in the *Confessio* tells the Jephte story. He does so in Book IV, devoted to illustrating Sloth for Amans, and the dangers inherent in pursuing love indolently.

Through Genius Gower thus presents the tragedy of Jephte's daughter as the earned wages of Sloth. She has been dilatory in finding a mate—a sin against Love which Genius serves:

Lo, thus sche deiede a wofull Maide
For thilke cause which I [i.e., Genius] saide,
As thou has understonde above.

Yet colouring Genius' narration, though easily overlooked, is a subtler palette which we should attribute to the poet rather than to his invented narrator. Read through this lens, sorrow in the tale seems not to centre in the blunt fact of death but rather in its by-product, in lost time and irrecoverable opportunity: 'hir youthe [is] lore/ Which nevere sche recovere mai.' Jephte's daughter herself frames the tragedy precisely thus when she makes her request for space and time to mourn before dying:

That sche the whyle mai bewepe
Hir maidenhood, *which sche to kepe*
So longe hath had and noght beset; [never compromised]
Wherof her lusti youthe is let. (my italics)

Admittedly, it is difficult to distinguish with assurance whether the words italicised above are part of Jephte's daughter's appeal to her father, or whether they are Genius' commentary on the situation. The sorrow is greater, of course, if the girl is the speaker, her consciousness of loss cutting nearer the quick, but in a sense it does not matter. As Housman continually reminds us, it works either way.[9] Whoever the speaker is, the kind of pain Gower invokes here is more cerebral albeit no less emotionally honest or affective than anything in Chaucer's broader-stroked portrayal. What the voice proclaims is a peculiarly modern-seeming, existential angst for which the persistent maidenhead is merely a placeholder. It is a fear, deep-seated and evidently known to Gower in late medieval England too, of a transformation of the 'real' into another world altogether, where the comfortably normative (one might almost say 'bourgeois') rules no longer apply.[10] Jephte's daughter's tragedy in Gower's hands shares elements with Gregor Samsa's: following the best social code, she has preserved her virginity as her years mounted toward a marriage and motherhood that, suddenly and irrationally, are snatched beyond her reach, leaving her body transmogrified and her self without purpose. This is, quite simply, suffering produced by unfounded, but unshakable, 'modern' dread: of going to bed, *mutatis mutandis*, the daughter of a victorious general and waking to find one's self innocent but effectively a corpse.

Kafka provides a serviceable model to gauge the profoundly subversive possibilities Gower's presentation of suffering raises here, on several levels. At a time in England when a dogmatic and Caesarian Church was increasingly questioned by Wyclifite and Lollard critiques, Gower seems to have been aware that easy certitudes may be deceptive, and, like Kafka, he constructed fictions to problematise the conventional.[11] Thorough pursuit of this claim would take us far from a discussion of pain and suffering, but some sketch of how such a pursuit would be shaped is germane. The slippery dualism of Genius as priest of Venus who applies Christian confessional structure and moralities to desire's business is both relevant and often noted, as is the consequent tension between ecclesiastical and natural law that Gower exploits to advantage in the *Confessio Amantis*.[12] Both of these are in observable operation in his handling of the Jephte story as not only an exemplum of the consequences of 'Sloth in Love' but also as a revelation, a naming, of a category of suffering infrequently embodied in medieval literatures.

We see this most clearly in Gower's treatment of Jephte and his daughter as they each realise, and respond to the appalling price Jephte has promised to pay to obtain victory for the Lord. Their reactions are a study in contrast. As noted above, in the Judges account the daughter's dutiful words—'My father, if thou hast opened thy mouth to the Lord, do unto me whatsoever thou hast promised'—betray no emotion, no pain, but merely a girl's humble acquiescence to the greater wills of her father and her God. Gower's account closely follows the Bible:

The Maiden, whan sche wiste of this, [knew]
And sih the sorwe hir fader made, [saw; sorrow]
So as sche mai with wordes glade [might]
Conforteth him, and bad him holde [bade]
The covenant which he is holde [had made]
Towardes god, as he behihte. [promised]

Flawless behaviour according to Christian tradition as this may be, it is troublesome to an empathetic heart and raises unavoidable questions about the purposes, if any, of suffering, in a universe that may or may not be just. Like Chaucer, Gower highlights these queries by giving Jephte a heart, and a voice to reveal it:

…and whan he com therate, [there]
And sih his douhter, he tobreide [saw; shredded]
Hise clothes and wepende he seide: [weeping]
'O mihti god among ous hiere, [us]
Nou wot I that in no manere [I know; no way]
This worldes joie mai be plein. [may worldly joy be complete]
I hadde al that I coude sein [ask for]
Ayein mi fomen be thi grace, [Against; foes]
So what I cam toward this place [that when]
Ther was non gladdere man than I:
But now, mi lord, al sodeinli
Mi joie is torned into sorwe

There is, to be sure, much about Jephte's speech that echoes standard, post-Boethian laments for Fortune's fickleness widely circulated in the Middle Ages. Gower's formulation, however, transcends the commonplace in the succeeding five lines, where with a few blunt words he forces his readers to confront the deed Jephte must perform, in all its agonizing physicality:

For I mi dowhter schal tomorwe
Tohewe and brenne in thi servise [cut to bits; burn]
To loenge of thi sacrifise [As a sacrifice to you]
Thurgh min avou, so as it is. [Because of my vow]

Where Chaucer characteristically gives us an image, a 'fadres pitee stikynge thurgh his herte,' Gower—equally characteristically—selects a pair of words to drive the same horror home *sotto voce*, but no less forcefully. 'Tohewe' and 'brenne' are verbs few fathers wish ever to apply to a daughter—and to know themselves the cause of such an innocent dying, as Jephte does ('thurgh min avou'), magnifies the suffering indeed.

How far ahead of their readerships in their explorations of suffering Chaucer and Gower might have been is difficult to determine—particularly in Gower's case, when his hand is generally very light, as here in his portrayal of Jephte. Nonetheless, to draw any kind of general conclusions from their work regarding attitudes toward pain and suffering in late medieval England, would require evidence of consciously concurring readers. In fact, we have reason to think that neither Chaucer nor Gower overshot their audience by much. At least one reader of the *Confessio Amantis*, indeed, seems to have understood Gower's complex handling of Jephte and his daughter fully: the late fifteenth-century illuminator (New York, Pierpont Morgan Library MS 126).[13]

All the elements are present in the painter's dramatic rendering (Fig. 1), which has the split-second immediacy of a snapshot. Jephte's sword has just swept through his daughter's neck so recently that her decapitated body, not yet collapsed, still kneels, her hands clasped in prayer, her severed head caught just as it strikes the floor in a bloody splash that contrasts arrestingly with the expression of resigned serenity on the face. The artist thus imagines Jephte's daughter's passing as Gower offered it: she dies as a body does, not free from gore which we as witnesses (or readers) must confront, but also as martyrs are enabled to do, cocooned from pain by holy agency (hence her serenely closed eyes).[14] And yet, because the artist seems to have comprehended Gower so keenly, Jephte's daughter is visually connected through the Marian blue of her gown to the two weeping Marys flanking the suffering, crucified Christ added above the (also interpolated) altar. Both details are absent from, but are wholly consistent with, Gower's narrative. Indeed, they re-enforce its larger, polyvalent exploration of suffering, both overt and suppressed.[15]

But to see how far the artist understood Gower's poem, we must look at the face and the raised left hand of Jephte himself. Both are intended to register emotional complexity glimpsed only at the far perimeter of experience. Consider the problem: how does a father appear, swinging a scimitar to behead his only daughter without desert, except to fulfil his own rash vow? What must he look like, no matter what rationalisations have sustained him up to the brink, at the moment her head and body separate because of his blow? Shocked and amazed (Jephte's face); denying and rejecting what he has done (the off-putting left hand): Jephte as painted here owes everything to Gower's sensibility, and words. The Morgan manuscript illuminator and Gower, although a generation apart, evince an affective affinity both profound and instructive.

Most instructive, perhaps, is how the poets Chaucer and Gower, and to a different degree the anonymous painter of MS Morgan 126, help advance what we know about how pain and suffering were experienced and portrayable in England at the close of the Middle Ages. Recent work has effectively traced the intellectual framework of pain—what it was, whether and whence it emanated in life and after death, the nature and degree of Christ's suffering—to scholastic debate at the University of Paris in the thirteenth century, and correspondingly in ecclesiastical circles pressed to establish levels of penance appropriate to various culpable acts and velleities following the institution of confession by the Fourth Lateran Council in 1215.[16] In their handling of the Jephte story—perhaps even by the act of choosing it—Chaucer and Gower provide us with tangible evidence of how sensitive thoughtful laymen could be to suffering beyond the bodily. Clearly, fourteenth- and fifteenth-century writers and readers recognised emotional registers of pain at least equivalent to corporeal forms, such as torture, that dominated the concerns of the scholastics. At least, if not more than: undoubtedly we should not overlook that, as we have seen, both Chaucer and

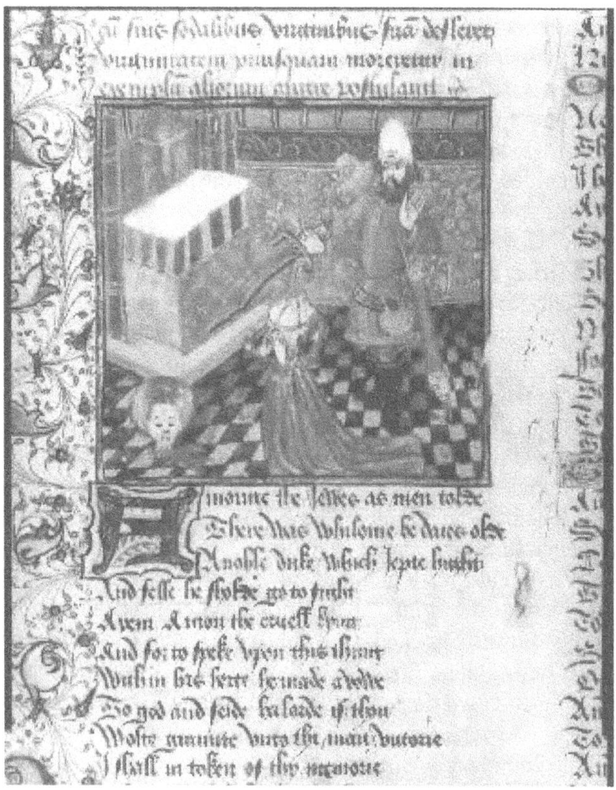

Fig. 1. John Gower, *Confessio amantis*, detail of miniature. The Pierpont Morgan Library, New York. MS M.126, fol. 76r. Purchased by J. Pierpont Morgan (1837-1913) in 1900. Photographic Credit: The Pierpont Morgan Library, New York

Gower devote significant attention to delineating affective suffering, but one is hard-pressed to uncover instances in their works where the physical pain of a character is given similarly complex shrift. Perhaps this is so because, as seems likely, neither poet deemed pain of the body unfamiliar enough—interesting enough—in a high-tolerance society to demand more than its mention for readers to comprehend. More intriguing, however, is another possibility, worth suggesting here: that the work of Chaucer and Gower manifest a developing social awareness of the emotional as a broad landscape, dim as yet but noticeably broadening, and deepening to account for complexity of feelings irrelevant to questions of sin or salvation yet too intense, and too universally present, to be left any longer unexplored in art.

Notes

[1] All quotations from the Bible are taken from the Douai-Rheims edition.
[2] All quotations from the works of Chaucer are taken from the *Riverside Chaucer*, 3rd edition, ed. Larry D. Benson (Boston: Houghton Mifflin, 1986).
[3] All quotations from the poetry of Gower are taken from *The Complete Works of John Gower*, ed. G. C. Macaulay, 4 vols. (Oxford: Clarendon, 1899-1902); English works, vols. 2 and 3.
[4] Very little critical/scholarly attention has been paid to how Gower and Chaucer thought about, or depicted, pain and suffering. One of the few is D. Thomas Hanks, Jr., although as his title suggests, pain is an ancillary subject (and is frequently used by Hanks as a synonym for 'grief'); see his 'Chaucer, *Auctoritas*, and the Problem of Pain,' in *'Seyde in forme and reverence': Essays on Chaucer and Chaucerians in Memory of Emerson Brown, Jr.*, ed. T. L. Burton and John F. Plummer (Adelaide: The Chaucer Studio, 2005), 219-236.
[5] See Edgar F. Shannon, 'The Physician's Tale,' in *Sources and Analogues of Chaucer's Canterbury Tales*, ed. W. F. Bryan and Germaine Dempster (New York: Humanities Press, 1958), 398-408.
[6] The tale of the Physician has prompted comparatively little scholarly/critical commentary over the years—just a few essays per decade—and not all of them are concerned with Jephte. Notable (if not always perceptive) are Richard R. Hoffman, 'Jephthah's Daughter and Chaucer's Virginia,' *Chaucer Review* 2 (1967): 20-31; Jeanne T. Mathewson, 'For Love and Not for Hate: The Value of Virginity in Chaucer's *Physician's Tale*,' *Annuale Mediaevale* 14 (1973): 35-42; Brian S. Lee, 'The Position and Purpose of The Physician's Tale,' *Chaucer Review* 22 (1987): 140-160 (suggests Virginius's resemblance to Apius); and more recently Daniel T. Kline, 'Jephthah's Daughter and Chaucer's Virginia: The Critique of Sacrifice in The Physician's Tale,' *JEGP* (2008): 77-103. Donald R. Howard

perhaps still speaks for most when he likens it to the Prioress's as 'moral tales whose morality seems questionable'; *The Idea of the Canterbury Tales* (Berkeley: University of California Press, 1978), 54; and similarly Anne Middleton, 'The *Physician's Tale* and Love's Martyrs: 'Ensamples mo than ten' as a Method in the *Canterbury Tales*,' *Chaucer Review* 8 (1973-1974): 9-32; and most recently V. A. Kolve, *Telling Images: Chaucer and the Imagery of Narrative II* (Stanford: Stanford University Press, 2009), 52-53, which sees 'the martyrdom of Virginia in *The Physician's Tale'* as 'suffering without purpose and without redemptive potential.' Others, including Robert Longworth, 'The Doctor's Dilemma: A Comic View of the *Physician's Tale*,' *Criticism* 13 (1971): 223-233, the title speaking for itself, take a diametrically different view. Perhaps Henry Ansgar Kelly best sums up collective critical response when speaking of 'the *Physician's Tale*, which Harry Bailly liked, but most subsequent auditors and readers have not;' see *Chaucerian Tragedy* (Cambridge: D. S. Brewer, 1997), 193.

[7] Hence Kolve compares the fate of Virginia with those of the heroines of the *Legend of Good Women*, whom Chaucer found in Ovid's *Heroides*; see his chapter 2, 'From Cleopatra to Alceste: An Iconographic Study of *The Legend of Good Women*,' *Telling Images*, 28-66. The *Heroides*, for Robert Worth Frank, Jr., 'is itself an exercise in pathos, and must have educated [Chaucer] in the method and encouraged him in the practice,' as evident in Chaucer's treatments of 'Custance, Griselda, Virginia, Lucrece, Philomela'; see *Chaucer and The Legend of Good Women* (Cambridge, MA: Harvard University Press, 1972), 95.

[8] As Gregory M. Sadlek has noticed, Gower's reasons for this emphasis include the advanced age of Amans, who has himself (apparently) waited too long to commit to love, and is no longer capable of procreation; see *Idleness Working: The Discourses of Love's Labor from Ovid through Chaucer and Gower* (Washington, D.C.: Catholic University of America Press, 2004), 200-201.

[9] Cf. for example 'To an Athlete, Dying Young.'

[10] The horrifying expansion of this transformation in Gower's work is Book I of his long poem in Latin, the *Vox Clamantis*. A depiction of the Revolt of 1381 as a nightmare, the so-called 'Visio' section vividly portrays the familiar world overturned by the lower orders, who all turn into carnivorous animals and birds. Interesting to consider in this regard is Robert Mills's application of the term 'burgerlijk' as a repressive mode of apprehension in his discussion of the fifteenth-century Dutch masterpiece, 'The Flaying of Sisamnes'; see *Suspended Animation: Pain, Pleasure and Punishment in Medieval Culture* (London: Reaktion Books, 2005), 79-80; and see also

Howard's comment on Chaucer's view of the 'bourgeois mentality' (*Idea*, 54).

[11] Much has been written on this conflict, but see recently (and variously) Ann W. Astell, *Political Allegory in Late Medieval England* (Ithaca: Cornell University Press, 1999), esp. 44-94; David Aers, *Faith, Ethics and Church: Writing in England, 1360-1409* (Cambridge: D. S. Brewer, 2000), esp. Chapter 1, 'Faith, Ethics, and Communities,' 1-25; Terry Jones, R. F. Yeager, Terry Dolan, Alan Fletcher and Juliette Dor, *Who Murdered Chaucer? A Medieval Mystery* (London: Methuen, 2003), esp. 60-96; Matthew Giancarlo, *Parliament and Literature in Late Medieval England* (Cambridge: Cambridge University Press, 2007), esp. 209-259; John M. Bowers, *Chaucer and Langland: The Antagonistic Tradition* (South Bend, IN: University of Notre Dame Press, 2007), esp. 103-156; and in particular *Wyclif: Political Ideas and Practice*: *Papers by Michael Wilks*, ed. Anne Hudson (Oxford: Oxbow Books, 2000), esp. chapters 1 ('John Wyclif, Reformer, c. 1327-1384'), 4 ('Reformatio Regni: Wyclif and Hus as Leaders of Religious Protest Movements'), and 6 ('Royal Priesthood: The Origins of Lollardy').

[12] An excellent overview is offered by Hugh White, *Nature, Sex, and Goodness in Medieval Literary Tradition* (Oxford: Oxford University Press, 2000).

[13] See the excellent study of Patricia Eberle, 'Miniatures as Evidence of Reading in a Manuscript of the *Confessio Amantis* (Pierpont Morgan MS M.126)' in *John Gower: Recent Readings*, ed. R. F. Yeager (Kalamazoo, MI: Medieval Institute Press, 1989), 311-364.

[14] Esther Cohen traces the late medieval representation of martyrs' apparent serenity while dying to William of Auxerre and other thirteenth-century scholastics, who held that martyrs transcended pain 'because they used their reason, or the upper part of their souls, to ward off the onslaught of passions provoked by external attacks. Alternatively, their souls were strong enough to feel and internalise the pain but behave as though they felt nothing.' See *The Modulated Scream: Pain in Late Medieval Culture* (Chicago: University of Chicago Press, 2010), 244. And see further Mills, *Suspended Animation*, who contrasts torment on the faces of suffering sinners with 'martyrdom and passion iconography [that] often depicts the saint's face as unmoved…or looking up to heaven..., and as such conveys a 'lack of fit' between the tortures being carried out and the psychological consequences of those tortures' (163). Mills suggestively compares martyrs to Deleuze's positive assessment of the masochists as those expecting 'pain as the condition that will bring about future pleasure' (159).

[15] I am grateful to one of the readers of this essay for reminding me that 'the Physician's Tale arguably draws some of its affective force' from the

hagiography of the virgin martyr legend—and that in the *Canterbury Tales* Virginia has 'sisters' in Griselda, Custance and St. Cecelia.

[16] Most recent is Cohen, *Modulated Scream*, especially chapters 6 ('The Christian History of Humanity') and 7 ('Human and Divine Passion'); but see also Elaine Scarry, *The Body in Pain: The Making and Unmaking of the World* (New York: Oxford University Press, 1985), and Donald Mowbray, *Pain and Suffering in Medieval Theology: Academic Debates at the University of Paris in the Thirteenth Century* (Woodbridge: Boydell Press, 2009).

Bibliography

Aers, David. *Faith, Ethics and Church: Writing in England, 1360-1409.* Cambridge: D. S. Brewer, 2000.

Astell, Ann W. *Political Allegory in Late Medieval England.* Ithaca: Cornell University Press, 1999.

Bowers, John M. *Chaucer and Langland: The Antagonistic Tradition.* South Bend, IN: University of Notre Dame Press, 2007.

Chaucer, Geoffrey. *The Riverside Chaucer.* 3rd edition. Edited by Larry D. Benson. Boston: Houghton Mifflin, 1986.

Cohen, Esther. *The Modulated Scream: Pain in Late Medieval Culture.* Chicago: University of Chicago Press, 2010.

Eberle, Patricia. 'Miniatures as Evidence of Reading in a Manuscript of the *Confessio Amantis* (Pierpont Morgan MS M.126).' In *John Gower: Recent Readings.* Edited by R. F. Yeager, 311-364. Kalamazoo, MI: Medieval Institute Press, 1989.

Frank, Jr., Robert Worth. *Chaucer and the Legend of Good Women.* Cambridge, MA: Harvard University Press, 1972.

Giancarlo, Matthew. *Parliament and Literature in Late Medieval England.* Cambridge: Cambridge University Press, 2007.

Gower, John. *The Complete Works of John Gower.* Edited by G. C. Macaulay, 4 vols. Oxford: Clarendon Press, 1899-1902.

Hanks, Jr., D. Thomas. 'Chaucer, *Auctoritas*, and the Problem of Pain.' In *'Seyde in forme and reverence': Essays on Chaucer and Chaucerians in Memory of Emerson Brown, Jr.* Edited by T. L. Burton and John F. Plummer, 219-236. Adelaide: The Chaucer Studio, 2005.

Hoffman, Richard R. 'Jephthah's Daughter and Chaucer's Virginia.' *Chaucer Review* 2 (1967): 20-31.

Howard, Donald R. *The Idea of the Canterbury Tales*. Berkeley: University of California Press, 1978.

Hudson, Anne, ed. *Wyclif: Political Ideas and Practice: Papers by Michael Wilks*. Oxford: Oxbow Books, 2000.

Jones, Terry, R. F. Yeager, Terry Dolan, Alan Fletcher and Juliette Dor. *Who Murdered Chaucer? A Medieval Mystery*. London: Methuen, 2003.

Kelly, Henry Ansgar. *Chaucerian Tragedy*. Cambridge: D. S. Brewer, 1997.

Kline, Daniel T. 'Jephthah's Daughter and Chaucer's Virginia: The Critique of Sacrifice in The Physician's Tale.' *JEGP* (2008): 77-103.

Kolve, V. A. *Telling Images: Chaucer and the Imagery of Narrative II*. Stanford: Stanford University Press, 2009.

Lee, Brian S. 'The Position and Purpose of The Physician's Tale.' *Chaucer Review* 22 (1987): 140-160.

Longworth, Robert. 'The Doctor's Dilemma: A Comic View of the *Physician's Tale*.' *Criticism* 13 (1971): 223-233.

Mathewson, Jeanne T. 'For Love and Not for Hate: The Value of Virginity in Chaucer's *Physician's Tale*.' *Annuale Mediaevale* 14 (1973): 35-42.

Middleton, Anne. 'The *Physician's Tale* and Love's Martyrs: 'Ensamples mo than ten' as a Method in the *Canterbury Tales*.' *Chaucer Review* 8 (1973-1974): 9-32.

Mills, Robert. *Suspended Animation: Pain, Pleasure and Punishment in Medieval Culture*. London: Reaktion Books, 2005.

Mowbray, Donald. *Pain and Suffering in Medieval Theology: Academic Debates at the University of Paris in the Thirteenth Century*. Woodbridge: Boydell Press, 2009.

Sadlek, Gregory M. *Idleness Working: The Discourses of Love's Labor from Ovid through Chaucer and Gower*. Washington, DC: Catholic University of America Press, 2004.

Scarry, Elaine. *The Body in Pain: The Making and Unmaking of the World.* New York: Oxford University Press, 1985.

Shannon, Edgar F. 'The Physician's Tale.' In *Sources and Analogues of Chaucer's Canterbury Tales.* Edited by W. F. Bryan and Germaine Dempster, 398-408. New York: Humanities Press, 1958.

White, Hugh. *Nature, Sex, and Goodness in Medieval Literary Tradition.* Oxford: Oxford University Press, 2000.

Pain as Emotion: The Role of Emotional Pain in Fifteenth-Century Italian Medicine and Confession

Na'ama Cohen-Hanegbi

Abstract
Pain and the healing of pain are found at the basis of the two healing professions of the Middle Ages: medicine, responsible for the preservation of the body from illness, and the clergy which claimed authority over the medicine of the soul and the healing of sins. Both disciplines were concerned with defining pain and understanding its role in the process of healing, not merely for theoretical purposes but for the sake of practice as well. In this essay I focus on the notion of pain (*dolor*) as an emotion, pain of the soul (*dolor animi*) and the pain of remorse (*contrition*) within both contexts. These forms of pain present a substantial methodological issue regarding the definition of pain and its nature since they are found on the periphery of the established definition of pain. In an attempt to contribute to our understanding of this rather large problem, ethe chapter provides a detailed case study of the terminology of emotional pain employed by physicians and confessors, its theoretical underpinnings and its use for assertion of professional authority.

Key Words: *Anima*, *animus*, *dolor*, *contritio*, pain of remorse, pain of the soul, accidents of the soul, sacrament of confession, emotional pain, physical pain, penance.

*****

Pain and the healing of pain were of fundamental interest to both medical and religious practices of the Middle Ages. Medicine sought to treat suffering patients and/or to alleviate their pain; the Church incorporated pain into its devotional practices as a means of reaching spiritual healing and salvation. The ways physicians and priests approached pain were interwoven with the conceptions of pain formulated by the disciplines in which they were active. Thus the definitions of pain and its supposed physical, mental and spiritual roles determined the methods professionals used in caring for and treating pain. Yet pain in itself was not an isolated phenomenon and since there were many definitions of pain, one can also speak of a variety of pains. Consider the distinct qualities of each of the following pains: the pain of crucifixion or self-flagellation and the pain caused by demonic possession, pain of surgery or disease, pain of childbirth. As Esther Cohen has recently argued, the plurality of pains determined the plurality of methods for dealing with pain.[1]

This essay is devoted to a type of pain which can be defined as emotional; it is principally felt in the psyche/soul and has either secondary or no physical manifestation.[2] This kind of pain requires the adoption of a different methodological approach with regard to the historical continuity of the notion of pain. Emotional pain introduces the psychological and mental components of pain which are often cast aside as secondary to physical/sensory pain. In their emotional orientation, these pains point to the boundaries of the definition of pain as a physical or sensory experience, placing a much stronger emphasis on the role of feelings such as sorrow and sadness and of more amorphous states such as suffering and afflictions. This holistic and non-dualistic consideration is especially relevant for studying the pre-modern world, but it can also shed light on contemporary thought about pain more generally. By considering this somewhat borderline phenomenon, emotional pain, which provides another angle on the subject of pain, it enables us to identify central issues in pain studies.

With this wide-ranging methodological issue in mind, the chapter focuses on two late medieval disciplines in which emotional pain is formulated: medicine and the theology of penance. The chapter analyses the terminology and theoretical underpinning of emotional pain employed in works of both disciplines—namely, writings of Italian physicians and confessors of the fifteenth century. In order to set the contours of the analysis, specific terms have been chosen: *pain* (*dolor*) appearing in passages on emotions, *pain of the soul* (*dolor animi*) and *pain of remorse* (*contritio*). Examining the use of these words and the meaning conveyed by them, I discuss the affinity and distinction between emotional pains, or pains of the soul, in such works. I argue that pain was conceptualised in the thought of both professions through an on-going negotiation concerning the rapport between the physical, psychological and mental dimensions of the human being. Furthermore, this negotiation allowed for a re-formulation of professional authority to treat emotional pain and consequently, more broadly, the souls of patients and penitents.

1. Physical and Emotional Pains

The study of pain in history inevitably investigates the definition of pain. In *The History of Pain*, Roselyne Rey regards pain as a physical, objective and biological state, consistent throughout history.[3] This default definition of pain, or the aspect of pain under focus, is widespread in much of the scholarship on the topic. In order to understand medieval pain, however, a less rigid distinction between the physical and the emotional should be implemented. As recent scholarship on pain in the Middle Ages has shown, it is nearly impossible to distinguish the physical state from the psychological and mental one in the thought of the period: sensation was viewed as a faculty of the soul. Theological, natural philosophical and medical theories turned to psychological faculties of perception and estimation in order to explain how pain was felt.[4] Impassibility and indifference to pain, seen in martyrs or holy people, were also usually attributed to the capacities of the soul and its ability to comprehend or resist pain.[5] The wounds of Christ were relived through intense mental exercises performed by mystics such as Bernard of Clairvaux and St Francis as well as through the celebration of the Eucharist.[6] Medieval pain was thus understood as a physical phenomenon configured by psychological processes.

In a similar vein, the pain or *dolor* of the soul, an aspect or a type of pain which is primarily psychological and involves little or no physical sensation, is most often discussed in relation to physical pain. David B. Morris, for example, points out that for Catherine of Siena the desired devotional suffering and spiritual pains were modelled on physical pains.[7] Rachel Fulton discusses the utilisation of emotional pain and anguish in devotional practices, showing that such pains were firmly linked to physical ones. According to her analysis of *passio*, medieval authors saw the pains of the soul as a simulation of the passion of Christ and of the crucifixion. Pain of the soul was thus attained through empathy or *compassio* with physical pain and was understood and construed through the prism of physical pain.[8] Still, the dependence of emotional pain on physical pain, which Morris and Fulton illustrate, touches on a fundamental problem in understanding medieval approaches to emotional pain. Theoretically, while physical pain was inherently dependent on operations of the soul and could not be felt without them, emotional pains did not require an involvement of the body. And yet, most accounts of emotional or psychological pain assume some kind of relationship with the body: they either mimic the pain of the body or draw analogies to it.

The strong correlation between physical, emotional or spiritual pain is exemplified in the vocabulary of pain. The two primary words for pain in medieval Latin, *dolor* and *passio*, signify both physical pain and pain of the soul. It is therefore not always clear and sometimes impossible to ascertain which pain is being referred to in a given text. Indeed, these terms can also conflate: as Donald Mowbray's analysis of the writings of thirteenth-century scholastics shows, theologians considered physical and emotional pain in close proximity and at times almost interchangeably.[9] For example, in his discussions of the passions Thomas Aquinas devotes seven articles to explicating the definition of pain as a passion of the soul, in relation to both physical and spiritual pain.[10] The consideration of pain and sorrow together (at times through the word *dolor* and sometimes by adding the word *tristitia*) and the identification of sorrow as a species of pain substantiate an integrated approach to pains of the body and of the soul.[11] However, reading Aquinas's discussion, it becomes clear that this integration did not overcome necessary distinctions between pain and sorrow and between physical and emotional states. Thus Aquinas describes a divergent cognitive path for pain which is experienced in the body—affecting the external senses—and pain that is experienced in the soul—through the internal senses.

Similar attempts to draw distinctions are also apparent in medieval medical literature.[12] In these texts a differentiation is often present between *passiones* signalling physical pains and *passiones animae/animi*, pains of the soul usually referring more generally to the emotions (a similar distinction is found in a range of sources between *dolor* and *dolor animi*). The fact that these distinctions were drawn within the holistic approach of the late Middle Ages should not be overlooked. The degree of dependence/independence of the pains of the soul was therefore an issue that drew the attention of medieval physicians and theologians, and both the disciplines oscillated between notions of unity and separateness of body and soul when discussing and defining pain. Moreover, the definitions of pain formulated by the practitioners were, I argue, made to serve professional needs, participating in the formulation of their professional methods and roles in ascribing patients and penitents a regimen of emotions.

2. Pain as an *Accident of the Soul* in Medieval Medicine

Accidents of the soul, or emotions, appear in medical literature first and foremost as causes affecting the health of the body. A regimen of emotions was prescribed to patients as a means of curing illness and securing health; it was counted among the six non-natural factors which influence the state of a person's complexion (*res non-naturales* comprise air, sleep, food and drink, exercise, purgation and the emotions). The two major genres of practical medicine of the late Middle Ages, the regimens of health and the *consilia* (collections of medical cases) include passages directing patients towards a correct emotional regimen suitable to their health. A survey of the vocabulary of emotions found in such medical literature written in Latin and Italian from the late twelfth to the fifteenth century shows a recurrent use of several words denoting emotion, in particular joy, anger, sorrow, fear and worries. These vocabulary choices are well rooted in the medical tradition echoing Galen's passage on emotions in the third book of the *Tegni*, which instructs one to avoid anger, sorrow, joy, wrath, fear, envy and worries.[13] Neither pain nor pain of the soul were included in this list. In fact, the word *dolor* indicating an emotion is nearly absent from Italian medical accounts up to the fifteenth century. In the fifteenth century, however, physicians began to include pain in their instructions of correct emotional behaviour.

Fifteenth-century medical works mention the 'accident of the soul' or pain almost ubiquitously as harmful to health and as an occurrence that should be avoided. Nevertheless, the specific nature of pain and the reasons for its harmful consequences are not clearly evident. Most instructions to avoid pain are brief and offered almost carelessly, among instructions concerning other damaging emotions. In his *Consilia ad diversas aegritudines*, the physician Ugo Benzi of Siena (1376-1439) instructed a patient suffering from obstructed vision to refrain from pain, anxiety and thoughts, but to rejoice and delight in measured proportion.[14] Ugo instructed another patient, one suffering from a weakening of the stomach, to avoid anger, sorrow, *accidia* (a state combining sloth and despair), worries, too much thinking and pain.[15] Similar instructions were repeated to patients who suffered from a cough or from chronic nasal mucus deriving from a weak stomach: avoid anger, pain, sorrow, shouting and quarrels;[16] avoid pain, anger, sorrow, fear and quarrels.[17] Bartholomaeus de Montagnana (d. 1460), a physician and professor of medicine in Padua and author of *Consilia CCCV*, chose a similar format when advising a patient with various episodes of trembling and sensory disturbances:

> Concerning the accidents of the soul, all excesses must be avoided. Therefore, all that moves moderately the spirit and spreads it and gathers it is suitable since when spirit and heat are suddenly moved it is unhealthy. Hence, superfluous joy, laughter, sorrow, worry and anger, pain and similar things should be avoided.[18]

The inclusion of pain among emotions is not explained. Both physicians list it alongside other emotions without mentioning what they mean by pain—an elaboration would not suit this genre of practical writing. Since our information about the practice of medical consultation is only mediated to us through texts edited and shaped according to the contemporary medical ideal, it is impossible to ascertain if in actual encounters with patients, fifteenth-century Italian physicians discussed emotional pain. We may further suspect that the emergence of this issue did not seem particularly problematic to the authors. Yet it is an addition that does point to a more general shift evolving in the medical thought about emotions in the period.

3. The Role of the Physician in Treating Emotions

From the late twelfth century, medical theory discussed the proper manner and degree of physicians' involvement with the accidents of the soul. Treating emotions suggested crossing the conventional boundaries of medicine as it led physicians to care not only for the body (which was their professional mandate) but also for the soul. From the twelfth to the fourteenth century, authors proposed various rationalisations to settle this difficulty. They recurrently mention, rather apologetically, the convention that physicians should only consider emotions in so far as they influence the body and its humoural complexion, but then go on to argue that in order to secure the patient's health it is necessary that physicians treat emotions as well. A representative approach to this professional quandary is found in the influential commentary to Galen's *Tegni*, *Plusquam commentum in microtegni Galeni* written in the early fourteenth century by Pietro Torrigiano (d. ca. 1320), a Florentine physician who also taught in Paris. Pietro notes that the task of treating emotions is more appropriate to philosophy and law, professions which have the tools and knowledge to influence and enforce appropriate emotional habits. In contrast to medicine which treats the body, philosophy and law are directed at modifying the soul. However, Pietro proceeds to state that behaviour is determined by physical condition, quoting a phrase he attributes to Galen: 'evil deeds follow the *species* of distempered complexion.'[19] In this commentary Pietro suggests that caring for the body constitutes caring for the soul and human behaviour, thus setting the ground for physicians' activity in adding emotions to their province. The justification for discussing and treating emotions in medicine is therefore based on the assumption that body and soul influence each other. Emotions are relevant to medicine because they shape and are in turn shaped by physical complexion. This notion was also put forth in the recurrent explanations by physicians of the physical movement that accompanies each emotion: for example, anger heats the blood around the heart while joy spreads the heat from the heart to the extremities of the body. Clearly the identification of the physical changes that emotions incur justified medicine's meddling in the affairs of the soul. This line (or similar ones) of reasoning on the relevance of emotions to medicine is proposed in theoretical medical writings throughout the fifteenth century, albeit, as I argue elsewhere, in an increasingly adamant tone endorsing the care of emotions in medicine.[20]

In view of medical authors' assertions that their interest in emotions is primarily physical, the appearance of *dolor* as an accident of the soul in the practical works of the fifteenth century is telling. Almost no precedents are extant, and I have yet to find a precise account of influence of pain, as an accident of the soul, on the body. Moreover, the complexional characteristics of pain are never mentioned per se. In a literature that is as conventional, formulaic and genre-abiding as the medical literature of the period, a novelty which strays from the accepted structure requires explanation. What then was the premise that allowed this new insertion of pain into the discourse of emotions? And consequently, what does this new insertion signify and what purpose did it serve?

4. *Dolor* and Other Emotions

In trying to decipher the use of pain in the context of practical medical sources, we may retrieve clues from specific cases in which the word *dolor* appears. The Paduan physician Batholomaeus de Montagnana advised one of his patients to refrain from sad or painful things and from the anxiety of loss.[21] The general tone of this instruction, which relates to states of sorrow and grief, suggests that *dolor* should be understood as a similar emotion. Further support to this use of *dolor* appears in Benedetto Reguardati da Norcia's (1398-1469) *De conservatione sanitatis* in which the author explicitly regards the 'pain of the soul' (*dolor animi*) as synonymous to sorrow.

In this identification of the pain of the soul with sorrow, Benedetto also clarifies the influence of pain on the body. Pain of the soul acts in a manner similar to the way sorrow does: the heat of the body moves inwards and causes hiccups (!): 'for in sorrow or in the pain of the soul the natural heat is diminished (*ignoratur*) because of the drawing back and the joining of the spirit to the interior members. And it consumes these superfluous things which induce hiccups in the stomach.' More dangerously sorrow, and therefore pain of the soul as well, draw the heat into the heart causing all members of the body to freeze.[22]

If indeed *dolor* and sorrow (*tristitia*) should be understood as the same emotions, the sudden insertion of *dolor* into the sections devoted to the accidents of the soul does not constitute a challenge to the conventions of medical writing about emotions. Emotional pain, like sorrow, is not confined to the soul alone but rather produces a change in the body which harms health and therefore requires medical intervention. It also provides a certain response to our query about the nature of emotional pain. Yet other queries persist. It remains unclear why physicians, who in all other instances and for all other purposes prefer a brief text, choose in this case to repeat these synonymous words in their advice to patients. Furthermore, some cases suggest that the identification of pain with sorrow does not capture the broader nature of the notion of *dolor* and *dolor animi* and should be more accurately translated as suffering. Thus, for example, in his *regimen sanitatis* the Florentine physician Antonio Benivieni (1443-1502) suggested refraining from pain and all other passions of the soul—*dolor et aliae animi passiones.*[23] *Dolor* here is equivalent not to a specific emotion but to emotions in general. However, the ambiguity concerning the meaning of pain in this context is emblematic of one of the significant changes that occurred within the medical discussion of emotions during this period. In the fifteenth century we witness a striking expansion of the emotions included under the physician's care, not all of which are clearly relevant to the medical profession.

A review of the vocabulary of emotions in medical literature reveals that at the end of the fourteenth century and throughout the fifteenth the vocabulary underwent a distinct expansion: anxiety (*angustia*), hatred (*odium*) and hope (*spes*) emerged alongside other emotions which had appeared more traditionally in practical medical texts. Some of the words are synonymous (or almost parallel) with words which had already entered medical discourse: *metus* was added to *timor* (both words denoting fear), *angustia* (anxiety) parallels *sollicitudo* (worries), and melancholy is parallel to *tristitia* (sorrow). In addition, it seems that some of the synonymous words (like *accidia* or *rixa* [quarrel or strife]) were borrowed from religious discussions and imported into medicine in various ways. Some of these borrowed words introduced completely new emotional experiences to the medical emotional vocabulary, as is the case with *misericordia*, or compassion.[24] Pain was thus not the only word to enter medical discourse in the fifteenth century.

The appearance of the word 'pain' in medical literature belongs to this extensive phenomenon. A new vocabulary of emotions in medicine was formulated, richer and more elaborate than before. Most of these new words were introduced without an explanation for their influence on the body and the clinical picture they produced. In this sense pain was not a unique case. The word *dolor* could have been inserted into medical discourse as a means of expanding the vocabulary of emotions relating to sorrow or to other types of sadness and suffering. For this purpose the significance of a word or its exact influence did not matter, since what was at stake was the lavish vocabulary itself and not the mental and physiological impact that a specific word bore.

Yet this elaborate language had wider implications. The expansion of the vocabulary offered physicians a double service: on the one hand, it enriched and diversified medical writing, making its technical style more flexible and adding to its breadth. On the other hand, it broadened physicians' authority and strengthened their role as healers of emotions.

Physicians' authority to treat emotions was, as we have seen, disputed by physicians themselves and required recurrent justification. During the fourteenth and fifteenth centuries a slow but stable change was apparent in physicians' demand to acknowledge their authority to treat emotions as part of their medical role. The expansion of the vocabulary of the emotions can be viewed as a practical step on their part to enforce this demand. The inclusion of the words *dolor* and *dolor animi* without a defined theoretical anchor demonstrates the physicians' desire to embrace a wider scope of treatment of the emotions without providing a physiological justification for each emotion included. It was clearly a testimony to the physicians' aspiration to acknowledge that all accidents of the soul, all emotions, are relevant to human health, and thereby to medicine.

The introduction of *dolor* and *dolor animi* into the medical account of emotions aptly exemplifies the use physicians made of the dialectics found at the core of the debate regarding the relationship between body and soul. For physicians it was necessary to justify their interest in emotions by claiming that all emotional affairs related to the body as well, by means of mutual influence. However, this position was very restrictive and constraining. Inserting a vocabulary that was not associated with the body implied a broader interest and a more inclusive involvement with the affairs of the soul.

5. *Dolor animi* and Contrition

We have seen how the introduction of several words denoting emotions expanded the vocabulary of emotions in medicine and was at times the result of the transfer of these words from religious and theological discourse. This importation did not occur in a systematic manner and it is impossible to designate a particular text from which these words were borrowed. Rather, these words were very common in religious contexts and in some cases were restricted to them, and their usage necessarily implied a Christian tone. In the example of the usage of *dolor animi* in medical tracts, this assimilation is particularly interesting because it preserves or echoes terminology, but not necessarily the meaning that was ascribed to it in religious contexts.

The compound *dolor animi* or *animi dolor* appears in theological writing over the centuries as a pain of the soul and as a pain detached from the body. One particularly important arena in which the pain of the soul was discussed was in relation to the process of penance. I shall discuss here the discourse of *dolor animi* within the theology of penance and confession not as a direct source of medical use of the term (which it most probably was not) but because this discourse reveals elements that are comparable to the medical discourse on the topic, particularly in the growing detachment of emotional pain from the body in both disciplines and in their contribution to the role of the caregivers.

From a theological standpoint, the pain of the soul relates to feelings of regret (*compunctio/contritio*) which are an integral and necessary part of the sacrament of penance. Thus, in contrast to the unwonted appearance of this term in fifteenth-century medical discourse concerning emotions, *dolor* continued to be a fundamental element in the medicine of the soul and especially in one of its central methods—the sacrament of penance.

The power of the sacrament of penance to heal was understood to occur through a procedure in which the sinning person (with the aid of the confessor) exposes his/her sins/illnesses, expels them and is filled instead with contrition. These images of sin as sickness and of the sacrament as medicine were well entrenched in the literature of confession and are found in many sources, including the church's decree ordering annual confession to all believers.[25] Bearing in mind the pervasive metaphoric use of physical illness, wound and remedy, it is not surprising to find that pain was associated with the process of cure from sin. Indeed, contrition, or regret, was defined in the literature on confession from the twelfth century on as a form of pain—*dolor*. But this was not an ordinary pain and its essence was a topic discussed at length between the twelfth and fifteenth centuries, when greater emphasis was placed on the inner state of contrition.[26] Various definitions of contrition were offered and they refer to a number of issues such as the origin of this emotion, its degree, its expression and the ways it can be detected. Notably, one aspect that attracted much debate touched essentially on the physicality of this pain.

The term *dolor animi* was used by Abelard (1079-1142) to describe the sacrament of penance in its entirety—that is, the act of seeking amends for one's sins involves feeling pain, or is led by a pain of the soul.[27] Towards the end of the century another Parisian master, Alain of Lille (1128-1202), who wrote extensively on penance, stated more specifically that the state of contrition—that is, remorse—derives from pain.[28] In both of these cases, the notion of pain as a state is not elaborated. However, both Abelard and Alain define the pain of penance as *dolor animi*. The word *animi* (nom. *animus*) relates to the mind—the intellectual faculty of the soul. This faculty was considered to be detached from the body. Although it often seems that *animus* and *anima* (the life-giving soul) were used interchangeably, in the case of contrition theologians claimed that the pain of remorse was of an intellectual type. If in the writings of Abelard and Alain this notion is merely suggested, it was well developed by later theologians in the course of the following two centuries.

6. The Nature of the Pain of Contrition

With the growing demand to maintain a more exact notion of what would be a valid contrition, we find during the thirteenth century intricate accounts of the true (and false) nature of contrition. A range of views on this topic is known, but one definition of contrition emerged above all and became canonised. It is found in all manuals of confession written between the thirteenth and fifteenth century: 'Contrition is a pain (*dolor*) over one's sins assumed voluntarily with the intention of confessing and doing satisfaction.' The emphasis on the voluntary nature of the pain of contrition was central to understanding the type of pain confessors sought to find and perhaps evoke in their penitents.

Will and pain are opposite phenomena according to medieval thought. Pain, as noted above, was understood to 'happen' to a person; a person is passive to the state of pain—hence, the Latin *passio*. Will, in contrast, was the epitome of human agency. It was procured by the intellect, a faculty of the soul, which was perceived to be detached from the body. Will was the product of the mind—the *animus*. The notion of voluntary pain, on the contrary, implied that pain was not inflicted passively and was not felt by the body. In fact, Albert the Great, Thomas Aquinas and others following them insisted that the pain of contrition should be achieved through the intellect and not felt through the senses.[29] In endorsing intellectual pain they argued that, as it was obtained through reason (and supposedly understanding), it would always be 'perfect' and always sufficient to erase one's sins, whereas sensible pain may be sufficient but does not secure grace.[30] The strong emphasis on voluntary and rational pain led thirteenth-century theologians to resist sensory expression of pain, predominantly avoiding, or at least trying to avoid, seeing it as a sign of true contrition as was traditionally accepted.[31] In fact, if contritional pain would appear to overflow into the senses and also affect them, it could be defined, according to some thirteenth-century theologians, as excessive pain.[32] Ann Thayer points out that authors of sermons encouraged listeners to express contrition through tears and external expression. She argues, contrary to Tentler's findings, that this is evidence of the very emotional understanding of contrition in the period.[33] The contradiction is, however, found in the texts themselves. Contrition is described as both a very deep emotion and a non-sensitive, non-emotional state. This dialectic defined the unique state of contrition as the pain of remorse which was very moving but also a pure mental process. Nevertheless, only through the emphasis on the intellectual nature of contrition was the pain of contrition distinguished from all other types of pain. Thus, the resentment of signs of physicality in the feeling of *contritio* was resentment towards the association of this pain with more mundane feelings. In emphasising contrition as a pain of the intellectual soul, theologians depicted contrition as a very extraordinary state, difficult to attain. The formulation of contrition as such granted it special spiritual value.

The significance and implications of the rising prominence of contrition within the sacrament of penance from the twelfth century on has elicited diverse interpretations by scholars. While it is problematic to claim that it gave way to a new understanding of the inner self and a new form of interiority, as some have argued,[34] it is clear that theologians had a greater need to discuss the ways in which inner experiences were felt, projected and expressed.[35] One of the major problems addressed was how the confessor could decide whether the penitent felt true contrition and was eligible for forgiveness.[36] In order to provide priests with criteria for granting absolution some external measures were constructed. Thus, while early thirteenth-century theologians and canon lawyers, such as the Papal jurist Raymond de Peñafort, insisted that only perfect contrition could merit absolution,[37] in later decades theologians suggested ways to circumvent this harsh stipulation which could not be truly tested. In the early fourteenth century, the Franciscan Astesanus of Asti (d. ca. 1330), and later on Antoninus of Florence (1389-1459), argued that even the willingness to repent, acknowledged by the act of going to confession, should suffice as proof of the existence of contrition.[38] According to these thinkers, even if the penitent was not fully contrite, his willingness to repent would transform the imperfect and partial pain (often named *attritio*) into a complete and necessary one—contrition. In this way, despite the difficulty (or impossibility) of judging whether a penitent was contrite, confessors could offer penitents the cure of salvation of the soul.

Defining the pain of contrition as unknowable to penitent and confessor was also liberating for the individual penitent. Inner processes were now translated into actions. One was only required to attend confession with the intention of seeking penance, and contrition would follow. At the same time, the individual process was neglected while dependence on the confessor and on the institution of confession grew immensely. Nevertheless, this new way of thinking about contrition was not only a casuistic manoeuvre which drew penitents to the church—it constituted an original way of thinking about voluntary pain. True pain is hard to attain and almost impossible to measure. Neither the penitent himself nor the confessor may determine how full and thorough it is. Only God knows its depth, and only He is able to determine whether it is worthy of absolution. Thus, essentially, it is spiritual pain.

7. *Contritio* as Spiritual Pain

In the definition formulated by the Franciscan Angelus Carletus (1411-1495), the healing pain of contrition is described as a phenomenon contingent upon grace:

> How does contrition differ from attrition? I respond following Francis and other theologians that it differs in two ways. The first: that attrition is imperfect pain, contrition truly is perfect pain. The second: that attrition is pain without endowed grace, but not so contrition. And therefore, contrition and attrition are materially similar, in the same way that a house is either dark or illuminated. Attrition indeed is the light of dawn which, increasing, becomes contrition in midday.[39]

The state of contrition, according to Angelus's preferred opinion, is a miraculous occurrence empowered by God. The degree of perfection of remorse is dependent not upon the penitent but on the interjection of divine grace. Grace perfects the pain of the penitent. The *dolor animi* of contrition is one which is obtained through interaction with the divine; the body is irrelevant to this type of pain.

Angelus was also struck with the problem such spiritual pain posed for the confessor as for the penitent—it was impossible to know whether the penitent felt partial pain or whether he enjoyed God's intervention and was endowed with perfect contrite pain. He, too, resorted to the ritual of the sacrament for aid, but instead of saying that adherence to the sacrament functioned as a sign, he argued that it was the presence of the priests who facilitated the grace of God for the penitents. The priests, endowed with the power to care for souls (the office of *cura animarum* given to clergy enabling them to hear confessions), could transform the state of the penitent: '[turn] a person who is not contrite, to one who is contrite through the power of absolution.' And he added that the confessing priest, 'due to his office, or as a mediator, is able through attrition to remove the obstacle to the Holy Spirit. He removes the blemish of sin by assisting through his office to the divine power to erase the sin.'[40]

According to Angelus, the priest held the keys which assisted in turning partial pain of repentance into contrition through the grace of God. Thus, he acted as an agent through which the miraculous power instilling true contrition was transmitted. Although Angelus did not challenge the accepted definition of contrition as a voluntary pain, he did stress strongly the necessary function of grace. This emphasis on divine intervention repositioned the importance of the agency of the will. The active role of the penitent in achieving contrition, according to Angelus, required and depended more firmly on the particular healing essence of contrition transmitted from God through the priest. Furthermore, Angelus's emphasis on the function of grace defined contrition as a state which belongs not to the intellect but to external powers, powers much greater than the penitent himself. The transformation in the understanding of the nature of contrition also had professional implications. It was no longer possible to argue (if one accepted Angelus's thinking) that a person may receive absolution in any form of non-formal confession. The authority of the confessor in the sacrament was not only one of default, due to his knowledge and learning and thus his ability to pass judgment—it was a spiritual role essential to the procedure of the sacrament and to the true experience of pain.

8. Healing Authority and Pain

The appearance of the word *dolor* and even more clearly the combination *dolor animi* within medical discussions on emotions was not a unique or isolated phenomenon in the fifteenth century. It is part of an expansion of the vocabulary of emotions in medicine and of the tendency to instil in medical discourse (especially with regard to the body) terms which related to the soul. As suggested above, these changes were entrenched in the growing aspiration to expand and extend the authority of physicians to a consideration of emotions, also evident in the theoretical medical literature of the period. The claim to greater authority was common to both physicians and priests. Changes in the definition of the pain of remorse also reflected social developments and needs in the arena of confession: a need to expand the circle of penitents and make the medicine of the soul available to all believers, alongside a wish to place the role of the priest at the centre of the sacrament and crown his unquestioned power with the title of sole healer.

The introduction of the term *dolor animi* into medical texts is an example of assimilation of non-medical language, originally religious language, into medical discourse. However, it is an odd and imprecise assimilation. The literal meaning of the term, manifested in the choice of *animi* (*animus*) over anima, designates the pain as spiritual and disconnected from the body (which is the essential domain of the medical art). This precise definition of the soul is significant in view of the theological debate and its insistence on defining the pain of remorse, as a spiritual, intellectual and decisively non-sensory experience. The medical usage of the term, in contrast, suppresses this meaning and even reverses it by treating it as identical with other emotions that exist on the spectrum of the united body-soul. And yet, by borrowing from religious terminology and retaining the primary meaning, it allowed physicians to resemble, at least superficially, the priest and the confessor.

9. Conclusion

Emotional pains or pains of the soul were considered in the late Middle Ages to be distinct and at the same time inseparable from physical pains. Fifteenth-century Italian physicians utilised this duality to include pains of the soul within their purview; theologians (in a more gradual process) utilised the duality to state the uniqueness of the pain of contrition and still maintain the very primary (and primal) connotation of the physical sensation of pain. The efforts of late medieval physicians and theologians to frame the pain of the soul in a manner which enabled them to enlist it for their needs demonstrate the elasticity of the concept of pain. To a large degree these physicians and theologians found self-serving answers to the questions raised at the beginning of this essay, answers through which they could identify themselves as healers of pain of the soul.

Notes

[1] Esther Cohen, *The Modulated Scream: Pain in Late Medieval Culture* (Chicago: University of Chicago Press, 2010), 7-8.
[2] Throughout the chapter I discuss the soul—*anima*—according to the medieval understanding of it as the locus of cognitive and some mental activities, those which in contemporary terms are considered psychological faculties. This is distinguished from the 'spiritual soul'—*animus*—which is the immortal soul, considered to be detached from the physical body.
[3] Roselyne Rey, *The History of Pain*, trans. Louise Elliott Wallace, J. A. Cadden and S. W. Cadden (Cambridge: Harvard University Press 1998), 3-5.
[4] Ibid., 170-175; Fernando Salmón, 'Academic Discourse and Pain in Medical Scholasticism (Thirteenth-Fourteenth Centuries),' in *Medicine and*

Medical Ethics in Medieval and Early Modern Spain: An Intercultural Approach, ed. Samuel S. Kottek and Luis García Ballester (Jerusalem: Magnes Press, 1996), 148; Salmón, 'From Patient to Text? Narratives of Pain and Madness in Medical Scholasticism,' in *Between Text and Patient: The Medical Enterprise in Medieval and Early Modern Europe*, ed. Eliza Glaze and Brian K. Nance (Florence: SISMEL, 2011), 378.

[5] See Cohen, *Modulated Scream*, 227-36; Barbara H. Rosenwein, 'The Mystical Skeleton in the Thomistic Closet: Aquinas's Impassibility,' *The Journal of Medieval Religious Cultures* 36 (2010): 233-246, esp. 241-242.

[6] Donna Trembinski, '*[Pro]passio doloris*: Early Dominican Conceptions of Christ's Physical Pain,' *The Journal of Ecclesiastical History* 59 (2008): 630-631; Miri Rubin, *Corpus Christi: The Eucharist in Late Medieval Culture* (Cambridge: Cambridge University Press, 1991), 319.

[7] David B. Morris, *The Culture of Pain* (Berkeley: University of California Press 1991), 135.

[8] Rachel Fulton, *From Judgment to Passion: Devotion to Christ and the Virgin Mary, 800-1200* (New York: Columbia University Press, 2002), 199-200.

[9] Donald Mowbray, *Pain and Suffering in Medieval Theology: Academic Debates at the University of Paris in the Thirteenth Century* (Woodbridge: Boydell Press, 2009), 23.

[10] Thomas Aquinas, *Summa theologiae: Latin Text and English Translation*, edited by Thomas Gilby (Cambridge: Blackfriars, 1964-1981), I^{a} II^{ae} q. 35.

[11] Ibid., I^{a} II^{ae} q. 35, a. 2.

[12] See, for example, the late thirteenth-century text by Arnaldus de Villanova, 'Speculum medicine,' in *Hec sunt opera Arnaldi de Villanova que in hoc volumine continentur...* (Lyon, 1504), fol. 28r.

[13] *Articella* (Venice, 1483), 187v.ii.

[14] Ugo Benzi, *Consilia ad diversis aegritudines* (Pavia, 1496-1499), fol. 22v.

[15] Ibid., fol. 45r.

[16] Ibid., fol. 34v.

[17] Ibid., fol. 50r.

[18] Bartholomaeus de Montagnana, *Consilia CCCV in quibus agitur de universis fere aegritudinibus, humano corpori evenientibus, & mira facilitate, curandi eas adhibetur modus* (Venice, 1497), fol. 349r.

[19] Pietro Torrigiano, *Plusquam commentum in microtegni Galeni* (Venice, 1498), fol. 87v.

[20] Na'ama Cohen-Hanegbi, *Accidents of the Soul: Physicians and Confessors on the Conception and Treatment of Emotions in Italy and Spain, 12th-15th Centuries* (PhD diss., Hebrew University of Jerusalem, 2011), 236-52.

[21] Batholomaeus de Montagnana, *Consilia*, fol. 200r.

[22] Benedetto Reguardati da Norcia, *De conservatione sanitatis* (Rome, 1475), np.
[23] Antonio Benivieni, *Antonii Benivienii de regimine sanitatis ad laurentium medicem* (Torino: Società Italiana di patologia, 1951), 45.
[24] Cohen-Hanegbi, *Accidents of the Soul*, 68-91.
[25] See *Decrees of the Ecumenical Councils*, ed. Norman P. Tanner, (London: Georgetown University Press, 1990), 1: 245; Nicole Bériou, 'La confession dans les écrits théologiques et pastoraux du XIIIe siècle: Médication de l'âme ou démarche judicaire?' in *L'aveu. Antiquité et Moyen-Âge: Actes de la table ronde organisée par l'École française de Rome avec la concours du C.N.R.S et de l'Université de Trieste*, (Rome: École française de Rome, 1986), 261-282.
[26] Peter Biller, 'Confession in the Middle Ages: An Introduction,' in *Handling Sin: Confession in the Middle Ages*, ed. Peter Biller and A. J. Minnis (York: York Medieval Press, 1998), 8. For a more detailed discussion of the period's new focus on contrition, see Alexander Murray, 'Counselling in Medieval Confession,' in *Handling Sin*, 63-78; Joseph Goering, 'The Scholastic Turn (1100-1500): Penitential Theology and Law in the Schools,' in *A New History of Penance*, ed. Abigail Firey (Leiden: Brill, 2008), 219-237.
[27] Peter Abelard, *Scito te ipsum*, edited by Rainer M. Ilgner, CCCM 190 (Turnhout : Brepols, 2001), 51.
[28] Alain de Lille, *Opusculum de sex alis cherubim*, PL 210, col. 274; Alain de Lille, *Liber Poenitentialis*, ed. Jean Longère (Louvain: Editions Nauwelaerts, 1965), 164.
[29] Thomas Tentler, *Sin and Confession on the Eve of the Reformation* (Princeton: Princeton University Press, 1977), 236-37; Mowbray, *Pain and Suffering*, 64-67.
[30] Antoninus of Florence, *Confessionale* (Strassburg, 1490), fol. 19r.
[31] Piroska Nagy, *Le don des larmes au moyen âge* (Paris: Bibliothèque Albin Michel Histoire, 2000), 364-380.
[32] Mowbray, *Pain and Suffering*, 70-72.
[33] Anne T. Thayer, *Penitence, Preaching and the Coming of the Reformation* (Aldershot: Ashgate, 2002), 53-55.
[34] For a summary of the debate see Emmet R. McLaughlin, 'Truth, Tradition, and History: The Historiography of High/Late Medieval and Early Modern Penance,' in *A New History of Penance*, 19-72, esp. 59-65.
[35] See Alister E. McGrath, *Iustitia Dei: A History of the Christian Doctrine of Justification.* Vol. 1: *From the Beginnings to 1500* (Cambridge: Cambridge University Press, 3rd edition, 2003), 85.

[36] See Dallas G. Denery, *Seeing and Being Seen in the Later Medieval World: Optics, Theology and Religious Life* (Cambridge: Cambridge University Press, 2005), 43.
[37] Raymond de Peñafort. *Summa sti. Raymundi de Peniafort Barcinonensis ord. Praedicator de poenitentia et matrimonio cum glossis Ioannis de Friburgo* (repr. Farnborough: Gregg Press, 1967 [1603]), 443-447.
[38] Astesanus de Asti. *Summa Astensis* (Lyon, 1519) 5.1.2.1; Antoninus of Florence, *Confessionale defecerunt* (Florence, 1467), ch. 7. See also Henry Charles Lea, *A History of Auricular Confession and Indulgences in the Latin Church* (Philadelphia: Lea Bros., 1896), 2 and 9.
[39] Angelus Carletus, *Summa de casibus conscientiae* (Strassburg, 1515), fol. 44r.
[40] Ibid., fol. 24v.

Bibliography

Abelard, Peter. *Scito te ipsum.* Edited by Rainer M. Ilgner. CCCM 190. Turnhout: Brepols, 2001.

Alain de Lille. *Liber Poenitentialis.* Edited by Jean Longère. Louvain: Editions Nauwelaerts, 1965.

———. *Opusculum de sex alis cherubim.* PL 210: cols 269-280.

Antoninus of Florence. *Confessionale.* Strassburg, 1490.

———. *Confessionale defecerunt.* Florence, 1467.

Aquinas, Thomas. *Summa theologiae: Latin Text and English Translation.* Edited by Thomas Gilby. Cambridge: Blackfriars, 1964-1981.

Arnaldus de Villanova. 'Speculum medicine.' In *Hec sunt opera Arnaldi de Villanova que in hoc volumine continentur...* Lyon, 1504.

Articella. Venice, 1483.

Astesanus de Asti. *Summa Astensis.* Lyon, 1519.

Bartholomaeus de Montagnana. *Consilia CCCV in quibus agitur de universis fere aegritudinibus, humano corpori evenientibus, & mira facilitate, curandi eas adhibetur modus.* Venice, 1497.

Benivieni, Antonio. *Antonii Benivienii de regimine sanitatis ad laurentium medicem*. Torino: Società Italiana di patologia, 1951.

Benzi, Ugo. *Consilia ad diversis aegritudines*. Pavia, 1496-1499.

Bériou, Nicole. 'La confession dans les écrits théologiques et pastoraux du XIIIe siècle: Médication de l'âme ou démarche judicaire?' In *L'aveu. Antiquité et Moyen-Âge: Actes de la table ronde organisée par l'École française de Rome avec la concours du C.N.R.S et de l'Université de Trieste*, 261-82. Rome: École française de Rome, 1986.

Biller, Peter. 'Confession in the Middle Ages: An Introduction.' In *Handling Sin: Confession in the Middle Ages*. Edited by Peter Biller and A. J. Minnis, 3-33. York: York Medieval Press, 1998.

Carletus, Angelus. *Summa de casibus conscientiae*. Strassburg, 1515.

Cohen, Esther. *The Modulated Scream: Pain in Late Medieval Culture*. Chicago: University of Chicago Press, 2010.

Cohen-Hanegbi, Na'ama. *Accidents of the Soul: Physicians and Confessors on the Conception and Treatment of Emotions in Italy and Spain, 12th-15th Centuries*. PhD diss., Hebrew University of Jerusalem, 2011.

Decrees of the Ecumenical Councils. Edited by Norman P. Tanner, 2 Vols. London: Georgetown University Press, 1990.

Denery, Dallas G. *Seeing and Being Seen in the Later Medieval World: Optics, Theology and Religious Life*. Cambridge: Cambridge University Press, 2005.

Fulton, Rachel. *From Judgment to Passion: Devotion to Christ and the Virgin Mary, 800-1200*. New York: Columbia University Press, 2002.

Goering, Joseph. 'The Scholastic Turn (1100-1500): Penitential Theology and Law in the Schools.' In *A New History of Penance*. Edited by Abigail Firey, 219-37. Leiden: Brill, 2008.

Lea, Henry Charles. *A History of Auricular Confession and Indulgences in the Latin Church*, 3 Vols. Philadelphia: Lea Bros., 1896.

McGrath, Alister E. *Iustitia Dei: A History of the Christian Doctrine of Justification.* Vol. 1: *From the Beginnings to 1500*. Cambridge: Cambridge University Press, 3rd edition, 2003.

McLaughlin, Emmet R. 'Truth, Tradition, and History: The Historiography of High/Late Medieval and Early Modern Penance.' In *A New History of Penance*. Edited by Abigail Firey, 19-72. Leiden: Brill, 2008.

Morris, David B. *The Culture of Pain.* Berkeley: University of California Press, 1991.

Mowbray, Donald. *Pain and Suffering in Medieval Theology: Academic Debates at the University of Paris in the Thirteenth Century.* Woodbridge: Boydell Press, 2009.

Murray, Alexander. 'Counselling in Medieval Confession,' in *Handling Sin: Confession in the Middle Ages*. Edited by Peter Biller and A. J. Minnis, 63-78. York: York Medieval Press, 1998.

Nagy, Piroska. *Le don des larmes au moyen âge*. Paris: Bibliothèque Albin Michel Histoire, 2000.

Raymond de Peñafort. *Summa sti. Raymundi de Peniafort Barcinonensis ord. Praedicator de poenitentia et matrimonio cum glossis Ioannis de Friburgo.* repr. Farnborough: Gregg Press, 1967 [1603].

Reguardati da Norcia, Benedetto. *De conservatione sanitatis*. Rome, 1475.

Rey, Roselyne. *The History of Pain.* Translated by Louise Elliott Wallace, J. A. Cadden and S. W. Cadden. Cambridge: Harvard University Press 1998.

Rosenwein, Barbara H. 'The Mystical Skeleton in the Thomistic Closet: Aquinas's Impassibility.' *The Journal of Medieval Religious Cultures* 36 (2010): 233-246.

Rubin, Miri. *Corpus Christi: The Eucharist in Late Medieval Culture*. Cambridge: Cambridge University Press, 1991.

Salmón, Fernando. 'Academic Discourse and Pain in Medical Scholasticism (Thirteenth-Fourteenth Centuries).' In *Medicine and Medical Ethics in Medieval and Early Modern Spain: An Intercultural Approach.* Edited by Samuel S. Kottek and Luis García Ballester, 136-153. Jerusalem: Magnes Press, 1996.

———. 'From Patient to Text? Narratives of Pain and Madness in Medical Scholasticism.' In *Between Text and Patient: The Medical Enterprise in Medieval and Early Modern Europe.* Edited by Eliza Glaze and Brian K. Nance, 373-395. Florence: SISMEL, 2011.

Thayer, Anne T. *Penitence, Preaching and the Coming of the Reformation.* Aldershot: Ashgate, 2002.

Tentler, Thomas. *Sin and Confession on the Eve of the Reformation.* Princeton: Princeton University Press, 1977.

Torrigiano, Pietro. *Plusquam commentum in microtegni Galeni.* Venice, 1498.

Trembinski, Donna. '*[Pro]passio Doloris*: Early Dominican Conceptions of Christ's Physical Pain.' *The Journal of Ecclesiastical History* 59 (2008): 630-656.

Part II

RECONCEPTUALISATIONS

The Changing Faces of Love Torments: Continuity and Rupture in the Medical Diagnosis of Lovesickness in the Modern West

Michal Altbauer-Rudnik

Abstract
The connection between love and states of illness or madness has existed since antiquity and is demonstrated in both medical and non-medical literature. While early modern descriptions of the clinical picture of lovesickness remained faithful to their classic and medieval predecessors, the volume of writing about lovesickness increased dramatically, with physicians devoting hundreds of pages to the specific diagnosis and prognosis, but most of all to the social aetiology and therapy of 'love melancholy.' This medical discussion reached a high point during the sixteenth and seventeenth centuries and then gradually faded out. Though there are clear references to this pathological condition in later medical texts, the writing changed dramatically: first declining in scope and coherence and then, in the nineteenth century, being replaced by the diagnosis 'erotomania.' The chapter views the continuity of the medical diagnosis on the one hand and its ruptures on the other, focusing on the changes in the European medical world and on the changes in the notion of romantic love in European society.

Key Words: Emotions, erotomania, humours, love, love melancholy, lovesickness, melancholy, social aetiology.

*****

> My sister has been diagnosed with this delusional disorder at the beginning of the year 2007. It is very sad to watch her turn into someone she is not. To see her family tear apart, and my parents' hearts broken is so painful. … the specialist diagnosed her with erotomania … she has lost a lot of weight, stays in her bedroom a lot and really doing some strange things. She really is a worry to us all. I am putting this on my page because I am hoping that someone out there knows more about this condition and can give me and my family some answers on what we can do to help her. … It is a 'delusional romantic preoccupation with a stranger.' … They [the patients] believe that they will be with that person one day and won't accept rejection.[1]

This painful confession, posted on a Facebook community page, is taken from an account of the suffering of unfulfilled love. But what turns love torments into an abnormal condition, defined by a distinct diagnosis? Do contemporary definitions such as the common 'four D's'[2]—*d*eviant behaviour that is *d*istressful to the individual, results in daily *d*ysfunction and presents *d*anger—encompass lovesickness as a physiological or a psychological disorder? When madly in love or desperately heart-broken, many of us manifest unusual behaviour or experience upsetting episodes that are disruptive to our daily routine and sometimes even present danger. 'In some ways,' claims Charles Rosenberg, 'disease does not exist until we have agreed that it does, by perceiving, naming and responding to it': a disease is a repertoire of verbal constructs reflecting the history of medicine as a discipline as well as a potential public policy.[3] This chapter offers a framework for studying the social context of lovesickness from the early modern diagnosis of 'love melancholy' to modern 'erotomania.' I focus on the continuity of this medical diagnosis on the one hand and its significant changes on the other, in respect to two axes: changes in the European medical world regarding diagnostic and explanatory systems (the decline of the humoural system, changing prospects of mind-body and the rise of psychiatry) and changes in the notion of romantic love and its place in conjugal relationships in the modern West. Both axes, I believe, influenced the prevalence of the diagnosis and its changing features.

The history of the modern diagnostic category of lovesickness has received little scholarly attention; it is traditionally dealt with from a psychiatric point of view, without actually referring to social factors.[4] Though psychiatrists G. E. Berrios and N. Kennedy assert that the disease is 'a *construct*, a secular conceptual mirror on which successive views of love, sex, and mental disorder are reflected,'[5] they pay little attention to the uniqueness of the consolidation of the disease in the early modern period. Nor do they offer social explanations of the changing historical convergences that they have identified.

The connection between love and states of illness and madness has existed since antiquity and is evident in both medical and non-medical literature.[6] As with all diseases, aetiological explanations of lovesickness were based upon the humoural theory, according to which the human body is made up of four humours—blood, yellow bile, black bile and phlegm—each characterised by different qualities of heat and moisture. Good health was the result of an optimal balance among the four humours. The earliest and most orderly discussions on the subject of lovesickness can be found in the writings of Aretaeus the Cappadocian (practised first century CE) and Galen (ca. 129-after 210 CE), both of whom described the disease as a depressive illness with symptoms that matched those of melancholy yet not with its aetiology.[7] According to the Hippocratic Corpus, the symptoms associated with melancholy include depression, fear, eating disorders, insomnia, irritability and restlessness.[8] However, in the case of melancholy, depression and fear have no apparent cause, whereas the onset of lovesickness has such a cause—separation from the object of love.[9] In the classical world medical discussions of lovesickness were few, but literary representations were abundant; suffice it to recall the notorious and raging madness of Euripides's Medea, Sappho's love poetry, or Ovid's *Metamorphoses* and *Remedia amoris*. These works can be read as representing the anamnesis of tormented lovers, without referring to concrete medical interference.[10]

The common medical view of lovesickness during the Middle Ages was not dramatically different from that of the ancient medical diagnoses. Oribasius (ca. 325-400) and Paul of Aegina (ca. 625-690) were among those who described lovesick persons as displaying symptoms of melancholy.[11] In the ninth and tenth centuries Arabic medicine contributed to the understanding of lovesickness by consolidating the symptoms into a specific diagnosis of 'love melancholy.' The clinical picture remained relatively unchanged, though recurrent therapeutic advice included recommendation of sexual intercourse for purposes of evacuating excessive semen and regaining the humoural balance, as is evident for example in the writings of Rhazes (865-925).[12] Thus, the disease was attributed mainly to men and was associated with sexual desire not necessarily accompanied by emotional involvement.[13]

Medical descriptions of lovesickness from the mid-sixteenth to the mid-seventeenth centuries remained faithful to their classic and medieval precursors, in terms of the diagnostic system and clinical picture. However, the volume of writings in that period increased dramatically, with eminent physicians, mainly but not exclusively French, such as Du Laurens, Aubrey, Valleriola, de Veyries, Ferrand, Montalto, Sennert or Zacutus Lusitanus,[14] devoting dozens of pages to this 'very ordinary and common' disease of love melancholy and regarding it as 'the greatest miserie.'[15]

Early modern medical presentations of lovesickness linked its predisposition to the dominance of blood, a sanguine tendency. High level of blood in the human body was believed to produce a natural inclination to the passions, especially erotic love. Sanguinity would upset the humoural balance of the body but would not, on its own, cause any agony or physical distress.[16] Though 'spermatic' men were mentioned as being at high risk of infection since excess of semen was ascribed to excess of blood,[17] none of the physicians attribute the disease exclusively to either men or women, as is clear from the discussions of the various symptoms as well as the presentation of case histories. A beautiful object attracting attention, most specifically of the eye, is necessary to bring about the infection.[18] Melancholy was believed to take over only in the second stage of the disease, when for some reason the person was separated from his or her beloved and could not consummate his love. Excessive mental action, due to constant meditation on the love object, dried and cooled the body, causing the dominance of black melancholy bile and deepening the person's despair and physical suffering.[19] French physician Jacques Ferrand (ca.1575-after 1623) listed the symptoms briefly, before providing details of each: 'Pale and wan complexion, joined by a slow fever … palpitations of the heart, swelling of the face, depraved appetite, a sense of grief, sighing, causeless tears, irresistible hunger, raging thirst, oppression, suffocation, insomnia, headaches, melancholy, epilepsy, madness, uterine fury, satyriasis, and other pernicious symptoms.'[20]

The medical treatment provided was mainly classical. After an accurate diagnosis, made only by an authorised physician, the regaining of humoural balance was sought, by means of a special diet, pharmaceutical prescriptions and bloodletting, almost identical to the therapeutic advice 'appoynted for the melancholike.'[21] This view was based upon earlier medical and literary traditions, yet the belief that it 'remained untouched until the middle of the seventeenth century'[22] is inaccurate. Not only did the scope of the writing on the subject increase dramatically by the sixteenth and seventeenth centuries but specific new points in regard to the aetiology and therapy were made. These were common to all the medical discussions of lovesickness during this period and did not reappear in later writings. They imply that the root causes of the disease were social in nature and associated with specific historical and cultural contexts.

What originally appeared to be an inclination of young wealthy men and women to this disease because of rich diet or idle lifestyle (that promoted heat and moisture and aroused lust) revealed itself as a disease of a social origin, as one can learn from the physicians' discussion of its prognosis. Alongside varied medical solutions, physicians agreed that it would only be possible to avoid a fatal prognosis and achieve complete recovery of the lovesick patient through union with the love object. This union did not merely refer to the sexual consummation of the patient's erotic desire; the emotional facets of the patient's suffering and the anchoring of the yearned-for relationship in marriage were likewise considered important. Several physicians stated that this union could be realised only in accordance with divine and human laws.[23] However, in discussions of love melancholy among married couples, an unprecedented subject that was specific to early modern medical writings, physicians showed full awareness that these divine and human rules were in many cases the cause for distress among the young.[24] Ferrand, for example, noted that marriage was no proof against the disease, admitting that love melancholy among married couples was usually the result of animosity arising in a couple who was coerced to marry and who consequently sought love outside marriage.[25] Others directly attacked the legal and social impediments that prevented young couples from being joined in marriage. Robert Burton (1577-1640), an English divine with an amateur interest in medicine, criticised parents, teachers and guardians who withheld their consent to a match because of the limitations imposed by law and custom, especially on account of an inequality of status between the lovers. He further deplored an 'iron age' that respected 'riches alone,' and condemned the cruelty of parents who caused despair by forcing arranged marriages on their children.[26]

This medical manifestation of social distress was based on the contemporary social reality of a patriarchal authoritarian upper-class in which the choice of a partner was made entirely by the parents, and in which most of the marriage arrangements were made between families of the same socio-economic status.[27] This was especially true in countries where political centralisation trends were redrawing the boundaries between public and private and transforming internal dynamics of the family, as reflected in both contemporary legislation and literature. In light of the evidence concerning consensual and clandestine marriages, one can argue that the bluntness of medical discourse correlated with specific social circumstances. In France, for example, where the limitations on love relationships were more strictly enforced, as late sixteenth-century and early seventeenth-century royal legislation against clandestine marriages exemplifies,[28] there were fewer literary examples of love torments. It was more convenient to deal with the problem from a medical perspective, suggesting surgical and pharmaceutical therapies for lovesickness. In England, however, the adoption of such methods was part of the critique of arranged marriages that flourished in Elizabethan and early Stuart literature and was influenced mainly by Puritanism which valorised affection between husband and wife as the foundation of marriage.[29]

The humoural model and traditional medical references to a pathology associated with love were substantial to this highly politicised realm of discourse. The popularity of the discussions of love melancholy starting from the mid-sixteenth century can be seen as another example of what Vivian Nutton described as the 'reversion' to Hippocrates which characterised European medical discourse during the second half of the sixteenth century.[30] Nor can one dismiss the systematic association of the disorder with melancholy at a time when melancholy was considered, both medically and legally, as a form of dotage or partial insanity (rather than madness or frenzy). English law, for example, defined melancholy as partial insanity, based on arguments made in 1592 by the jurist Richard Cosin who claimed that a person could be insane with respect to specific issues while remaining perfectly sane with respect to others for which he would be held legally accountable.[31] In the seventeenth century, melancholy was used as an apt example of partial insanity. It was claimed that the melancholic patients' imagination was only partially harmed, as exemplified by their specific hallucinations.[32] Melancholy gained not only medical but also intellectual and literary popularity, leading to the period being considered *l'âge d'or de la mélancolie* [the golden age of melancholy], and accounting for the exceptional artistic traits and divine inspiration associated with it.[33] Consequently, the susceptibility of a small but significant segment of society—young upper-class men and women—was anchored in a medical framework that did not label them as insane but called for a physical and social solution to their malady by prescribing love marriages.

This medical diagnosis reached the peak of its frequency during the second half of the sixteenth and the first half of the seventeenth centuries and then gradually declined, never to attain this dominance again. Though references to this pathological condition in later medical texts exist, the writing changed dramatically. The scope of writing and the amount of references to lovesickness in medical discourse decreased from the mid-seventeenth century onwards. In the period from the mid-seventeenth century to the beginning of the nineteenth century the disorder lost its distinct diagnosis, and its discussion again became vague.

Thus in the second half of the seventeenth century, the English physician Thomas Willis (1621-1675) claimed that uncontrollable love was only one of several causes of melancholy.[34] During the first half of the eighteenth century, Richard Mead (1673-1754) asserted that love could cause madness, either melancholy or mania.[35] Defining *amor* in his *Medicinal Dictionary*, the English physician Robert James (1703-1776) explained that love 'is productive of many Disorders, especially Madness.'[36] Such references were scarce and short. Love appeared in medical textbooks as a possible aetiological explanation for madness, manifested in either melancholic or manic symptoms, but not as a specific diagnostic category. Further and more importantly, it was not the torments of unrequited love but rather the very nature of love which was regarded as the pathogen.

It is important to note that even though William Harvey's seminal work on blood circulation was published as early as in 1628, and Marcello Malphighi's work published in 1661 presented the correct modern description of blood circulation, it was only during the eighteenth century that this account managed to overthrow the humoural model which had reigned supreme in the European medical discourse. Mechanistic philosophy that rejected the humoural model likewise spread throughout Europe by the end of the seventeenth century.[37] This process entailed a gradual decrease of references to love melancholy, whose clinical existence was dependent on the idea of humoural imbalance. Unlike mania, whose clinical definition remained practically unchanged until the end of the nineteenth century, the concept of melancholy was related not to a form of behaviour but rather to an aetiological hypothesis based on the humoural theory—excessive black bile, *melaina chole*, characterised by sadness and fear.[38] Another expression of this process was the penetration of updated terms into the discussion (no longer particularly vivid) of love's pathological dimensions. Thus, German physician Friedrich Hoffmann (1660-1742) mentioned love as one of the causes of 'irregular motions of the circulation' associated with melancholy.[39] The emotional despair of love melancholy, however, no longer fit either Willis's neurology that situated passions in certain parts of the brain or Hoffmann's solidistic explanations focusing on pores and vessels.[40]

In his 1811 *Dissertation on Insanity*, William Black mentioned that love was the sixth most common cause for admission in the London asylum of Bedlam—74 patients of a total 863 patients were hospitalised on account of love-related pathologies. Black differentiated these patients from those hospitalised as a consequence of 'misfortunes, troubles, disappointments and grief,' focusing on love's nature rather than on the emotional despair entailed in unrequited love.[41] Detailed descriptions of some of these admissions can be found in the writings of John Haslam (1764-1844), an apothecary at Bedlam. Love was a common aetiology of insanity, but the diagnosis of love melancholy was absent from Haslam's account, and his descriptions focused on the severity of madness rather than on the melancholic symptoms.[42] The French physician Jean-Etienne-Dominique Esquirol (1772-1840) regarded love as the third most common reason for admission of patients suffering from melancholy in Parisian asylums but described love-related conditions as 'erotic monomania' or 'erotomania.' This innovative concept was in part a reflection of a terminological discussion regarding melancholy and the attempt to update its diagnosis by focusing on symptomatic explanations rather than aetiological ones—an attempt that resulted in the proposed diagnosis of 'monomanic sadness.'[43] Erotomania marked a further dramatic change in the medical discourse of lovesickness.[44] Esquirol depicted a delusional disorder, characterised by the patients' fantasy that their desire for their love object was reciprocated. Though the patients' emotion towards their love objects was of a sexual kind, Esquirol differentiated this state from physical disorders that originated from the genital organs, and stated that this was a strictly mental affection caused by impaired imagination and judgment.[45]

Esquirol's description set the tone for the construction of the disorder as a delusional one, of a manic and sexual kind, in modern psychiatric literature. Emil Kraepelin's (1856-1926) reference to erotomania as a subdivision of delusional disorders in his famous 1883 *Manic-Depressive Insanity and Paranoia* offered a systematic description of this pathology.[46] His consolidation of the material resulted in the understanding that '[e]rotomania is a syndrome whose hallmark is an elaborate, systematised delusion; specifically, the erotomanic patient becomes convinced that she or he is passionately loved by another person.'[47] The patients were mostly women.

The colourful accounts of the French psychiatrist Gaëtan de Clérambault (1872-1934) left a noticeable effect on modern psychiatric discourse. The French psychiatrist described women who suffer delusional attacks of a sexual nature, falsely believing they are being distinguished and loved by an older man of a higher social status. They were not only convinced that their love object was the one who initiated the relationship but also mistook random gestures for intentional communication and interpreted direct rejections as signs of affection.[48] Though contemporary popular psychiatric discourse refers to 'syndrome de Clérambault' as a synonym for 'erotomania,' starting from the third and revised edition of the *Diagnostic and Statistical Manual of Mental Disorders* the syndrome is defined as an 'erotomanic type,' a sub-type of delusional disorder, along the lines of Kraepelin's descriptions.[49]

What do the young lovesick patients of the early modern period, who manifested a melancholic clinical picture due to their parents' lack of consent to follow their heart's desire, share with de Clérambault's famous description of a 53-years-old Frenchwoman whose manic repertoire includes a conviction that King George V of England is in love with her? They all experience love and manifest its pathological dimension to different extents as evaluated in terms of changing contemporary medical discourse and social norms. One might argue that early modern love-melancholy patients would today have been diagnosed as suffering from major depressive episodes[50] rather than erotomania, and that, clinically speaking, we should look for the continuity of symptoms rather than focus on the pathological dimension of love characterised by ruptures. Though scholars believe that erotomanic delusion 'seemed to fill a vacuum in these patients' lives and so masked depression,'[51] the depressive clinical picture of the early modern period has practically disappeared from the clinical explanations associated with pathological dimensions of love.

Both axes mentioned at the beginning of the chapter are crucial in determining the prevalence of the diagnosis and its changing features. First, changes in the medical discourse following the scientific revolution prevented the existence of the diagnostic category of love melancholy. In this sense, starting in the mid-seventeenth century, the 'scientific revolution' and the 'modern' medicine did indeed create new conventional explanations (despite the anachronistic and teleological nature of these terms.[52]) Second, changes in the notion of romantic love were of course not only crucial to the popularity of the notion of 'love melancholy' in the early modern period but also to its fading and the rise of modern 'erotomania.' The more prevalent the ideas of romantic love and the fulfilment of romantic union became, during the eighteenth century and onwards, the less need there was to deal with social distress through medical tools. I am not implying that socio-economical considerations did not remain factors in modern love, as is well exemplified in contemporary sociological studies.[53] However, as Peter Stearns justly claims, even though the actual emotional experience may have changed less dramatically than emotionally prescribed norms,[54] those norms changed substantially, especially in regard to the relationship of love and body, as the medical literature reflects.

The expression of sexual desire became the target of moral criticism of both the social and the religious establishments, and thus was included in the medical discourse as well; 'indeed, many forms of sexuality *were* madness' and were identified with either perversion or prostitution.[55] Moreover, there was a fundamental shift in the view of women in psychological and medical discourse: madness came to be associated predominantly with women in both medical and non-medical literature.[56] Even though many sixteenth- and seventeenth-century physicians claimed, following the classical medical tradition, that women deprived of sexual activity turned ill and mad, this was differentiated from the discussion on love melancholy.[57] The tendency to ascribe unrequited desire for the most part to women grew from the end of the eighteenth century. While one of the shapes that this process took is seen in the diagnosis of modern female hysteria,[58] it is also exemplified in the diagnosis of erotomania, turning the condition of lovesickness into a manic and erotic pathology attributed mainly to women.

Considering the ruptures and continuities in diagnosing lovesickness through the early modern and modern periods, one may conclude with Ian Hacking's concept of 'transient mental illness.' Hacking coined the term in regard to madness 'that appears at a time, in a place, and later fades away,' disorders that might be 'selective for social class or gender.'[59] Hacking asserts that what enables these kinds of disorders to thrive is the existence of an 'ecological niche.' This niche allows fitting the patient's suffering to an existing medical diagnostic system. At the basis of this niche there ought to be, according to Hacking, a 'certain cultural polarity: two elements of contemporary culture, one romantic and virtuous, the other vicious and tending to crime,'[60] such as the dichotomous representation of, for example, glorious romantic love as opposed to sinful desire. These ecological niches are, indeed, the cornerstones of this chapter: while recognizing the universal and timeless nature of love torments, one should acknowledge the cultural components of a disease, which both shapes society and is shaped by it.

Notes

[1] The text is taken from a Facebook community page titled 'Erotomania, or de Clérambault's Syndrome' initiated by Karen Gilly from Dartford, UK. Whether this is an authentic piece of life-evidence or a fabricated testimony,

it stresses the relevance of these psychiatric terms to contemporary Western society.
[2] Ronald J. Comer, *Abnormal Psychology* (New York: W. H. Freeman, 1995), 3-5.
[3] Charles E. Rosenberg, 'Framing Disease: Illness, Society, and History,' in *Framing Disease: Studies in Cultural History*, ed. Charles E. Rosenberg and Janet Golden (New Brunswick: Rutgers University Press, 1997), xiii.
[4] Stanley Jackson, *Melancholia and Depression: From Hippocratic Times to Modern Times* (New Haven: Yale University Press, 1986), 356-365; G. E. Berrios and N. Kennedy, 'Erotomania: A Conceptual History,' *History of Psychiatry* 13 (2002): 381-400; Frank Tallis, *Love Sick: Love as Mental Illness* (New York: Thunder's Mouth Press, 2005).
[5] Berrios and Kennedy, 'Erotomania,' 397.
[6] For general surveys on medical and literary representations of lovesickness, see Lawrence Babb, *The Elizabethan Malady: A Study of Melancholia in English Literature, 1580-1642* (East Lansing: Michigan State College Press, 1951), 128-42; Jackson, *Melancholia and Depression*, 356-365. Donald A. Beecher and Massimo Ciavolella, 'Jacques Ferrand and the Tradition of Erotic Melancholy in Western Culture,' in *A Treatise on Lovesickness*, trans. and edited with an introduction by Donald A. Beecher and Massimo Ciavolella (Syracuse: Syracuse University Press, 1990), 39-97. Jacalyn Duffin, *Lovers and Livers: Disease Concepts in History* (Toronto: University of Toronto Press, 2005), 43-65.
[7] Aretaeus, *The Extant Works of Aretaeus the Cappadocian*, trans. and ed. Francis Adams (Boston: Milford House, 1972), 300; Galen, *On Prognosis*, trans. and edited Vivian Nutton (Berlin: Akademie-Verlag, 1979), 103.
[8] The Hippocratic Corpus is a compilation of over sixty medical writings tradition-ally attributed to Hippocrates of Cos. The Corpus dates back to 420-350 BCE. There is no consensus as to which parts of the Corpus (if any) were actually written by Hippocrates. See Vivian Nutton, 'Medicine in the Greek World, 800-50 BC,' in *The Western Medical Tradition, 800 BC to AD 1800*, ed. Lawrence I. Conrad, Michael Neve, Vivian Nutton, Roy Porter and Andrew Wear (Cambridge: Cambridge University Press, 1995), 19-22.
[9] For a more comprehensive discussion of ancient medical discourse of lovesickness see Peter Toohey, *Melancholy, Love and Time: Boundaries of the Self in Ancient Literature* (Ann Arbor: University of Michigan Press, 2004), 71-74; Mary F. Wack, *Lovesickness in the Middle Ages: The Viaticum and its Commentaries* (Philadelphia: University of Pennsylvania Press, 1990), 3-18.
[10] This is the basis for Marie-Paule Duminil's claim that ancient lovesickness was mainly a romantic literary construct rather than a prevalent medical

phenomenon; see: Marie-Paule Duminil, 'La mélancholie amoureuse dans l'Antiquité,' in *La folie et le corps*, ed. Jean Céard, Pierre Naudin and Michel Simonin (Paris: Presses de l'École normale supérieure, 1985), 109. A similar claim was made by Peter Toohey, based on the difference between the melancholic manifestation of lovesickness in medical discussions and the manic manifestation of it in the literary descriptions; see: Peter Toohey, 'Love, Lovesickness and Melancholia,' *Illinois Classical Studies* 17 (1992): 275-282.

[11] Oribase, *Oeuvres*, trans. and ed. Ulco Cats Bussemaker and Charles Daremberg (Paris: Imprimerie nationale, 1853), 413-14; Paulus Aegineta, *The Seven Books of Paulus Aegineta*, trans. Francis Adams (London: The Sydenham Society, 1844), 390-391.

[12] Al-Rāzī, *Kitab al-Hawi fi al-tibb* (Ḥaydarābād al-Dakkan, Maṭba'at Majlis Dā'irat al-Ma'ārif al-'Uthmānīyah, 1955), 61-86. For a discussion of therapeutic intercourse in later Latin translations, see Wack, *Lovesickness in the Middle Ages*, 66-70.

[13] For a comprehensive discussion of medieval medical discourse of lovesickness, see Wack, *Lovesickness in the Middle Ages*, 18-176. For a survey of Arabic medical discourse of lovesickness, see Michael W. Dols, *Majnun: The Madman in Medieval Islamic Society* (Oxford: Clarendon Press, 1992), 313-348.

[14] André du Laurens, *Discours de la conservation de la veue: des maladies melancholiques: des catarrhes: & de la vieillesse* (Paris: Théodore Samson, 1598), 164-75; Jean Aubery, *L'antidote d'amour* (Paris: chez Claude Chappelet, 1599); Farancisci Valleriola, *Observationum Medicinalium libri VI* (Lyon: Franciscum Fabrum, 1605), 140-66; Jean de Veyries, *La genealogie de l'amour divisée en deux livres* (Paris : chez Abel l'Angelier, 1609); Jacques Ferrand, *De la maladie d'amour ou mélancholie érotique* (Paris: Denis Moreau, 1623); Philothei Eliani Montalto, *Archipathologia in qua internarum capitis affectionum essentia, causæ, signa, præsagia & curatio accuratißima indagine edisseruntur* (Paris: Apud F. Jacquin, 1614), 381-89; Daniel Sennert, *Medicina practica* (Lyon: G. Ravaud, 1629), 430-441; Zacuti Lusitani, *Praxis Historiarum* (Lyon: Joannis Antonii Huguetan and Marci Antonii Ravaud, 1657), 211-213. Discussions of lovesickness in that period appeared both in treatises devoted solely to the subject and in general textbooks describing pathologies in *de capite ad pedem* scheme, in contemporary *Observationes medicae* literature, and in medical dissertations at the various European faculties of medicine; see Michal Altbauer-Rudnik, 'Love, Melancholy and Social Order: Lovesickness in France, England and the Italian Jewish Communities, 1550-1650' (PhD diss. The Hebrew University of Jerusalem, 2010), 72-73 (in Hebrew). For purposes of reading

fluency, in this chapter I used English translations of medical treatises when available, or translated the passages myself.

[15] André du Laurens, *A Discourse of the Preservation of the Sight; of Melancholike Diseases; of Rheumes, and Old Age*, trans. Richard Surphlet (London: Felix Kingston for Ralph Iacson, 1599), 117.

[16] Valleriola, *Observationum Medicinalium*, 157; Ferrand, *De la maladie d'amour*, 51-53; Robert Burton [Democritus Junior, pseudo.], *The Anatomy of Melancholy* (Oxford: Henry Cripps, 1651), 660.

[17] Ferrand, *De la maladie d'amour*, 51 and 194; Burton, *Anatomy of Melancholy*, 661; Petri Foresti, *Observationum et curationum medicinalium ac chirurgicarum* (Rotterdam: Joan and Davidis Berthelin, 1653), 445.

[18] Du Laurens, *Discours de la conservation*, 308-10; Burton, *Anatomy of Melancholy*, 664; Ferrand, *De la maladie d'amour*, 10; Montalto, *Archipathologia*, 381-382. Donald Beecher discusses lovesickness as an example of contagion from a distance, focusing on the importance of sight and imagination in the disease's aetiology, see Donald Beecher, 'Windows on Contagion,' in *Imagining Contagion in Early Modern Europe*, ed. Claire L. Carline (New York: Palgrave Macmillan, 2005), 32-46.

[19] This is an all too brief presentation of the subject. In an illuminating paper Donald Beecher identifies three distinct aetiological systems for lovesickness in Renaissance medical treatises. However, the focal point of this chapter is the social and emotional interpretation of the medical discourse: see Donald Beecher, 'The Lover's Body: The Somatogenesis of Love in Renaissance Medical Treatises,' *Renaissance and Reformation* 24 (1988): 1-11.

[20] Jacques Ferrand, *A Treatise on Lovesickness*, trans. and ed. Donald A. Beecher and Massimo Ciavolella (Syracuse: Syracuse University Press, 1990), 229.

[21] Du Laurens, *Discourse of the Preservation of the Sight*, 124.

[22] Berrios and Kennedy, 'Erotomania,' 384. A similar tendency characterises Jacalyn Duffin's short discussion of early modern lovesickness, see Duffin, *Lovers and Livers*, 55.

[23] Du Laurens, *Discours de la conservation*, 318-321; Ferrand, *De la maladie d'amour*, 207.

[24] Ferrand, *De la maladie d'amour*, 210-221; Burton, *Anatomy of Melancholy*, 821-866.

[25] Ferrand, *De la maladie d'amour*, 210-211.

[26] Burton, *Anatomy of Melancholy*, 803-808.

[27] Sarah Hanley, 'Engendering the State: Family Formation and the State Building in Early Modern France,' *French Historical Studies* 16 (1989): 6-15; David Cressy, *Birth, Marriage and Death: Ritual, Religion and the Life-Cycle in Tudor and Stuart England* (Oxford: Oxford University Press, 1997),

316-335. This does not necessarily support the main thesis of the School of Sentiment regarding the invention of sentiment, especially romantic love, during the eighteenth century, see for example: Philippe Ariès, *L'Enfant et la vie familiale sous l'Ancien Regime* (Paris: Librairie Plon, 1960); Jean-Louis Flandrin, *Families in Former Times: Kinship, Household and Sexuality*, trans. Richard Southern (Cambridge: Cambridge University Press, 1979); Lawrence Stone, *Family, Sex and Marriage in England: 1500-1800* (New York: Harper and Row, 1977); Edward Shorter, *The Making of the Modern Family* (New York: Basic Books, 1975). Critique of this standpoint concerns the School's disregard of geographical and socio-economical variance and focus on freedom of choice and mutual affection in marriages as one goes down the social scale, as well as on literary descriptions that flourished prior to the eighteenth century of the misery entailed in unfulfilled love; see, for example, Michael Anderson, *Approaches to the History of the Western Family, 1500-1914* (London: Macmillan Press, 1980), 39-64; Donna T. Andrew, 'Marriage History as Social History,' *Canadian Journal of History* 24 (1989): 381-385; Ralph A. Houlbrooke, *The English Family, 1450-1700* (London: Longman, 1984), 14-15. However, in regard to marriages among the European upper class, the School's descriptions of 'parental absolutism' is still widely accepted—see Lawrence Stone, 'Social Mobility in England, 1500-1700,' *Past and Present* 33 (1966): 38.

[28] See Barbara B. Diefendorf, *Paris City Councillors in the Sixteenth Century: The Politics of Patrimony* (Princeton: Princeton University Press, 1983), 155-170; Hanley, 'Engendering the State,' 4-27.

[29] See Daniel Rogers, *Matrimoniall Honour* (London: Th. Harper for Philip Nevel, 1642), 80-81; Richard L. Greaves, *Society and Religion in Elizabethan England* (Minneapolis: University of Minnesota Press, 1981), 155-162. The foundations of this interpretive line of thinking were laid in a previous paper of mine: Michal Altbauer-Rudnik, 'Love, Madness and Social Order: Love Melancholy in France and England in the Late Sixteenth and Early Seventeenth Centuries,' *Gesnerus* 63 (2006), 33-45.

[30] Vivian Nutton, 'Hippocrates and the Renaissance,' in *Die Hippokratischen Epidemien: Theorie-Praxis-Tradition*, ed. Gerhard Baader and Rolf Winau (Stuttgart: Franz Steiner Verlag, 1989), 435.

[31] Richard Cosin, 'Conspiracie, for Pretended Reformation,' in *Three Hundred Years of Psychiatry*, ed. Richard Alfred Hunter and Ida Macalpine (New York: Carlisle, 1982), 43-45.

[32] Stanley Jackson, 'Melancholia and Partial Insanity,' *Journal of the History of the Behavioral Sciences* 19 (1983): 173-184.

[33] Jean Delumeau, 'L'âge d'or de la mélancolie,' *L'Histoire* 42 (1982): 26-37; Winfried Schleiner, *Melancholy, Genius, and Utopia in the Renaissance*

(Wiesbaden: O. Harrassowitz, 1991), 19-29; Noel L. Brann, *The Debate over the Origin of Genius During the Italian Renaissance* (Leiden: Brill, 2002), 247-332.

[34] Thomas Willis, *Two Discourses Concerning the Soul of Brutes* (London: Thomas Dring, 1683), 199.

[35] *The Medical Works of Dr. Richard Mead* (Edinburgh: Alexander Donaldson, 1765), 3: 40.

[36] Robert James, *A Medicinal Dictionary*, 1 (London: T. Osborne, 1743).

[37] For a good survey on the loss of orthodoxy of Galenic medicine, see Roy Porter, 'The Eighteenth Century,' in *The Western Medical Tradition, 800 BC to AD 1800*, ed. Lawrence I. Conrad et al., 371-475.

[38] Jean Starobinsky, 'Mania and Depression,' in *General Psychopathology*, ed. Michael Shepherd and Oliver Louis Zangwill (Cambridge: Cambridge University Press, 1983), 43.

[39] Friedrich Hoffmann, *A System of the Practice of Medicine*, trans. William Lewis and Andrew Duncan, 2 vols. (London: J. Murray and J. Johnson, 1783), 2: 300.

[40] A similar process can be detected in relation to aetiological explanations of religious enthusiasm, which in the seventeenth century were associated with melancholy. While late sixteenth-century and early seventeenth-century medical discussion explained religious melancholy in terms of excessive black bile, mechanistic explanations concentrated on obstruction in blood vessels and recurrent impulses of the brain; see Michael Heyd, *'Be Sober and Reasonable': The Critique of Enthusiasm in the Seventeenth and Early Eighteenth Centuries* (Leiden: Brill, 1995), 191-196; Roy Porter, *Madness: A Brief History* (Oxford: Oxford University Press, 2002), 28-29.

[41] William Black, *A Dissertation on Insanity* (London: Ridgway, 1811), 22.

[42] John Haslam, *Observations on Madness and Melancholy* (London: J. Callow, 1809), 139-40, 175-180.

[43] Starobinsky, 'Mania and Depression,' 43.

[44] Though the term 'erotomania' appeared in medical texts as early as the seventeenth-century, as in the title of the English translation of Jacques Ferrand's treatise on love melancholy (1640), up until Esquirol's use of the term in the eighteenth century it referred to a pathology characterised by depressive symptoms.

[45] Jean-Étienne-Dominique Esquirol, *Des Maladies mentales considérées sous les rapports médical, hygienique et médico-legal* (Paris: J. B. Baillière, 1838), 1-130.

[46] Emil Kraepelin, *Manic-Depressive Insanity and Paranoia*, trans. R. Mary Barclay, ed. George M. Robertson (Edinburgh: E. & S. Livingstone, 1921), 245-249.

[47] Jonathan H. Segal, 'Erotomania Revisited: From Kraepelin to DSM-III-R,' *American Journal of Psychiatry* 146 (1989): 1261.
[48] Gaëtan Gatian de Clérambault, *Oeuvres psychiatriques* (Paris: Presses Universitaires des France, 1942).
[49] American Psychiatric Association (APA), *Diagnostic and Statistical Manual of Mental Disorders, Third Edition-Revised, DSM-III-R* (Washington: American Psychiatric Association Press, 1987).
[50] APA, *Diagnostic and Statistical Manual of Mental Disorders, Third Edition-Revised, DSM-IV* (Washington: American Psychiatric Association Press, 1994), 320-23.
[51] David E. Raskin and Kathleen E. Sullivan, 'Erotomania,' *The American Journal of Psychiatry* 131 (1974): 1035.
[52] Lorraine Daston, 'The Nature of Nature in Early Modern Europe,' *Configurations* 6 (1998), 149-154.
[53] See Eva Illouz, *Consuming the Romantic Utopia* (Berkeley: University of California Press, 1997); Zygmunt Bauman, *Liquid Love* (Cambridge: Polity, 2003).
[54] Peter N. Stearns, 'History of Emotions: Issues of Change and Impact,' in *Handbook of Emotions*, ed. Michael Lewis and Jeannette M. Haviland-Jones (New York: Guilford Press, 2004), 20.
[55] Roy Porter, 'Love, Sex, and Madness in Eighteenth Century England,' *Social Research* 53 (1986): 223.
[56] Michael MacDonald, 'Women and Madness in Tudor and Stuart England,' *Social Research* 53 (1986): 261-281; Helen Small, *Love's Madness: Medicine, the Novel and Female Insanity, 1800-1865* (Oxford: Clarendon Press, 1996).
[57] See Altbauer-Rudnik, 'Love, Melancholy and Social Order,' 94-96.
[58] See Elaine Showalter, *The Female Malady: Women, Madness, and English Culture, 1830-1980* (New York: Penguin, 1985); Mark S. Micale, *Approaching Hysteria: Disease and Its Interpretations* (Princeton: Princeton University Press, 1995); Andrew Scull, *Hysteria: The Biography* (Oxford: Oxford University Press, 2009).
[59] Ian Hacking, *Mad Travelers: Reflections on the Reality of Transient Mental Illness* (Cambridge, MA.: Harvard University Press, 1998), 1.
[60] Ibid., 1-2.

Bibliography

Al-Rāzī. *Kitab al-Hawi fi al-tibb*. Ḥaydarābād al-Dakkan, Maṭba'at Majlis Dā'irat al-Ma'ārif al-'Uthmānīyah, 1955.

Altbauer-Rudnik, Michal. 'Love, Madness and Social Order: Love Melancholy in France and England in the Late Sixteenth and Early Seventeenth Centuries.' *Gesnerus* 63 (2006): 33-45.

———. 'Love, Melancholy and Social Order: Lovesickness in France, England and the Italian Jewish Communities, 1550-1650.' PhD diss. The Hebrew University of Jerusalem, 2010 (in Hebrew).

American Psychiatric Association (APA). *Diagnostic and Statistical Manual of Mental Disorders, Third Edition-Revised, DSM-III-R*. Washington: American Psychiatric Association Press, 1987.

———. *Diagnostic and Statistical Manual of Mental Disorders, Third Edition-Revised, DSM-IV*. Washington: American Psychiatric Association Press, 1994.

Anderson, Michael. *Approaches to the History of the Western Family, 1500-1914*. London: Macmillan Press, 1980.

Andrew, Donna T. 'Marriage History as Social History.' *Canadian Journal of History* 24 (1989): 381-387.

Aretaeus. *The Extant Works of Aretaeus the Cappadocian*. Translated and edited by Francis Adams. Boston: Milford House, 1972.

Ariès, Philippe. *L'enfant et la vie familiale sous l'Ancien Regime*. Paris: Librairie Plon, 1960.

Aubery, Jean. *L'antidote d'amour*. Paris: chez Claude Chappelet, 1599.

Babb, Lawrence. *The Elizabethan Malady: A Study of Melancholia in English Literature, 1580-1642*. East Lansing: Michigan State College Press, 1951.

Bauman, Zygmunt. *Liquid Love*. Cambridge: Polity, 2003.

Beecher, Donald. 'The Lover's Body: The Somatogenesis of Love in Renaissance Medical Treatises.' *Renaissance and Reformation* 24 (1988): 1-11.

———. 'Windows on Contagion.' In *Imagining Contagion in Early Modern Europe*. Edited by Claire L. Carline, 32-46. New York: Palgrave Macmillan, 2005.

Beecher, Donald A. and Massimo Ciavolella. 'Jacques Ferrand and the Tradition of Erotic Melancholy in Western Culture.' In *A Treatise on Lovesickness*, by Jacques Ferrand, translated and edited with an introduction by Donald A. Beecher and Massimo Ciavolella, 1-202. Syracuse: Syracuse University Press, 1990.

Berrios, G. E. and N. Kennedy. 'Erotomania: A Conceptual History.' *History of Psychiatry* 13 (2002): 381-400.

Black, William. *A Dissertation on Insanity*. London: Ridgway, 1811.

Brann, Noel L. *The Debate over the Origin of Genius during the Italian Renaissance*. Leiden: Brill, 2002.

Burton, Robert [Democritus Junior, pseudo.] *The Anatomy of Melancholy*. Oxford: Henry Cripps, 1651.

Comer, Ronald J. *Abnormal Psychology*. New York: W. H. Freeman, 1995.

Cosin, Richard. 'Conspiracy for Pretended Reformation.' In *Three Hundred Years of Psychiatry*. Edited by Richard Alfred Hunter and Ida Macalpine, 43-45. New York: Carlisle, 1982.

Cressy, David. *Birth, Marriage and Death: Ritual, Religion and the Life-Cycle in Tudor and Stuart England*. Oxford: Oxford University Press, 1997.

Daston, Lorraine. 'The Nature of Nature in Early Modern Europe.' *Configurations* 6 (1998): 149-172.

De Clérambault, Gaëtan Gatian. *Oeuvres psychiatriques*. Paris: Presses Universitaires des France, 1942.

Delumeau, Jean. 'L'âge d'or de la mélancolie.' *L'Histoire* 42 (1982): 26-37.

Diefendorf, Barbara B. *Paris City Councillors in the Sixteenth Century: The Politics of Patrimony*. Princeton: Princeton University Press, 1983.

Dols, Michael W. *Majnun: The Madman in Medieval Islamic Society*. Oxford: Clarendon Press, 1992.

Duffin, Jacalyn. *Lovers and Livers: Disease Concepts in History*. Toronto: University of Toronto Press, 2005.

Du Laurens, André. *Discours de la conservation de la veue: des maladies melancholiques: des catarrhes: & de la vieillesse*. Paris: Théodore Samson, 1598.

—. *A Discourse of the Preservation of the Sight; of Melancholike Diseases; of Rheumes, and Old Age*. Translated by Richard Surphlet. London: Felix Kingston for Ralph Iacson, 1599.

De Veyries, Jean. *La genealogie de l'amour divisée en deux livres*. Paris: chez Abel l'Angelier, 1609.

Duminil, Marie-Paule. 'La mélancholie amoureuse dans l'Antiquité.' In *La folie et le corps*. Edited by Jean Céard, Pierre Naudin and Michel Simonin, 91-109. Paris: Presses de l'École normale supérieure, 1985.

Esquirol, Jean-Étienne-Dominique. *Des Maladies mentales considérées sous les rapports médical, hygienique et médico-legal*. Paris: J. B. Baillière, 1838.

Ferrand, Jacques. *De la maladie d'amour ou mélancholie érotique*. Paris: Denis Moreau, 1623.

———. *Erotomania or a Treatise Discoursing of the Essence, Causes, Symptomes, Prognosticks, and Cure of Love or Erotique melancholy*. Translated by Edmund Chilmead. Oxford: L. Lichfield, 1640.

———. *A Treatise on Lovesickness*. Translated and edited with an introduction by Donald A. Beecher and Massimo Ciavolella. Syracuse: Syracuse University Press, 1990.

Flandrin, Jean-Louis. *Families in Former Times: Kinship, Household and Sexuality*. Translated by Richard Southern. Cambridge: Cambridge University Press, 1979.

Foresti, Petri. *Observationum et curationum medicinalium ac chirurgicarum*. Rotterdam: Joan and Davidis Berthelin, 1653.

Galen. *On Prognosis*. Translated and edited by Vivian Nutton. Berlin: Akademie-Verlag, 1979.

Greaves, Richard L. *Society and Religion in Elizabethan England*: Minneapolis: University of Minnesota Press, 1981.

Hacking, Ian. *Mad Travelers: Reflections on the Reality of Transient Mental Illness*. Cambridge, MA: Harvard University Press, 1998.

Hanley, Sarah. 'Engendering the State: Family Formation and the State Building in Early Modern France.' *French Historical Studies* 16 (1989): 4-27.

Haslam, John. *Observations on Madness and Melancholy*. London: J. Callow, 1809.

Heyd, Michael. *'Be Sober and Reasonable': The Critique of Enthusiasm in the Seventeenth and Early Eighteenth Centuries*. Leiden: Brill, 1995.

Hoffmann, Friedrich. *A System of the Practice of Medicine*. 2 vols. Translated by William Lewis and Andrew Duncan. London: J. Murray and J. Johnson, 1783.

Houlbrooke, Ralph A. *The English Family, 1450-1700*. London: Longman, 1984.

Illouz, Eva. *Consuming the Romantic Utopia*. Berkeley: University of California Press, 1997.

Jackson, Stanley. *Melancholia and Depression: From Hippocratic Times to Modern Times*. New Haven: Yale University Press, 1986.

———. 'Melancholia and Partial Insanity.' *Journal of the History of the Behavioral Sciences* 19 (1983): 173-184.

James, Robert. *A Medicinal Dictionary*, 3 vols. London: T. Osborne, 1743-1745.

Kraepelin, Emil. *Manic-Depressive Insanity and Paranoia*. Translated by R. Mary Barclay. Edited by George M. Robertson. Edinburgh: E. & S. Livingstone, 1921.

MacDonald, Michael. 'Women and Madness in Tudor and Stuart England.' *Social Research* 53 (1986): 261-81.

Mead, Richard. *The Medical Works of Dr Richard Mead.* 3 vols. Edinburgh: Alexander Donaldson, 1765.

Micale, Mark S. *Approaching Hysteria: Disease and Its Interpretations.* Princeton: Princeton University Press, 1995.

Montalto, Philothei Eliani. *Archipathologia in qua internarum capitis affectionum essentia, causæ, signa, præsagia & curatio accuratißima indagine edisseruntur*. Paris: Apud F. Jacquin, 1614.

Nutton, Vivian. 'Hippocrates and the Renaissance.' In *Die Hippokratischen Epidemien: Theorie-Praxis-Tradition.* Edited by Gerhard Baader and Rolf Winau, 420-39. Stuttgart: Franz Steiner Verlag, 1989.

———. 'Medicine in the Greek World, 800-50 BC.' In *The Western Medical Tradition, 800 BC to AD 1800.* Edited by Lawrence I. Conrad, Michael Neve, Vivian Nutton, Roy Porter and Andrew Wear, 11-38. Cambridge: Cambridge University Press, 1995.

Oribase. *Oeuvres.* Translated and edited by Ulco Cats Bussemaker and Charles Daremberg. Paris: Imprimerie nationale, 1853.

Paulus Aegineta. *The Seven Books of Paulus Aegineta.* Translated by Francis Adams. London: The Sydenham Society, 1844.

Porter, Roy. 'The Eighteenth Century.' In *The Western Medical Tradition, 800 BC to AD 1800.* Edited by Lawrence I. Conrad, Michael Neve, Vivian Nutton, Roy Porter and Andrew Wear, 371-475. Cambridge: Cambridge University Press, 1995.

———. 'Love, Sex, and Madness in Eighteenth Century England.' *Social Research* 53 (1986): 211-242.

———. *Madness: A Brief History*. Oxford: Oxford University Press, 2002.

Raskin, David E. and Kathleen E. Sullivan. 'Erotomania.' *The American Journal of Psychiatry* 131 (1974): 1033-1035.

Rogers, Daniel. *Matrimoniall Honour*. London: Th. Harper for Philip Nevel, 1642.

Rosenberg, Charles E. 'Framing Disease: Illness, Society, and History.' In *Framing Disease: Studies in Cultural History*, xiii-xxvi. New Brunswick, N. J.: Rutgers University Press, 1997.

Schleiner, Winfried, editor. *Melancholy, Genius, and Utopia in the Renaissance*. Wiesbaden: O. Harrassowitz, 1991.

Scull, Andrew. *Hysteria: The Biography*. Oxford: Oxford University Press, 2009.

Segal, Jonathan H. 'Erotomania Revisited: From Kraepelin to DSM-III-R.' *American Journal of Psychiatry* 146 (1989): 1261-1266.

Sennert, Daniel. *Medicina practica*. Lyon: G. Ravaud, 1629.

Shorter, Edward. *The Making of the Modern Family*. New York: Basic Books, 1975.

Showalter, Elaine. *The Female Malady: Women, Madness, and English Culture, 1830-1980*. New York: Penguin, 1985.

Small, Helen. *Love's Madness: Medicine, the Novel and Female Insanity, 1800-1865*. Oxford: Clarendon Press, 1996.

Starobinsky, Jean. 'Mania and Depression.' In *General Psychopathology*. Edited by Michael Shepherd and Oliver Louis Zangwill, 42-44. Cambridge: Cambridge University Press, 1983.

Stearns, Peter N. 'History of Emotions: Issues of Change and Impact.' In *Handbook of Emotions*. Edited by Michael Lewis and Jeannette M. Haviland-Jones, 16-29. New York: Guilford Press, 2004.

Stone, Lawrence. *Family, Sex and Marriage in England: 1500-1800*. New York: Harper and Row, 1977.

———. 'Social Mobility in England, 1500-1700.' *Past and Present* 33 (1966): 16-55.

Tallis, Frank. *Love Sick: Love as Mental Illness*. New York: Thunder's Mouth Press, 2005.

Toohey, Peter. 'Love, Lovesickness and Melancholia.' *Illinois Classical Studies* 17 (1992): 265-286.

———. *Melancholy, Love and Time: Boundaries of the Self in Ancient Literature*. Ann Arbor: University of Michigan Press, 2004.

Valleriola, Farancisci. *Observationum Medicinalium libri VI*. Lyon: Franciscum Fabrum, 1605.

Wack, Mary F. *Lovesickness in the Middle Ages: The Viaticum and its Commentaries*: Philadelphia: University of Pennsylvania Press, 1990.

Willis, Thomas. *Two Discourses Concerning the Soul of Brutes*. London: Thomas Dring, 1683.

Zacuti Lusitani. *Praxis Historiarum*. Lyon: Joannis Antonii Huguetan and Marci Antonii Ravaud, 1657.

The Rhetoric of Pain: Religious Convulsions and Miraculous Healings in the Jansenist Parish of Saint Médard, Paris (1727-1732)

Michèle Bokobza Kahan

Abstract
This chapter explores the documentation of depositions regarding the experience of pain in the context of religious convulsions and miraculous healings. The author uses the corpus of testimonies related to the Convulsionaries of Saint Médard associated with Parisian Jansenism in eighteenth-century France in order to analyse the discursive procedures and rhetorical strategies concerning the new phenomenon of anatomic exhibition through the medium of detailed and redundant descriptions of the suffering body. It demonstrates how the dominance of medical terminology, combined with realistic descriptions of pain and suffering, works both to guarantee the reliability of the testimony and to create an emotional effect. Furthermore, it claims that both religious and cultural aspects have an impact on this exploration of the extreme limits of the sick body. Finally, this process of appropriation of methodological tools and new philosophical and ideological concepts points to the incorporation of commonplace knowledge into a discourse whose objective clashes with the liberal secular ideals of the Enlightenment.

Key Words: Jansenism, convulsionaries, thaumaturgic miracles, miracle registration, body, disease, Archdeacon Pâris, pain description, eighteenth-century religiosity.

*****

The spiritual and religious movement known as Jansenism is considered a crucial agent of influence in seventeenth- and eighteenth-century French history. Throughout the reign of Louis XIV, the period of the Regency, and up to the French Revolution, key Jansenist figures, such as Abbé de Saint-Cyran, Antoine Arnauld, Blaise Pascal, the nuns of the convent of Port-Royal and later on Pasquier Quesnel, the deacon François Pâris, established new forms of political resistance in their defiance of papacy, episcopacy and monarchy. The development of this movement is punctuated by the brief period between 1727 and 1732, during which we find a sudden proliferation of written testimonies of Jansenist miracles and convulsions at the tomb of the Jansenist deacon François de Pâris in the cemetery of Saint-Médard. This documentation is widespread and heterogeneous: accounts of illness and recovery, testimonies dictated by the people who miraculously cured themselves—signed and certified before a notary, eyewitness reports of convulsionary manifestations, as well as theoretical essays on testimony and on the reasons for the necessity either to accredit testimonies or denounce their falseness.

The convulsionary movement was intrinsically linked to Parisian Jansenism, and so it quickly became part of a resistance movement, exceeding the context of the religious and political quarrel. Moreover, it subsequently transformed into the most spectacular example of the popularisation and democratisation of later Jansenism: traveling down the century of Enlightenment all the way to the Revolution, it became a means of legitimising the Jansenist cause in a turbulent cultural and philosophical context.[1]

At first glance, the miraculous cures seemed in no way different from similar events that swept through the French populace at irregular intervals throughout the medieval and early modern period. But due to the unusual combination of circumstances, the cures attributed to Deacon Pâris were drawn into the stormy arena of contemporary ecclesiastical politics. As such, they constituted a turning point not only in terms of the history of religions and ideas, but also, due to the specific material involved and its significance, in historical approaches to literary and testimonial practices.

In addition to the religious controversy involved, the witnessing phenomenon raises broader questions concerning testimonial discourses and the procedures employed in its validation and accreditation within the context of eighteenth-century France. It highlights the use of a range of discursive modalities, such as the choice of rhetorical strategies in order to legitimize the irrational testimony within a hostile context that privileges a model of evidence that is rational and objective; the aesthetic dimension of the various processes of compilation;[2] the conditions of testimony accreditation that closely depend on the *ethos* of the witness (i.e., the target audience remains strongly influenced by its perception of the witness in deciding whether to accredit the testimony later offered by him[3]), and the procedures of fictionalisation as part of the strategy of popularising testimonial religious discourse.[4]

In this chapter, I shall focus on the testimonies gathered in a book entitled *La Vérité des Miracles opérés à l'intercession de M. de Pâris et autres Appellants, démontrée contre M. l'Archevêque de Sens* (*The Truth of the Miracles Worked by the Intercession of Mr. de Pâris and other Appellants Demonstrated in Opposition to the Archbishop of Sens*). This work was compiled and redacted by Louis-Basile Carré de Montgeron, magistrate and councillor at the second *Chambre des Enquêtes*, a former libertine and deist who converted to the cause of the convulsionaries after a visit to the cemetery of Saint-Médard on September 7, 1731. It was published in December 1736 in two simultaneous printings, one in Utrecht under the care of Abbé Nicolas Le Gros, the other in an underground printing house in Paris.[5] The main issue to note is the repetitive specificity of the content, combined with the different procedures for describing the suffering of the sick body before its miraculous release. Although narratives of pain and bodily distress relating to miraculous healings exist since the Middle Ages,[6] the detailed and repetitive descriptions of the suffering body occupy such a predominant place in the Jansenist testimonies that we seem to be confronted with a new phenomenon, a late stage in the evolution of a long cultural strand.

Jansenism is considered a dominant force in seventeenth- and eighteenth- century French history. Indeed, when exploring the evolving controversy concerning the interpretation of Augustinianism, one must take into account the institutional structures peculiar to France, and the complex relations between the Gallican church, the papacy and the French crown. These specific political and sociological factors brought a decisive change that reverberated all the way to the French Revolution. In the series of increasingly intransigent bulls promulgated by the pope during the seventeenth century we can follow the power negotiations between the Gallican Church, which was concerned with its autonomy, the Holy See, which wanted to exercise universal jurisdiction, and the French monarchy, which tended to eradicate any form of political subversion—all colluding to limit Jansenism. However, at the end of the seventeenth century, when the decline of Jansenism seemed irreversible, two royal decisions, whose arbitrary nature could not escape notice, triggered a resurgence and restructuring of Jansenism on a very different scale. The first of these decrees ordered the razing of the Port-Royal monastery between 1711 and 1713 and the removal of the massacred bodies which were thrown into a common grave. The second asked the pope to issue the bull *Unigenitus*. The bull, published in September 1713, officially condemned Jansenism by banning Oratorian Pasquier Quesnel's *Réflexions morales sur le Nouveau Testament* (*Moral Reflections on the New Testament*), which was highly popular among French Catholic families. It had been approved in 1696 by the Archbishop of Paris, Louis-Antoine de Noailles, but was later considered heretical. These two royal actions united the Jansenists of the early eighteenth century, around the memory and ideal of Port-Royal. They emphasised the divine mission incumbent upon them to remember and to bear witness in order to protect the truth within a Church that had become steeped in error, as evidenced by the bull *Unigenitus*. A massive anti-establishment movement composed mainly of the lower order of the clergy formed around a work entitled *Le témoignage de la vérité dans l'Eglise* (*Testimony on the Truth in the Church*; 1714) by Father Vivien de la Borde, published in Holland. De la Borde reflected on Saint Paul's precept that one ought to obey God rather than men, and advocated a return to the egalitarian spirit of the early Church. Parish clergy from the countryside and from Paris issued repeated appeals to rescind the papal order, transforming their refusal of the bull into a supreme act of faith.[7]

It is not a coincidence that precisely at this time, a proliferation of miracles occurred around the grave of the Deacon François de Pâris. The young man intended to make his life an imitation of the martyrdom of the saints of Port-Royal, but in 1727 his ideal of poverty led to his premature death at the age of thirty-seven. His tomb became an object of devotion, through which popular response to the Figurist doctrine, a mixture of monotheistic and pagan faith, conflating orthodox and 'superstitious' activities and beliefs, found expression.[8]

In addition to displaying Figurist values, the testimonies of convulsions and healing miracles contain a new element of aggressive publicity. They were first published and distributed separately and later republished as collections. Accounts of the convulsions and miraculous cures appeared notably in pamphlets, dissertations and short articles published in the underground Jansenist periodical *Nouvelles écclésiastiques*. An enormous amount of writings was devoted to the subject with the purpose to introduce the Jansenist cause to the community, creating a favourable public opinion. Although still hesitant, it was likely to affect the position of the institutions in power.

Carré de Montgeron was one of the chief players among Jansenism's partisans. A parliamentarian, he devoted himself to the distribution and legitimisation of the miracles of Deacon Pâris; he risked his fortune and social status for the sake of the Jansenist enterprise. His sole objective was to publicize the truth of the miracles of Pâris and their divine nature. To this purpose, he devoted five years of his life and a large part of his fortune to gathering evidence supporting the irrefutable occurrence of the miracles. He corresponded intensely with Jansenist sympathizers: priests, bishops, theologians, doctors, magistrates, lawyers and notaries in Europe, particularly in France. He sought out documents—depositions taken before notaries, medical certificates, or professional assessments—finally publishing them in the aforementioned *La Vérité des Miracles opérés à l'intercession de M. de Pâris et autres Appellants, démontrée contre M. l'Archevêque de Sens*.

The entire work, its internal organisation and structure, its rhetoric and aesthetic strategies, its logic of increment and iteration, is devoted to the depiction of the body suffering from all manner of ailments and from terrible catastrophes that hurt and destroy it. All this leads to the unique moment when the body is cured through divine help and the sainthood of Deacon Pâris. The full rhetorical and literary skills of these transcriptions become apparent only when we take into account the consistent assertion that physical pain is an inevitable martyrdom that the true Christian must undergo. This goes beyond the Figuriste Catholic vision of the body as the main tool for identification with the person of Jesus (relics, Eucharistic, flagellations, etc.). Such a focus exceeds the intention to repeat the same miracle in multiple variations in order to transform it into evidence of the divine greatness faithfully represented by Jansenist believers. Rather, the exhibition of the atrocities perpetrated on the body is meant to provoke shock and horror by showing everything: the vulnerability, the destructibility, the decrepitude of the sick body.

The reasons for such a compulsive involvement are various: cultural factors such as the proliferation of libertine and pornographic literary texts that were perceived as conveying ideas concerning the naturalness of bodily sensations and pleasures; the vulgarisation and diffusion of medical dissertations with the medical and anatomical naming of diseases and body parts. In addition, the flourishing of a materialist thesis that concentrated on the body as an organic machine played a significant role in the fascination with the human body during the Enlightenment.[9] The dominance of medical terminology combined with realistic descriptions functions both to guarantee the reliability of the testimony and to create an emotional impact. The expressiveness of the terms of pain is connected to its immediate and strong effect on the audience, on the one hand, and to the credibility earned by the account of physiological proofs on the other hand. One can assume that the purpose of this anatomic exhibition lay also in the need to clearly dissociate the sickness and its miraculous healing from the common accusations of feminine hysteria and/or spasms and neurotic behaviour.[10] Nevertheless, there was always a risk that the excess and the coarseness of the verbal treatment would provoke a contrary effect and lead to the collapse of the argument.

A quick glance at the first volume of the *Témoignages*[11] reveals a methodical principle governing the composition of the book, a structure that underlines the programmed and premeditated aspect of the testimony; it is therefore implausible that the violence of the descriptions was uncontrolled. The book opens with the volume called *Epitre au Roi* (*Letter to the King*), Montgeron's personal testimony of the miracle of his conversion, combined with a short dissertation on moral issues concerning the duty of the witness. It presents eight cases of illness and miraculous healing, all of which are narrated in the third person. Then descriptions of those who experienced the illness and its miraculous cure follow: certifications of identity and social and moral profiles expected to guarantee the witnesses' respectability. Afterwards, Montgeron presents official documents testifying to the miracles: medical consultants' reports, surgeons' and pharmacists' validations of miraculous healing, notaries' records of testimonies and attestations. The volume closes with a collection of essays and letters dealing mainly with the controversial arguments on the issue of the miracles. Despite their varied nature and the heterogeneity of the voices invoked, the texts form a single entity whose logical structure relies on a very clear principle of unification: the introductions, the stories, the documents, and the dissertations are combined in such a way as to create the sense of one organic discursive piece rather than that of a compilation of items. Montgeron's book is thus a coherent entity which is still open to additions of an unlimited number of miracles.

The effect of unity is mainly due to the regularity of the typographical set-up and the inner and external symmetry of the cases, which use the same narrative structure, are of the same approximate length, and include similar literary and stylistic components. Each testimony opens with two engravings depicting the sufferer, one before and one after the miracle, drawn by the well-known engraver Jean Restout.[12] These pictures body forth the written word and draw the reader's eye to the concrete reality of illness. The use of illumination has been an integral element of religious-miracle literature since the birth of the printed text. The visual evidence that reinforces the verbal testimony aims to provoke an immediate effect on the reader, demanding that he become involved sensorily and affectively. This systematic use of the visual reveals the aesthetic consciousness of the author, as well as his concern with publicity. It represents a premeditated publishing strategy rather than a faithful transcript of the events, as is claimed. The concomitance of the visual and the verbal that must affect the reader sensually is a rhetorical device for incorporating the miracle both into the realm of daily life and into the aesthetic realm appealed to by the quality and precision of the engraving.

Beneath each engraving, a short explanation introduces the reader to the specific story. It enumerates the details depicted in the picture, which will appear in written form later in the chapter. For example, demonstration VII related to Demoiselle Coirin presents the illness in the following terms under the first picture:

> Rongée par un cancer au sein du côté gauche, qui depuis 12 ans lui avait fait tomber le bout de la mamelle, et percluse par une paralysie sur tout ce même côté qui depuis le même temps avait entièrement retiré et desséché les muscles de sa cuisse et de sa jambe, applique avec foi le 12 Août 1731 sur ces maux incurables de la terre prise auprès du Tombeau de M. de Pâris.
>
> [Gnawed by breast cancer on her left side that twelve years ago had caused the tip of her nipple to fall off, and simultaneously crippled by a paralysis on the same side that for the same period of time had contracted and withered the muscles of her thigh, on the twelfth of August 1731 she

applies with faith some earth taken from the grave of M. de Pâris to her incurable illnesses.]

Beneath the second picture is the following caption:

Est guérie subitement la nuit du 12 au 13 Août de sa paralysie et de son cancer, elle se lève et s'habille. Sa servante qui lui apporte un bouillon est étonnée de la voir levée et droite dans son fauteuil, qu'elle ne peut croire que ce soit elle, et qu'elle va la chercher dans le lit quoi qu'elle soit devant ses yeux.

[She was miraculously healed on the night between the twelfth and the thirteenth of August. Her paralysis and her cancer vanished, she got up and dressed. When the maid brought the soup, she was surprised to find her mistress sitting straight in her armchair. She could not believe that it was true, and searched the bed for her, even though she was sitting there before her eyes.]

Montgeron admirably integrates the visuals into the reading experience by choosing different typographic characters for the title, the subtitle, the abstract and the narrative. Following the pictures and their captions, a second abstract, printed in italics, introduces the full testimony. The first word of each sentence appears in block characters, while the sentences are arranged one beneath the other. The result is a list of epithets printed in bold creating a double effect of accumulation and horror: BROKEN, ATTACKED, TORMENTED, EXHAUSTED, SHAKEN, SHOCKED, CURED, (*Demonstration* IV, p. 1). Each epithet is followed by a description of the symptoms of the illness:

BRISEE par differentes chutes qui lui ont causé, entre autres maux, une rupture de vaisseaux dans l'estomac, et l'on rendue sujette à des hémorragies journalières.

ATTAQUEE d'un mal de tête continuel pendant cinq ans, joint à une fièvre ardente avec frissons et redoublements.
TOURMENTEE d'une douleur de côté insupportable et d'une insomnie continuelle.

EPUISEE par une inanition de plusieurs années pendant lesquelles elle était forcée de rejeter sur le champ avec un affreux vomissement de sang toutes les nourritures qu'elle prenait, ayant même passé les derniers six mois sans presque rien avaler.

LIVREE à des attaques fréquentes d'apoplexie qui la jetaient dans un état léthargique, où elle restait sans mouvement et presque sans vie des dix jours de suite.

ACCABLEE par une hydropisie générale qui la suffoquait et qui lui permettait à peine de respirer.

FRAPPEE de paralysie sur tout le côté gauche et principalement sur le bras.

GUERIE subitement chaque jour de quelqu'une de ces maladies et successivement de toutes en cinq jours, sur le tombeau de M. de Pâris les 16, 17, 18, 19 et 20 juillet 1731, et recouvrant la santé la plus parfaite le 21 du même mois.

[BROKEN by many falls that caused, among other pains, vessels of the stomach to burst, provoking daily bleedings.

SUBJECTED to continuous headaches combined with burning fever and violent shivers for five full years.

PLAGUED by an unbearable pain in her side and continuous sleeplessness.

EXHAUSTED by lassitude, of many years' duration, during which she immediately and violently vomited any foods she ate, bringing up blood. She has barely eaten anything for nearly six months.

OVERCOME by frequent apoplectic attacks, she fell into a state of lethargy, could not move, and was nearly lifeless for ten contiguous days.

SMITTEN by general dropsy, she was suffocating and could barely breathe.

STRUCK by paralysis on her left side, mainly in her arm.

CURED suddenly of her various sicknesses during five successive days by the grave of M. de Pâris, the sixteenth,

> seventeenth, eighteenth, nineteenth, and twentieth July 1731, she recovered her full health on the twenty-first of the same month.]

These visual tools (block letters, variations in type face, sophisticated editing) emphasise the extraordinary aspects of the event while simultaneously working together with the engravings to provoke an immediate response in the reader, even before he has absorbed the full story. The various medical terms—which include both symptoms and diagnosis—emphasise the objective aspect of the report. Since medical terms such as 'apoplexy,' 'dropsy' and 'paralysis' describe objective malfunctions of the organism, the reader immediately relates to the discourse as scientific, and interprets the contents as factual. The pains spring from identifiable illnesses, have bodily referents and are therefore considered authentic, validated by the causality established in illness and injury. Furthermore, the severity of the symptoms eliminates any potential controversy regarding the diagnosis, reinforcing the testimony's impact by tapping into a discourse of indisputable knowledge.

However, the tone changes at the beginning of the actual body of the demonstration, moving from medical to literary discourse. The expressiveness and the pathos of the plot, which relates terrible accidents and catastrophic injuries, trap the reader within a world of horror and fear. In the fourth demonstration, related by Marguerite Françoise Duchesne, the narrator constructs the testimonial discourse in a manner very similar to that of suspense narrative, combining the commonly used ingredients of fantasy and tension.

Several dramatic accidents happen in a very short period of time, with almost no intervals:

> Le 4 octobre, étant au haut de son escalier, elle tomba jusqu'à la moitié de l'étage sur des boites qu'elle portait.
>
> [On the fourth October 1727, while standing at the top of the staircase, she fell halfway down, landing on the boxes she had been carrying.]
>
> Au mois de Mai de 1728, étant montée pour détendre la toile cirée qui sert de couverture à l'échoppe où elle étale, attenant la grille de l'Abbaye, le pied lui glisse, elle tombe sur l'appui de sa boutique, le coup porte encore entre la poitrine et l'estomac, et lui répend entre les deux épaules, ce qui la fait évanouir. Revenue à elle-même, loin de perdre courage, elle remonte pour continuer à défaire la toile de sa

> boutique; mais étant encore toute éblouie et toute hors d'elle-même par la chute qu'elle venait de faire, elle retombe une seconde fois encore plus rudement, se blesse au même endroit, mais si cruellement qu'elle rend aussitôt le sang par la bouche avec une affreuse abondance.
>
> [On May 1728, having climbed up in order to loosen the oilcloth which serves to cover the booth where she offers her wares by the gate to the abbey, her foot slips and she falls onto the base of the booth. The blow injures her between her chest and stomach, the damage spreading between her shoulders, so that she faints. When she recovers, instead of giving up, she climbs again in order to continue loosening the oilcloth; but she is so stunned and disoriented by the previous fall that she trips a second time, even more grievously, and is wounded in the same place to such a cruel degree that she starts to bring up a dreadful quantity of blood.]
>
> Ce n'est pas tout, une dernière chute achève encore de la briser. A peine quinze jours s'étaient-ils écoulés depuis les deux chutes précédentes, qu'étant montée sur l'appui extérieur de sa boutique, elle se laisse tomber sur la barre de fer qui soutient la grille de l'Abbaye, et de là sa tête se précipite la première sur le pavé avec une telle violence qu'elle la crut entièrement fracassée.
>
> [This is not the end: a final fall ends up shattering her. Less than fifteen days after the two prior falls, she climbs up the external support of her booth and falls upon the iron bar of the abbey gate, her head hitting the pavement with such violence that it is nearly smashed.]

The dates and the temporal details place the discourse in the historical realm, and function as a guarantee to the story, while the metamorphosis of Marguerite from a simple, lower-class girl to a heroine—courageous and strong, faithful to her belief, optimistic, hard-working, non-complaining—serves to heighten the tension. The eloquence of pain combined with an unnatural degree of pain-tolerance transform the young woman into the emblematic figure of the Christian martyr. However, the crescendo of destruction, along with the accumulation of horrifying consequences, the spectacle of the gradual disintegration of the damaged body, creates a tension in the reader, who is torn between pity and rejection of the events as too ghastly to be true. The focus on the collapse of the broken body highlights a process of corruption, physical putrescence. It creates a vision of the body emptying itself, heading toward total disappearance:

> un vomissement de sang très abondant fait comprendre qu'il s'était rompu quelques veines dans la poitrine ou l'estomac. … les vomissements de sang ne peuvent être arrêtés, ils deviennent habituels: le pus des vaisseaux déchirés, dont les cicatrices tombent en suppuration, se mêlant avec le sang, augmente infiniment la force de la fièvre continue dont elle était déjà tourmentée. (2)
>
> [the vomiting of a large quantity of blood reveals that some of the vessels in the chest and stomach had broken. … the vomiting of blood cannot be stopped, and becomes chronic. The pus from the damaged vessels, whose scars begin to suppurate, mix with the blood, greatly intensifying the continuous fever that has already been tormenting her.]
>
> Or
>
> c'est un si grand relâchement des fibres de l'estomac, qu'il ne peut plus supporter aucune nourriture; c'est une corruption qui lui infecte si fort l'organe du goût, que la seule odeur du bouillon lui excite des soulèvements de cœur auxquels elle ne peut résister; c'est une abondance d'humeurs glaireuses, qui arrêtant et liant l'action des ressorts, lui cause des étouffements que la saignée ne paraît suspendre pendant quelques instants, que pour donner lieu à une toux âcre causée par l'irritation des fibres musculeuses de l'estomac, et toujours suivie d'un affreux vomissement de sang. (3)
>
> [there is such an extreme loosening of the stomach fibres, that it cannot retain any food. It is such a corruption of the organs of taste that even the smell of soup provokes unbearable nausea; there is an excess of loose humours, which blocks and entangles the channels, causing suffocation. Bleeding her provides relief for only a few moments, and causes a dry cough, which in conjunction with the irritation of the stomach's muscular fibres, instigates horrible vomiting of blood.]

The narrator relates the intensifying progress of the disease with an abundance of images linked to excess and chaos, turning the body into a space of desolation and destruction. The excretions, blood and vomit trigger disgust by transforming the sick body into a rotten entity in the process of disintegration. All these details are presented in both a medical and ordinary lexicon; therefore, the non-specialist reader can understand every element and experience the metamorphosis of a woman into a monster with a distorted face:

> Quel plus effrayant spectacle que de voir son visage dans le temps de ces accidents, n'offrir plus qu'une couleur terreuse, rehaussée d'un violet obscur; sa langue épaissie et d'un noir foncé, rester immobile et comme collée à son palais; sa bouche se contourner en des figures forcées; sa gorge s'enfler à vue d'œil, ses lèvres bleuâtres et livides être marquées de vestiges même de la mort, quelques gouttes de somme égarées dans les extrémités lui sortir sous les angles et par l'angle des yeux! Quelle horreur (4)
>
> [What a horrible sight to see her face during one of these attacks. Her colour is ashen, with a purplish overlay. Her tongue is thickened, dark black, and unmoving, as though stuck to her palate; her mouth is forced into strange contortions; her throat is swelling visibly, and her lips are a sickly blue, marked by the shadows of death. Some drops of muck are trickling out of the corners of her eyes! What a horror]

In the passage above, we can trace the move from an objective to a subjective tone, when the putative medical report is interrupted by exclamation marks addressed to the reader.

The description of the bodily breakdown and suffering comes hand in hand with a rhetorical move towards subjectivity and expressiveness. Both contents and form work to construct a very particular kind of testimony, which appeals to the visceral response of the reader, rather than to his intellect.

Thus literary techniques play an important role in the processes of validating the testimony in *La Vérité des Miracles*: the fictionalisation of testimony works as a supplementary strategy of seduction. The very specific and detailed demonstration of the various stages of illness; the construction of suspense by presenting an accumulation of disasters and consequent gradual deterioration of health; the cumulative excess of terrifying details of bodily disintegration and degeneration—all these discursive procedures help to immerse the reader in the story, forcing a corporeal involvement. The reader cannot but react emotionally in a dual movement of connection and identification.

It seems that such an empathic process has little to do with the accreditation of facts. But there is a merging between the citation of expert scientific authorities on the one hand and subjectively expressive voices communicating personal experiences of pain on the other. The combination serves as a rhetorical tool aimed at resolving the problem of subjectivity within a discourse that aims to objectively validate testimony of a miracle.

The obsessive focus on pain and suffering serves to produce a particular kind of knowledge, because the discourse on pain places the reader in a unique space of variable trust and distrust. As is known, not all reports of pain are taken seriously, and credibility depends on cultural expectations and ideological contexts. For example, women's complaints were often associated with a 'female syndrome,' such as hysteria, depression or the so-called 'vapours.' Notable among the doctors who contributed to the gendered approach to illness and the suffering body are Nicolas Venette, well-known for his *The Mysteries of Conjugal Love Reveal'd*, 1686 (*Tableau de l'amour humain considéré dans l'état du mariage*) and Bienville, who wrote a treatise on *Nymphomania* (1789). Montgeron's focus on physical agony and injury dissociates the bodily experience from mental forms of pain typically associated with women at the time. Furthermore, a strong presence of medical voices gathered together from verifiable personal experience was necessary in order to avoid the widespread criticism of belief in the miraculous and the prevalent distrust of enthusiasm and the malady of imagination.[13]

There are both religious and cultural aspects in the exploration of the sick body to its most extreme limits. A pragmatic dimension exists in this kind of testimonial discourse. Repeating the same miracle in multiple variations produces two crucial effects on the written text: it strengthens its authenticity because of its simultaneous and collective aspect, and it endows it with a structure of authority because of its empirical character. It implicitly conforms to the predominant positivist method of constituting facts in early Enlightenment France, and to the new organisation of thought through Cartesian paradigmatic processes.[14] If the testimonies of Montgeron go beyond the reasonable scientific description of the sick body and border on the discourse of obscenity and horror, it is because they aim at a general mobilisation of public opinion. The appropriation of methodological tools belonging to the Enlightenment and the seizure of materialist and libertine concepts concentrated on the 'Homme Machine,' the famous title of La Mettrie's materialist book (1748), indicate the incorporation of commonplace knowledge and shared beliefs into a discourse whose objective clearly stands against the liberal secular ideals of the Enlightenment.

The testimonies regarding the sick body registered both an opposition to and an incorporation of the other discourses. The incongruous juxtaposition of multiple discourses, the combination of the expressiveness of pain with the scientific listing of symptoms, and the placement of the suffering body at the pivot of testimonial discourse, displays the paradoxical ways in which the most rational thoughts of the Enlightenment era are penetrated by irrational streams.

Notes

[1] Dale K. Van Kley, *The Religious Origins of the French Revolution from Calvin to the Civil Constitution, 1590-1791* (New Haven: Yale University Press, 1996); William Doyle, *Jansenism Catholic Resistance to Authority from the Reformation to the French Revolution* (New York: St Martin's Press, 2001).
[2] Michèle Bokobza Kahan, 'Recueil de miracles: les convulsionnaires de Saint-Médard (1727-1732),' in *Esthétique du témoignage*, ed. Renaud Dulong and Carole Dornier (Paris: Editions des Sciences de l'Homme, 2005), 301; Bokobza Kahan, 'Les témoignages des convulsionnaires de Saint-Médard: l'entreprise des Lumières au service de la vérité divine,' *Dix-Huitième Siècle* 39 (2007): 180.
[3] See Bokobza Kahan, 'Ethos in Testimony: The Case of Carré de Montgeron, a Jansenist and a Convulsionary in the Century of Enlightenment,' *Eighteenth Century Studies* 43 (2010): 431.
[4] Bokobza Kahan, 'Mise en fiction des témoignages des convulsionnaires de Saint-Médard (1727-1732), vers une poétique de l'horreur,' *Revue Romane* 44 (2009): 324-328.
[5] Robert Kreiser, *Miracles, Convulsions and Ecclesiastical Politics in Early Eighteenth-Century Paris* (Princeton: Princeton University Press, 1978), 375-394; Catherine Maire, *De la cause de Dieu à la cause de la Nation* (Paris: Gallimard, 1998), 265-304.
[6] Esther Cohen, 'Thaumatology at One Remove: Empathy in Miraculous-Cure Narratives in the Later Middle Ages,' *Partial Answers* 7 (2009): 190-195.
[7] Jean-Pierre Chantin, *Le Jansénisme* (Paris: Cerf, 1996), 32-34.
[8] Bryan E. Strayer, *Suffering Saints: Jansenists and Convulsionnaires in France, 1640-1799* (Portland: Sussex Academic Press, 2008).
[9] Roselyne Rey, *The History of Pain*, trans. Louise Elliott Wallace, J. A. Cadden, and S. W. Cadden (Cambridge, MA: Harvard University Press, 1993).
[10] Lindsay Wilson, *Women and Medicine in the French Enlightenment* (Baltimore: John Hopkins University Press, 1993), 17-33.

[11] The citations refer to the edition of Utrecht, Chez les Libraires de la Compagnie, 1737, 2 vols.
[12] Christine Gouzi, *L'Art et le Jansénisme au 18e siècle* (Paris: Nolin, 2007), 154.
[13] Lorraine Daston and Katharine Park, *Wonders and the Order of Nature 1150-1750* (New York: Zone Books, 1998), 329-363.
[14] Jean-Robert Armogathe, 'A propos des miracles de Saint-Médard: les preuves de Carré de Montgeron et le positivisme des Lumières,' *Revue de l'histoire des religions* 180 (1971): 156.

Bibliography

Armogathe, Jean-Robert. 'À propos des miracles de Saint-Médard: les preuves de Carré de Montgeron et le positivisme des Lumières.' *Revue de l'histoire des religions* 180 (1971): 135-160.

Bokobza Kahan, Michèle. 'Ethos in Testimony: The Case of Carré de Montgeron, a Jansenist and a Convulsionary in the Century of Enlightenment.' *Eighteenth Century Studies* 43 (2010): 419-433.

———. 'Mise en fiction des témoignages des convulsionnaires de Saint-Médard (1727-1732), vers une poétique de l'horreur.' *Revue Romane* 44 (2009): 313-331.

———. 'Recueil de miracles: les convulsionnaires de Saint-Médard (1727-1732).' In *Esthétique du témoignage*. Edited by Renaud Dulong and Carole Dornier (Paris: Editions des Sciences de l'Homme, 2005), 287-302.

———. 'Les témoignages des convulsionnaires de Saint-Médard: l'entreprise des Lumières au service de la vérité divine.' *Dix-Huitième Siècle* 39 (2007): 175-188.

Chantin, Jean-Pierre. *Le Jansénisme.* Paris: Cerf, 1996.

Cohen, Esther. 'Thaumatology at One Remove: Empathy in Miraculous-Cure Narratives in the Later Middle Ages.' *Partial Answers* 7 (2009): 189-200.

Daston, Lorraine and Katharine Park. *Wonders and the Order of Nature 1150-1750*. New York: Zone Books, 1998.

Doyle, William. *Jansenism Catholic Resistance to Authority from the Reformation to the French Revolution.* New York: St. Martin's Press, 2001.

Gouzi, Christine. *L'Art et le Jansénisme au 18e siècle.* Paris: Nolin, 2007.

Kreiser, Robert. *Miracles, Convulsions and Ecclesiastical Politics in Early Eighteenth-Century Paris.* Princeton: Princeton University Press, 1978.

Maire, Catherine. *De la cause de Dieu à la cause de la Nation.* Paris: Gallimard, 1998.

Rey, Roselyne. *The History of Pain.* Translated by Louise Elliott Wallace, J. A. Cadden and S. W. Cadden. Cambridge, MA: Harvard University Press, 1993.

Strayer, Bryan E. *Suffering Saints: Jansenists and Convulsionnaires in France, 1640-1799.* Portland, OR: Sussex Academic Press, 2008.

Van Kley, Dale K. *The Religious Origins of the French Revolution from Calvin to the Civil Constitution, 1590-1791.* New Haven: Yale University Press, 1996.

Wilson, Lindsay. *Women and Medicine in the French Enlightenment.* Baltimore: Johns Hopkins University Press, 1993.

The Limits of Enlightenment Sensitivity To the Suffering of Animals

Nathaniel Wolloch

Abstract
This article examines the nature and limits of eighteenth-century ethical sensitivity to the suffering of animals. It claims that, contrary to common scholarly interpretations, rising humanitarian concern with animal rights in the eighteenth century was in fact limited. When it appeared to collide with human interests, it was habitually downplayed. Enlightenment thought emphasised the need to avoid causing unnecessary suffering to animals but at the same time developed a new conception of the vital role that command of natural resources, including animals, played in the development of human culture. The result was an anthropocentrically-motivated limited sensitivity to animal suffering, prefiguring the mainstream modern attitude toward them. The discussion examines these developments while considering the views of various thinkers, in particular Georges-Louis Leclerc, the Comte de Buffon, and J. Hector St. John de Crèvecoeur.

Key Words: Animals, Enlightenment, ethics, theriophily, anthropocentrism, historiography, literature, Buffon, Adam Smith, Crèvecoeur.

*****

The convergence of the terms 'knowledge' and 'pain' is bound to remind one of animals. Debates regarding the cognitive and sensual characteristics of animals, and the ethical implications of their treatment, have received consistent attention for centuries. Intellectuals in antiquity, the middle ages, early modern and modern times were all interested in animals, although from very different cultural perspectives.[1] Historians have often attempted to describe changes in the history of Western attitudes toward animals. This chapter argues, however, that throughout history there has been a remarkable overall consistency in human attitudes toward animals, particularly in terms of the ethical sensitivity to animal suffering, or rather, the limits of this sensitivity. Despite changes in language and cultural underpinnings, consideration of animal suffering remained confined within clearly marked anthropocentric bounds.

This limited sensitivity was particularly pronounced in the eighteenth century. Scholars have often seen this as the time when a new, more modern and humanitarian concern with animal suffering emerged. An early exponent of this outlook, Henry Salt, wrote that 'it was not until the eighteenth century, the age of enlightenment and 'sensibility,' of which

Voltaire and Rousseau were the spokesmen, that the rights of animals obtained more deliberate recognition.'[2] This assertion has become ubiquitous in modern scholarship, which has often included an emphasis on Jeremy Bentham as a signal figure in the rise of a new moral sensitivity to animal suffering irrespective of the animals' cognitive inferiority to human beings. This is evident in Bentham's claim: 'The question is not, Can they [animals] reason? nor, Can they talk? but, Can they suffer?'[3] Bentham, in fact, was not as original on this point as is often assumed. Jean-Jacques Rousseau had made similar claims and was much more influential.[4] Yet early modern theriophiles (lovers of animals) almost always evinced a clearly limited concern with animal suffering. For example, Michel de Montaigne outlined emphatic arguments for sensitivity to animals but also admitted, in a self-reproaching tone, his enjoyment of hunting despite his aversion to the animal suffering involved.[5] Later, Rousseau recommended that Émile practice hunting, despite the cruelty involved, since it served as a distraction from improper adolescent sexual passions.[6] Both Montaigne and Rousseau were typical in this respect. Early modern sensitivity to animals almost never overstepped clear anthropocentric limits, particularly when this might have required serious practical steps. Philosophical remonstration was one thing; practical change was quite another.

Erica Fudge has recently located the transition from the early modern to the modern consideration of animals at an earlier stage, specifically regarding the seventeenth-century Cartesian 'beast-machine' theory of animal automatism. The Cartesian position excluded animals from the discourse on the nature of reason, and animals were consequently discussed separately from the emerging modern notion of the human. The seemingly simple differentiation between human and animal rational abilities resulted, however, in blurred categorisation, ultimately forcing early modern thinkers to recognise the possibility of animal rationality and sentience. According to Fudge, by imposing the Cartesian notion of the distinctly non-animal human on pre-Cartesian culture, scholars have mistakenly disregarded the presence of animals in earlier debates about reason.[7] In any event, Fudge's analysis demonstrates that in early modern debates the ethical dimension was usually subservient to the assertion of the animals' cognitive and emotional characteristics.

From an ethical point of view, the Cartesian beast-machine theory was compelling precisely because it explained away the ethical qualms involved in causing pain to animals. Its rapid downfall by the beginning of the eighteenth century was due primarily to its counter-intuitive nature. In the intellectual climate of the Enlightenment, with its preference for common-sense reasoning, especially concerning ethical issues, the Cartesian consideration of animals was bound to seem like unpalatable casuistry. The reason for this was not necessarily a concern for the well-being of animals but rather a more general change in intellectual types of reasoning between the seventeenth and the eighteenth centuries. The eighteenth-century impatience with older types of philosophical discourse about animals was ironically noted in Georg Christoph Lichtenberg's observation: 'That man is the noblest creature may also be inferred from the fact that no other creature has yet contested this claim.'[8] Because of this change in modes of philosophical argumentation, intellectuals were forced to face the possibility that animal suffering could not be 'solved' either as a practical or a theoretical problem. The result was twofold: on the one hand, this led to a seemingly growing concern with animal suffering, which has often been described as a forerunner of the enhanced form of 'humanitarian' concern for animal welfare beginning in the eighteenth century. On the other hand, this new approach opened the way for the often uninhibited mass utilisation of animals in the wake of the Industrial Revolution. The eighteenth-century rise in sensitivity to animals was often expressed in the context of fictional literature, for example in the famous 'lesson of universal good-will' which Tristram Shandy learns from his uncle Toby's kindness to a fly.[9] Yet in non-fictional types of discourse it seemed more difficult to present sensitivity to animal suffering in such a straightforward manner.

Scholars have often concentrated on early modern philosophical, scientific and literary discussions of animals. They have usually overlooked other types of debate, which evinced a different outlook, much less concerned with the cognitive capacity of animals or their suffering. This attitude did not mean a lack of concern with animal pain, quite the contrary. Yet particularly in the late Enlightenment, such ethical sensitivity customarily took a back seat to a growing awareness that cultural progress required the utilisation of animals. The debate about animal pain seemed a moot point. The animals' capacity for suffering was commonly recognised, as was the need to avoid inflicting *unnecessary* pain upon them. The infliction of pain, however, often seemed all too necessary. The discarding of the beast-machine theory notwithstanding, eighteenth-century intellectuals still faced the problem of the incongruity between the ethical consideration of animal suffering and the general overriding priority of human interests.

Nowhere was this outlook more evident than in late eighteenth-century historiographical discourse. A historiographical element was common to many contemporaneous discussions, not all of them belonging strictly to historical literature in the modern sense.[10] Key to such debates was the rise, in the second half of the century, of the early type of nascent theoretical anthropology termed 'conjectural history.' This genre offered surmises about the origins of human material and social culture.[11] It was no coincidence that many of Rousseau's remarks were made in his famous second discourse, which was in many ways concerned with conjectural history. Nevertheless, Rousseau's uncommon primitivism should be contrasted with more typical contemporaneous outlooks. A prime example was the famous naturalist the Comte de Buffon, who also used conjectural history in his depiction of the rise of human societies, intimately connected with the gradual control of nature. This control included such things as the creation of new species of plants and animals, the warming of the climate due to deforestation, the control of rivers, the use of fire, the settlement of specific geographical regions, and other forms of development of natural resources.[12] Buffon was aware of the climate's influence on human culture, which was a common theme in Western thought since antiquity. Yet in contrast with Montesquieu, another famous contemporary to discuss this issue, Buffon also emphasised the human ability to change nature.[13] He repeatedly noted the unique position of human beings in nature and their power to improve their natural surroundings.[14]

How was this outlook reflected in his ethical consideration of animals? Above all, Buffon exhibited a distinctly anthropocentric attitude, emphasising human superiority and the right of humans to use animals. Nevertheless, he seemed quite aware of the capacity of animals to suffer, and of the need to consider this characteristic from a moral perspective.[15] He opposed unnecessary harm to animals, but regarded consumption of animal flesh as part of the natural order, helping for example to control the relative populations of various animal species. Human beings physically required a carnivorous diet, and Buffon opposed the primitivistic notion of vegetarian humanity in the state of nature, criticizing philosophers (mainly Rousseau) who supported this 'fiction, in which man is regarded as an animal' (fable, où l'on emploie l'homme comme un animal').[16] Human beings destroyed more animals than all other carnivorous beasts, more due to intemperance than real want. Yet, however great the waste created by humans, the total quantity of life never diminished: 'reproduction is born of destruction' ('la reproduction naisse de la destruction').[17] In short, Buffon regarded the human manipulation of nature as an ongoing trend necessary for human progress, morally permissible both because of innate human qualities and because nature was able to sustain any amount of human manipulation. Like most of his contemporaries, he would probably have found subsequent modern notions such as over-population quite surprising.[18]

The human use of animals also seemed justified because of the latter's inferiority to the former. At one point Buffon claimed, in a seemingly Cartesian fashion (unusual at a time when the beast-machine theory had already been discredited) that animals acted in purely mechanical fashion, while spirituality was conferred only on human beings.[19] Slightly later, however, he insisted that he did not reduce animals to insensible automata. On the contrary, he claimed that their sensations were perhaps even more acute than human ones, but they lacked thought or reflection. Animals were conscious of their present existence, yet not of the past. They had sensations but lacked the ability to compare them or form ideas:

> The animals are therefore capable, like us, of both pain and pleasure; they do not recognise good or evil, yet they feel them: that which is agreeable to them is good, that which is disagreeable is bad; the one and the other are only suitable or contrary connections with their nature, and their organisation.[20]

Animals, like humans, were not equal. Both among animals and among humans there was a scale of feeling ranging from automaton-like behaviour to great sensitivity. Just as there was a difference in this respect between savages and civilised human beings, so there was a difference between wild animals with natural sensibility and domestic animals with improved feelings.[21] Ultimately, this also had ethical consequences:

> The animals, at least those endowed with senses, flesh and blood, are sensible beings; like us they are capable of pleasure and subject to pain. It is therefore a type of cruel insensibility to unnecessarily sacrifice those especially who are similar to us, live with us, and who resemble us by displaying signs of pain; for those whose nature is different from ours, are hardly able to affect us.[22]

Natural pity was founded on an analogy with the suffering object, and therefore, while the suffering of a dog or a lamb excited human emotion, the destruction of a tree or an oyster did not. Buffon based his ethical outlook on the common eighteenth-century perception of 'sympathy,' which in contemporaneous terms meant the ability to commiserate with another's feelings. Most commonly this applied to other human beings, but it could also apply to animals, if only to a limited extent. The typical Enlightenment outlook, exemplified so clearly by Buffon, emphasised sensitivity to animal pain, but only so long as this did not collide with vital human interests, specifically as relating to the ongoing material and social progress of humanity. Despite his apparent interest in the traditional debate regarding the cognitive and sensual qualities of animals, Buffon was unwilling to let such concerns hamper his advocacy for the utilisation of animals.

The historiographical element in this *Weltanschauung* was evident in the most common version of conjectural history, the stadial theory, specifically the four-stages theory. This theory asserted that human societies almost universally developed according to a fixed pattern, beginning with a hunting stage, through a shepherding one (pastoralism), followed by agriculture (the crucial transition from a nomadic to a sedentary existence), and finally by the advanced stage of commercialism.[23] The four-stage theory was developed mainly by Scottish Enlightenment philosophers, most significantly by Adam Smith. Stadial theory emphasised the gradually rising sophistication of the means of acquiring subsistence by cultivating nature, including animals. This necessitated considering animals primarily as property—objects manipulated for the benefit of human beings—a view which was clearly expressed by Smith.[24] Yet Smith also recognised the capacity of animals for suffering, and the need to take this into ethical consideration. He wrote expressly about

> that fellow-feeling which Nature has, for the wisest purposes, implanted in man, not only towards all other men, but (though no doubt in a much weaker degree) towards all other animals. Having destined him to be the governing animal in this little world, it seems to have been her benevolent intention to inspire him with some degree of respect, even for the meanest and weakest of his subjects.[25]

Like Buffon, Smith admitted the need for sensitivity to animal suffering. This was a 'fellow-feeling' to the degree that animals were similar to human beings. However, since such similarity, based essentially on the perception of anthropomorphic animal qualities, was not unlimited, this moral sensitivity was comparably restricted.

The Scottish historian William Robertson had a similar outlook. He claimed that the American savages were insensible both to the suffering of animals and to that of other human beings, including their own family members. '[I]t is universally observed that they always treat them [the imported European domesticated animals] harshly, and never employ any method either for breaking or managing them, but force and cruelty.' The American savage, according to Robertson, had no sensitivity either to animals or to human beings, and he behaved 'with little attention or sensibility to the sentiments and feelings of the beings around him.'[26] Yet Robertson perceived no problem with the human utilisation of animals, repeatedly commenting on its importance for cultural progress:

> Whenever any people have experienced the advantages which men enjoy, by their dominion over the inferior animals, they can neither subsist without the nourishment which these afford, nor carry on any considerable operation independent of their ministry and labour.[27]

The eighteenth-century historiographical consideration of animals was elaborated particularly by the century's greatest historian, Edward Gibbon. A story, perhaps apocryphal, related how the young Gibbon, hearing the cries of a dog one of the servants was beating, intervened on behalf of the dog by beating the servant.[28] He

> shudder[ed] at the recollection of the bloody spectacles of the Romans; those savage combats of wild beasts, which Cicero so much despised and detested. Solitude and silence were by him preferred to these master-pieces of magnificence, horrour, and wretchedness of taste. In fact, to take delight in blood-shed is only worthy an herd of savages.[29]

Nevertheless, despite their vanity and cruelty, these spectacles had had their value for 'naturalists,' and were unequalled historically as an expenditure and artistic effort for amusing a people.[30] Ultimately, Gibbon emphasised the importance of the human utilisation of nature in general, and of animals in particular. This control was vital for sustained human progress, and Gibbon therefore did not refer to any serious ethical problem which it involved, noting that 'Our toil is lessened, and our wealth is increased, by our dominion over the useful animals.'[31] Not surprisingly, he also consistently subscribed to the stadial theory, with its emphasis on the use of animals.[32] The common Enlightenment outlook on animals was again plainly evident—needless cruelty was condemned, but all too often the suffering of animals seemed lamentably necessary, in which case it was tacitly overlooked.

The tension between praise of the human command of nature on the one hand and sensitivity to animals on the other received one of its most eloquent eighteenth-century expressions in the writings of J. Hector St. John de Crèvecoeur. Combining the traditional praise of the moral worth of agricultural pursuits with a sense of the importance of commanding the American wilderness, Crèvecoeur extolled the human endeavour exemplified by the settlers of the New World. At the same time, however, he was enthralled by the awesome quality of nature in America, which offered such ample room for humanity's efforts to build a civilisation on the basis of cultivation of natural resources. Animals, of course, were bound to be affected by this huge undertaking. Crèvecoeur, who became intimately aware of this influence, thus found himself probably unintentionally expressing the inherent Enlightenment tension between sensitivity to animals and the ineluctable need to harm them in order to provide for human necessities. In the case of the life of American farmers, these were indeed absolute necessities, without which survival in the harsh wilderness was impossible.

In *Letters from an American Farmer*, Crèvecoeur's protagonist and mouthpiece James describes his enjoyment of wild and domestic animals on his farm, combining appreciation of animals with thoughts of their utilisation for human benefit.[33] He was astonished at the sagacity of animals, which occasionally surpassed that of humans, and objected to derogatory views regarding animal instinct:

> I never see an egg brought on my table but I feel penetrated with the wonderful change it would have undergone but for my gluttony; it might have been a gentle, useful hen leading her chicken with a care and vigilance which speaks shame to many women. A cock perhaps, arrayed with the most majestic plumes, tender to its mate, bold, courageous, endowed with an astonishing instinct, with thought, with memory, and every distinguishing characteristic of the reason of man.[34]

James finds himself in an ethical bind, caught between his admiration of animals and his constant need to utilise them. For example, he regrets that the bees on his farm are destroyed by king-birds, but these birds guard his fields against the depredations of crows. He resists killing them till they overpopulate his property.[35] He goes on to write about his enjoyment of quails and his attempts to help them during winter: 'I do not know an instance in which the barbarity of man is so strongly delineated as in the catching and murthering those harmless birds, at that cruel season of the year.'[36]

Both in *Letters from an American Farmer* and in *Sketches of Eighteenth-Century America*, Crèvecoeur constantly struggles with this dilemma. He sees a connection between cruelty towards animals and human beings and political corruption.[37] At one point he writes how, out of a 'Pythagorean disposition,' he refused to destroy an ant colony to satisfy his 'impious' curiosity regarding its structure. But at another time he destroyed ants which had threatened a beehive. Pythagorean vegetarian allusions notwithstanding, when noting the consumption of snapping turtles, he claims that 'as long as we feed on what would feed on us, that seems to be founded on a just retaliation.'[38] Other animals, however, seemed harmless and therefore true victims of unjustified human barbarity. Beavers were of course one of the most common examples of hunted animals. They were

> the philosophers of the animals; the gentlest, the most humble, the most harmless. Yet brutal Man kills them. I was once a witness to the destruction of one of their

> associated confederacies. I saw many of them shed tears, and I wept also; nor am I ashamed to confess it.[39]

Nevertheless, the need to kill animals was at times a truly lamentable necessity. Regarding the regrettable need to hunt squirrels which harmed the crops, Crèvecoeur writes:

> For my part, I cannot blame them [the squirrels carrying away corn husks], but I should blame myself were I peaceably to look on and let them carry all. As we pay no tithes in this country, I think we should be a little more generous than we are to the brute creation.[40]

Even when one could not avoid harming animals, this had to be done while making an effort to mitigate their plight, as seen in the battle of farmers against birds which harmed their crops:

> But after all the effects of our selfishness, are they [the blackbirds] not the children of the great Creator as well as we? They are entitled to live and to get their food wherever they can get it. … But Man is a huge monster who devours everything and will suffer nothing to live in peace in his neighbourhood. … [The black-birds'] depredations proceeded from hunger, not from premedi-tateed malice . . . it is necessary that either Man or Nature should feed them.[41]

Nevertheless, Crèvecoeur does not at any point deny the evident necessity to make constant use of animals, and to destroy them whenever the need arises. Hunting animals does not necessarily involve inherent ethical qualms. Crèvecoeur's positive depiction of whaling in the Cape Cod islands is a case in point.[42] To modern sensitivities this might seem particularly blameworthy, although subsequent recognition of the mental capacities of cetaceans was still not available in the eighteenth century. This was not the case, however, regarding other animals. Thus, regret at the suffering of blackbirds notwithstanding, there is no hint of criticism of cruelty in the depiction of the hunting of pigeons with a net, 'to which they are allured by what we call tame wild pigeons, made blind and fastened to a long string.'[43] At this point of our discussion, however, this seeming inconsistency of Crèvecoeur should come as no surprise. It is perfectly in tune with the prevalent attitude of his contemporaries toward animals. Crèvecoeur's writing combines literary musings with realistic depictions of frontier life, the latter imbued with the Enlightenment praise of cultural progress. The literary aspect accommodates poignant sensitivity to animals, yet the overall realistic underpinning of the discussion leaves much less room for this ethical concern.

What were the reasons for this entrenched anthropocentrism, which we have encountered in different forms in the writings of various Enlightenment intellectuals?[44] As Lynn White noted in a famous article, biblical cosmology was the prime root of the Western view of human superiority in material creation.[45] Yet White's thesis constitutes a partial explanation. Another important intellectual legacy which helped entrench this anthropocentrism was manifested in certain aspects of classical philosophy, specifically those embodied by the famous theory of the Great Chain of Being, which enjoyed great popularity in early modern times. Moreover, the scientific revolution, despite its advocacy of rational procedures, did not relinquish traditional religious anthropocentrism but rather combined it with the new scientific method.[46] Therefore, when Enlightenment scholars praised the instrumental attitude toward mastery of nature propounded in the preceding century by Francis Bacon and others, they were consolidating an approach which combined the old anthropocentric cosmology with the powerful new tools of modern science. As subsequent history has proved, this did not bode well for animals, which since the Industrial Revolution have been utilised and manipulated to a qualitative and quantitative extent far exceeding anything in pre-modern times.

Nevertheless, there is no denying that, since the late eighteenth century and reaching an unprecedented pitch in our own times, modern culture has also consistently exemplified a distinct concern with what has come to be known as 'animal rights.' This moral solicitude did not stem just from the conservative concern with how mistreatment of animals might lead to insensitivity toward humans (a view outlined for example by Immanuel Kant)[47] but also often expressed a genuine concern for animals. Nevertheless, almost no one in the eighteenth century was willing to follow this line of ethical reasoning beyond clear anthropocentric bounds. How are we to explain this inconsistency? Keith Thomas has claimed that there was 'a growing conflict between the new sensibilities and the material foundations of human society.' This conflict 'is one of the contradictions upon which modern civilisation may be said to rest. About its ultimate consequences we can only speculate.'[48] Thomas's perceptive interpretation should be even more accentuated. Much of the modern sensitivity to animal suffering has been socially and culturally conditioned. Baiting, a common early modern practice, went out of fashion by the nineteenth century; hunting did not. Moreover, the rising eighteenth-century 'humanitarian' concern with animals was in many ways an early romantic reaction to the growing distance of modern humanity from the natural world. It is difficult to deny that in a quite thorough-going manner, the modern attitude towards animals exhibits a dialectical tension, attempting to reconcile moral sensitivities with material and social requirements. Yet one should remember in this context that the underlying anthropocentrism of Western cosmology a priori limited the extent to which new humanitarian concerns could affect the ethical consideration of animals. The rising modern idea of progress, which emerged during the long eighteenth century, was to a large extent concerned with practical moral improvement. Some of this concern influenced increased sensitivity to animal suffering. Indeed, mitigating the suffering of animals was often viewed as a requirement for improving the world in which human beings lived; it was part of the progress of civilisation in general. Yet modern humanitarianism, as it emerged during the eighteenth century and continues in our own time, is primarily concerned with ameliorating the human condition. When animal welfare conflicts with this overriding anthropocentric outlook, the result is predetermined.

The modern lifestyle, for better and for worse, is built upon the human utilisation of nature, and especially animals. The cruelty involved no doubt requires very serious consideration. Yet a world without human beings causing suffering to animals regrettably seems at present a matter of wishful thinking. Enlightenment intellectuals, at the historical point of transition between early modern and modern civilisation, exhibited this dialectic. Despite their sensitivity to animal suffering, when human and animal needs collided, they habitually sided with the former. In that respect they were already modern.

Notes

[1] On antiquity, see, for instance, Richard Sorabji, *Animal Minds and Human Morals: The Origins of the Western Debate* (Ithaca: Cornell University Press, 1993); on medieval culture, see Joyce E. Salisbury, *The Beast Within: Animals in the Middle Ages* (New York: Routledge, 1994); on the nineteenth century, see Kathleen Kete, *The Beast in the Boudoir: Petkeeping in Nineteenth-Century Paris* (Berkeley: University of California Press, 1994); Harriet Ritvo, *The Animal Estate: The English and Other Creatures in the Victorian Age* (Cambridge, MA: Harvard University Press, 1987). For the early modern era, in addition to the studies mentioned below, see e.g. George Boas, *The Happy Beast in French Thought of the Seventeenth Century* (New York: Octagon Books, 1966 [1933]); Bruce Boehrer, *Shakespeare Among the Animals: Nature and Society in the Drama of Early Modern England* (New York: Palgrave, 2002).

[2] Henry S. Salt, *Animals' Rights Considered in Relation to Social Progress* (New York: Macmillan, 1894), 3. For other varying emphases of the new eighteenth-century attitude toward animals, see, e.g., Dix Harwood, *Love for Animals and How It Developed in Great Britain* (PhD dissertation, Columbia

University, New York, 1928), 64, 74-75, 126 and passim; Hester Hastings, *Man and Beast in French Thought of the Eighteenth Century* (Baltimore: Johns Hopkins University Press, 1936), 16; John Passmore, 'The Treatment of Animals,' *Journal of the History of Ideas* 36 (1975): 195-218; Luciano Floridi, 'Scepticism and Animal Rationality: the Fortune of Chrysippus' Dog in the History of Western Thought,' *Archiv für Geschichte der Philosophie* 79 (1997): 27-57; Katherine Kerestman, 'Breaking the Shackles of the Great Chain of Being and Liberating Compassion in the Eighteenth Century,' *1650-1850, Ideas, Aesthetics, and Inquiries in the Early Modern Era* 3 (1997): 57-76.

[3] Jeremy Bentham, *An Introduction to the Principles of Morals and Legislation*, ed. J. H. Burns and H. L. A. Hart (London: Athlone Press, 1970), 282-83. On Bentham as a representative figure for late eighteenth-century rising sensitivity to animals, see, e.g., Andreas-Holger Maehle, 'Cruelty and Kindness to the 'Brute Creation': Stability and Change in the Ethics of the Man-Animal Relationship, 1600-1850,' in *Animals and Human Society: Changing Perspectives*, ed. Aubrey Manning and James Serpell (London: Routledge, 1994), 93; Keith Thomas, *Man and the Natural World: Changing Attitudes in England 1500-1800* (Harmondsworth: Penguin, 1984), 176; and even Jacques Derrida, 'The Animal that Therefore I Am (More to Follow),' *Critical Inquiry* 28 (2002): 395-397.

[4] See Jean-Jacques Rousseau, *Discours sur l'origine et les fondemens de l'inégalité parmi les hommes*, in *Oeuvres Complètes*, ed. Bernard Gagnebin and Marcel Raymond, 5 vols. (Paris: Gallimard, 1959-1995), 3: 126. Also see ibid., passim, especially the preface, and various sections of Part I, Notes V, VIII, X, XII. Rousseau also discussed animals in other works; see Nathaniel Wolloch, 'Rousseau and the Love of Animals,' *Philosophy and Literature* 32 (2008); 293-302.

[5] For his theriophily see Michel de Montaigne, 'On Cruelty' and 'An Apology for Raymond Sebond,' in *The Complete Essays*, trans. M. A. Screech (Harmondsworth: Penguin, 1991), 472-88 and 489-683, respectively. For the passage on hunting see Ibid., 480-482.

[6] *Émile, ou de l'éducation*, in Rousseau, *Œuvres*, 4: 644-645.

[7] Erica Fudge, *Brutal Reasoning: Animals, Rationality, and Humanity in Early Modern England* (Ithaca: Cornell University Press, 2006). On the beast-machine theory in general, see Leonora Cohen Rosenfield, *From Beast-Machine to Man-Machine: Animal Soul in French Letters from Descartes to La Mettrie* (New York: Octagon, 1968 [1940]).

[8] Georg Christoph Lichtenberg, *Aphorisms*, trans. R. J. Hollingdale (Harmondsworth: Penguin, 1990), 59. Yet Lichtenberg accepted that humans

were superior to animals. See also Ibid., 24, 31, 34 ('Of all the animals on earth, man is closest to the ape'), 85, 88, 95, 98, 108, 138, 143, 145, 192-193.

[9] See Laurence Sterne, *Tristram Shandy* (London: Everyman's Library, 1964), 82 (Bk. II, ch. 12); see also 116 (III.4), 381-83 (VII.32), 446-47 (IX.6).

[10] For Enlightenment considerations of nature in general, see Nathaniel Wolloch, *History and Nature in the Enlightenment: Praise of the Mastery of Nature in Eighteenth-Century Historical Literature* (Farnham: Ashgate, 2011).

[11] See H. M. Höpfl, 'From Savage to Scotsman: Conjectural History in the Scottish Enlightenment,' *Journal of British Studies* 17 (1978): 19-40; Christopher J. Berry, *Social Theory of the Scottish Enlightenment* (Edinburgh: Edinburgh University Press, 2001), 61-71; Aaron Garrett, 'Anthropology: The 'Original' of Human Nature,' in *The Cambridge Companion to the Scottish Enlightenment*, ed. Alexander Broadie (Cambridge: Cambridge University Press, 2003), 79-93.

[12] See Georges-Louis Leclerc, Comte de Buffon 'Septième et dernière époque. Lorsque la puissance de l'Homme a secondé celle de la Nature,' in *Histoire naturelle, générale et particulière*, 36 vols. (Paris: De l'imprimerie royale, 1749-1789, Supplément 1778), 5: 225-54.

[13] See Clarence J. Glacken, *Traces on the Rhodian Shore: Nature and Culture in Western Thought from Ancient Times to the End of the Eighteenth Century* (Berkeley: University of California Press, 1967), 565-581, 587-591, 655, 663-681, 704-705. See also Jacques Roger, *Buffon: A Life in Natural History*, trans. Sarah Lucille Bonnefoi, ed. L. Pearce Williams (Ithaca: Cornell University Press, 1997), 228-267, 418-421; E. C. Spary, *Utopia's Garden: French Natural History from Old Regime to Revolution* (Chicago: University of Chicago Press, 2000), 99-154.

[14] See 'De la Nature. Première Vue,' in Buffon, *Histoire naturelle* (1764), 12: i-xvi.

[15] On Buffon's attitude toward animals, see, for example, Michèle Duchet, *Anthropologie et Histoire au siècle des lumières: Buffon, Voltaire, Rousseau, Helvétius, Diderot* (Paris: François Maspero, 1971), 235-49; Louise E. Robbins, *Elephant Slaves and Pampered Parrots: Exotic Animals in Eighteenth-Century Paris* (Baltimore: Johns Hopkins University Press, 2002), passim; Diana Donald, *Picturing Animals in Britain, 1750-1850* (New Haven: Yale University Press, 2007), 23, 33, 67, 103, 106, 165-166; Spary, *Utopia's Garden*, 99-117.

[16] 'Les Animaux carnassiers,' in Buffon, *Histoire naturelle* (1758), 7: 3-38, at 4-9, 25-31.

[17] Ibid., 3-4.

---

[18] See Frederick G. Whelan, 'Population and Ideology in the Enlightenment,' *History of Political Thought* 12 (1991): 35-72; Sylvana Tomaselli, 'Moral Philosophy and Population Questions in Eighteenth Century Europe,' *Population and Development Review* 14 Supplement (1988): 7-29; Carol Blum, *Strength in Numbers: Population, Reproduction, and Power in Eighteenth-Century France* (Baltimore: Johns Hopkins University Press, 2002).

[19] 'Discours sur la nature des animaux,' in Buffon, *Histoire naturelle* (1753), 4: 3-110, at 22-23.

[20] Ibid., 40-42: 'Les animaux ont donc comme nous de la douleur & du plaisir; ils ne connoissent pas le bien & le mal, mais ils le sentent: ce qui leur est agréable est bon, ce qui leur est desagréable est mauvais; l'un & l'autre ne sont que des rapports convenables ou contraires à leur nature, à leur organisation.' All translations are my own unless otherwise noted.

[21] Buffon, 'Les Animaux carnassiers', 8-9.

[22] Ibid., 6-7: '[L]es animaux, du moins ceux qui ont des sens, de la chair & du sang, sont des êtres sensibles; comme nous ils sont capables de plaisir & sujets à la douleur. Il y a donc une espèce d'insensibilité cruelle à sacrifier, sans nécessité, ceux surtout qui nous approchent, qui vivent avec nous, & dont le sentiment se réfléchit vers nous en se marquant par les signes de la douleur; car ceux dont la nature est différente de la nôtre, ne peuvent guère nous affecter.'

[23] See Ronald L. Meek, *Social Science and the Ignoble Savage* (Cambridge: Cambridge University Press, 1976); Istvan Hont, 'The Language of Sociability and Commerce: Samuel Pufendorf and the Theoretical Foundations of the Four-Stages Theory,' in *The Languages of Political Theory in Early-Modern Europe*, ed. Anthony Pagden (Cambridge: Cambridge University Press, 1987), 253-276; Berry, *Social Theory*, 93-99; J. G. A. Pocock, *Barbarism and Religion*, 4: *Barbarians, Savages and Empires* (Cambridge: Cambridge University Press, 2005); Roger L. Emerson, 'Conjectural History and Scottish Philosophers,' *Historical Papers / Communications Historiques* 19 (1984): 63-90; Frank Palmeri, 'Conjectural History and the Origins of Sociology,' *Studies in Eighteenth-Century Culture* 37 (2008): 1-21.

[24] See his outline of stadial theory in Adam Smith, *Lectures on Jurisprudence*, ed. R. L. Meek, D. D. Raphael and P. G. Stein (Indianapolis: Liberty Classics, 1982), 14-16, and also 17-20, 459-460. For Smith's stadial theory see also the discussion in J. G. A. Pocock, *Barbarism and Religion*, 2: *Narratives of Civil Government* (Cambridge: Cambridge University Press, 1999), 309-29. Smith often considered animals as property. Among many examples, see in particular Adam Smith, *An Inquiry into the Nature and*

Causes of the Wealth of Nations, edited by R. H. Campbell, A. S. Skinner, and W. B. Todd (Oxford: Clarendon Press, 1979), 1: 235-55.

[25] See Adam Smith, 'Of the External Senses,' in *Essays on Philosophical Subjects*, edited by W. P. D. Wightman, J. C. Bryce and I. S. Ross (Indianapolis: Liberty Classics, 1982), 136. Also see the similar outlook evident in Adam Smith, *The Theory of Moral Sentiments*, ed. Knud Haakonssen (Cambridge: Cambridge University Press, 2002), 110-12.

[26] William Robertson, *The History of America*, 6th edition (London: A. Strahan and T. Cadell, 1792), 2: 216-217.

[27] Ibid., 2: 35-36. For more examples of Robertson's consideration of this issue see Ibid., 1: 171; 2: 122-125; 3: 12, 152-154, 217-218, 311-312.

[28] See Patricia B. Craddock, *Young Edward Gibbon, Gentleman of Letters* (Baltimore: Johns Hopkins University Press, 1982), 132-133.

[29] Edward Gibbon, *Essai sur l'étude de la littérature and An Essay on the Study of Literature* (Dublin: Guillaume Hallhead, 1777 [French edition]); (London: T. Becket and P. A. De Hondt, 1764 [English translation]; reprint London: Routledge and Thoemmes Press, 1994), 80 in the English translation. For the original see the French text at 64-65: 'Je rapelle en frémissant les spectacles sanglans des Romains. Le sage Ciceron les détestoit et les méprisoit. La solitude et le silence l'emportoient de beaucoup chez lui sur ces chefs-d'œuvre de magnificence, d'horreur et de mauvais gout. En effet, se plaire au carnage n'est digne que d'une troupe de sauvages.'

[30] Ibid., 79-82 (in the English edition), 64-66 (in the French edition).

[31] Edward Gibbon, *The History of the Decline and Fall of the Roman Empire*, ed. David Womersley, 3 vols. (Harmondsworth: Penguin, 1995), 3: 154. For the importance of the human control of nature, see, in particular, the famous essay 'General Observations on the Fall of the Roman Empire in the West,' Ibid., 2: 508-516. For more regarding Gibbon's emphasis on the importance of the human use of animals, despite the animal suffering involved, see ibid., 1: 1026-27, 1068-1069. Also see Nathaniel Wolloch, 'Edward Gibbon's Cosmology,' *International Journal of the Classical Tradition* 17 (2010): 165-177.

[32] See in particular Gibbon, *History of the Decline and Fall of the Roman Empire*, 2: 819-20; and 1: 238-39, 996-99, 1027-29; 3: 151-56, 449. See also J. G. A. Pocock, 'Gibbon and the Shepherds: The Stages of Society in the *Decline and Fall*,' *History of European Ideas* 2 (1981): 193-202; Pocock, *Barbarians, Savages and Empires*, passim.

[33] J. Hector St. John de Crèvecoeur, *Letters from an American Farmer and Sketches of Eighteenth-Century America*, ed. Albert E. Stone (Harmondsworth: Penguin, 1981), 51-65.

[34] Ibid., 55. On animal sagacity and other animal qualities, see also Ibid., 61-62, 120, 305-307.
[35] Ibid., 55-56.
[36] Ibid., 56-57.
[37] This seems to be the implication of the passages in Ibid., 418-19.
[38] See the remarks in, respectively, Ibid., 244-49, 295, 301. Also see 398, and for further appreciation of bees, 55-56, 315.
[39] Ibid., 301.
[40] Ibid., 294.
[41] Ibid., 292-94.
[42] Ibid., 163-64.
[43] Ibid., 61. For uncritical mentions of hunting see also Ibid., 92-93, 286. For more regarding Crèvecoeur's views on hunting see Gay Wilson Allen and Roger Asselineau, *St. John de Crèvecoeur: The Life of an American Farmer* (New York: Viking, 1987), 41-45. On his attitude toward animals, see also Thomas Philbrick, *St. John de Crèvecoeur* (New York: Twayne, 1970), 97-106.
[44] For detailed discussions of the connection between anthropocentrism and philo-sophical considerations of animals, see Gary Steiner, *Anthropocentrism and Its Discontents: The Moral Status of Animals in the History of Western Philosophy* (Pittsburgh: University of Pittsburgh Press, 2005); and Nathaniel Wolloch, *Subjugated Animals: Animals and Anthropocentrism in Early Modern European Culture* (Amherst: Humanity Books, 2006).
[45] Lynn White, Jr., 'The Historical Roots of our Ecological Crisis,' *Science* 155 (10 March 1967): 1203-1207.
[46] For the combination of the biblical and classical traditions in this context, see Francis Oakley, 'Lovejoy's Unexplored Option,' *Journal of the History of Ideas* 48 (1987): 231-245. For the scientific revolution see Peter Harrison, 'Subduing the Earth: Genesis 1, Early Modern Science, and the Exploitation of Nature,' *Journal of Religion* 79 (1999): 86-109; and Harrison, *The Fall of Man and the Foundations of Science* (Cambridge: Cambridge University Press, 2007).
[47] See Immanuel Kant, *Lectures on Ethics*, trans. Louis Infield (New York: Harper and Row, 1963), 239-241.
[48] See Thomas, *Man and the Natural World*, 303, and generally also 181-191, 300-303. See also D. G. Charlton, *New Images of the Natural in France: A Study in European Cultural History 1750-1800* (Cambridge: Cambridge University Press, 1984), 199-220 and passim.

Bibliography

Allen, Gay Wilson and Roger Asselineau. *St. John de Crèvecoeur: The Life of an American Farmer*. New York: Viking, 1987.

Bentham, Jeremy. *An Introduction to the Principles of Morals and Legislation*. Edited by J. H. Burns and H. L. A. Hart. London: Athlone Press, 1970.

Berry, Christopher J. *Social Theory of the Scottish Enlightenment*. Edinburgh: Edinburgh University Press, 2001.

Blum, Carol. *Strength in Numbers: Population, Reproduction, and Power in Eighteenth-Century France*. Baltimore: Johns Hopkins University Press, 2002.

Boas, George. *The Happy Beast in French Thought of the Seventeenth Century*. New York: Octagon, 1966 [1933].

Boehrer, Bruce. *Shakespeare among the Animals: Nature and Society in the Drama of Early Modern England*. New York: Palgrave, 2002.

Buffon, Georges-Louis Leclerc, Comte de. *Histoire naturelle, générale et particulière*. 36 vols. Paris: De l'imprimerie royale, 1749-1789.

Charlton, D. G. *New Images of the Natural in France: A Study in European Cultural History 1750-1800*. Cambridge: Cambridge University Press, 1984.

Craddock, Patricia B. *Young Edward Gibbon, Gentleman of Letters*. Baltimore: Johns Hopkins University Press, 1982.

Derrida, Jacques. 'The Animal that Therefore I Am (More to Follow).' *Critical Inquiry* 28 (2002): 369-418.

Donald, Diana. *Picturing Animals in Britain, 1750-1850*. New Haven: Yale University Press, 2007.

Duchet, Michèle. *Anthropologie et Histoire au siècle des lumières: Buffon, Voltaire, Rousseau, Helvétius, Diderot*. Paris: François Maspero, 1971.

Emerson, Roger L. 'Conjectural History and Scottish Philosophers.' *Historical Papers / Communications Historiques* 19 (1984): 63-90.

Floridi, Luciano. 'Scepticism and Animal Rationality: the Fortune of Chrysippus' Dog in the History of Western Thought.' *Archiv für Geschichte der Philosophie* 79 (1997): 27-57.

Fudge, Erica. *Brutal Reasoning: Animals, Rationality, and Humanity in Early Modern England.* Ithaca: Cornell University Press, 2006.

Garrett, Aaron. 'Anthropology: the 'Original' of Human Nature.' In *The Cambridge Companion to the Scottish Enlightenment.* Edited by Alexander Broadie, 79-93. Cambridge: Cambridge University Press, 2003.

Gibbon, Edward. *Essai sur l'étude de la littérature and An Essay on the Study of Literature.* Dublin: Guillaume Hallhead, 1777 (French edition); London: T. Becketand P. A. De Hondt, 1764 (English translation); reprint London: Routledge and Thoemmes Press, 1994.

———. *The History of the Decline and Fall of the Roman Empire.* Edited by David Womersley. 3 vols. Harmondsworth: Penguin, 1995 [1776-1788].

Glacken, Clarence J. *Traces on the Rhodian Shore: Nature and Culture in Western Thought from Ancient Times to the End of the Eighteenth Century.* Berkeley: University of California Press, 1967.

Harrison, Peter. *The Fall of Man and the Foundations of Science.* Cambridge: Cambridge University Press, 2007.

———. 'Subduing the Earth: Genesis 1, Early Modern Science, and the Exploitation of Nature.' *Journal of Religion* 79 (1999): 86-109.

Harwood, Dix. *Love for Animals and How It Developed in Great Britain.* PhD dissertation, Columbia University, New York, 1928.

Hastings, Hester. *Man and Beast in French Thought of the Eighteenth Century.* Baltimore: Johns Hopkins Press, 1936.

Hont, Istvan. 'The Language of Sociability and Commerce: Samuel Pufendorf and the Theoretical Foundations of the Four-Stages Theory.' In *The Languages of Political Theory in Early-Modern Europe*. Edited by Anthony Pagden, 253-76. Cambridge: Cambridge University Press, 1987.

Höpfl, H. M. 'From Savage to Scotsman: Conjectural History in the Scottish Enlightenment.' *Journal of British Studies* 17 (1978): 19-40.

Kant, Immanuel. *Lectures on Ethics*. Translated by Louis Infield. New York: Harper and Row, 1963.

Kerestman, Katherine. 'Breaking the Shackles of the Great Chain of Being and Liberating Compassion in the Eighteenth Century.' *1650-1850, Ideas, Aesthetics, and Inquiries in the Early Modern Era* 3 (1997): 57-76.

Kete, Kathleen. *The Beast in the Boudoir: Petkeeping in Nineteenth-Century Paris*. Berkeley: University of California Press, 1994.

Lichtenberg, Georg Christoph. *Aphorisms*. Translated by R. J. Hollingdale. Harmondsworth: Penguin, 1990.

Maehle, Andreas-Holger. 'Cruelty and Kindness to the 'Brute Creation': Stability and Change in the Ethics of the Man-Animal Relationship, 1600-1850.' In *Animals and Human Society: Changing Perspectives*. Edited by Aubrey Manning and James Serpell, 81-105. London: Routledge, 1994.

Meek, Ronald L. *Social Science and the Ignoble Savage*. Cambridge: Cambridge University Press, 1976.

Montaigne, Michel de. *The Complete Essays*. Translated by M. A. Screech. Harmondsworth: Penguin, 1991.

Oakley, Francis. 'Lovejoy's Unexplored Option.' *Journal of the History of Ideas* 48 (1987): 231-45.

Palmeri, Frank. 'Conjectural History and the Origins of Sociology.' *Studies in Eighteenth-Century Culture* 37 (2008): 1-21.

Passmore, John. 'The Treatment of Animals.' *Journal of the History of Ideas* 36 (1975): 195-218.

Philbrick, Thomas. *St. John de Crevecoeur*. New York: Twayne, 1970.

Pocock, J. G. A. *Barbarism and Religion*, vol. 2: *Narratives of Civil Government*. Cambridge: Cambridge University Press, 1999.

———. *Barbarism and Religion*, vol. 4: *Barbarians, Savages and Empires*. Cambridge: Cambridge University Press, 2005.

———. 'Gibbon and the Shepherds: the Stages of Society in the *Decline and Fall*.' *History of European Ideas* 2 (1981): 193-202.

Ritvo, Harriet. *The Animal Estate: The English and Other Creatures in the Victorian Age*. Cambridge, MA: Harvard University Press, 1987.

Robbins, Louise E. *Elephant Slaves and Pampered Parrots: Exotic Animals in Eighteenth-Century Paris*. Baltimore: Johns Hopkins University Press, 2002.

Robertson, William. *The History of America*. 6th edition, 3 vols. London: A. Strahan and T. Cadell, 1792.

Roger, Jacques. *Buffon: A Life in Natural History*. Translated by Sarah Lucille Bonnefoi. Edited by L. Pearce Williams. Ithaca: Cornell University Press, 1997.

Rosenfield, Leonora Cohen. *From Beast-Machine to Man-Machine: Animal Soul in French Letters from Descartes to La Mettrie*. New York: Octagon, 1968 [1940].

Rousseau, Jean-Jacques. *Oeuvres Complètes*. Edited by Bernard Gagnebin and Marcel Raymond. 5 vols. Paris: Éditions Gallimard, 1959-1995.

St. John de Crèvecoeur, J. Hector. *Letters from an American Farmer and Sketches of Eighteenth-Century America*. Edited by Albert E. Stone. Harmondsworth: Penguin, 1981.

Salisbury, Joyce E. *The Beast Within: Animals in the Middle Ages*. New York: Routledge, 1994.

Salt, Henry S. *Animals' Rights Considered in Relation to Social Progress*. New York: Macmillan, 1894.

Smith, Adam. *An Inquiry into the Nature and Causes of the Wealth of Nations*. Edited by R. H. Campbell, A. S. Skinner, and W. B. Todd. 2 vols. Oxford: Clarendon Press, 1979 [1776].

———. *Essays on Philosophical Subjects*. Edited by W. P. D. Wightman, J. C. Bryce and I. S. Ross. Indianapolis: Liberty Classics, 1982 [1795].

———. *Lectures on Jurisprudence*. Edited by R. L. Meek, D. D. Raphael, and P. G. Stein. Indianapolis: Liberty Classics, 1982.

———. *The Theory of Moral Sentiments*. Edited by Knud Haakonssen. Cambridge: Cambridge University Press, 2002 (1759).

Sorabji, Richard. *Animal Minds and Human Morals: The Origins of the Western Debate*. Ithaca: Cornell University Press, 1993.

Spary, E. C. *Utopia's Garden: French Natural History from Old Regime to Revolution*. Chicago: University of Chicago Press, 2000.

Steiner, Gary. *Anthropocentrism and Its Discontents: The Moral Status of Animals in the History of Western Philosophy*. Pittsburgh: University of Pittsburgh Press, 2005.

Sterne, Laurence. *Tristram Shandy*. London: Everyman's Library, 1964.

Thomas, Keith. *Man and the Natural World: Changing Attitudes in England 1500-1800*. Harmondsworth: Penguin, 1984.

Tomaselli, Sylvana. 'Moral Philosophy and Population Questions in Eighteenth Century Europe.' *Population and Development Review* 14 Supplement (1988): 7-29.

Whelan, Frederick G. 'Population and Ideology in the Enlightenment.' *History of Political Thought* 12 (1991): 35-72.

White, Lynn, Jr. 'The Historical Roots of our Ecological Crisis.' *Science* 155 (10 March 1967): 1203-207.

Wolloch, Nathaniel. 'Edward Gibbon's Cosmology.' *International Journal of the Classical Tradition* 17 (2010): 165-77.

———. *History and Nature in the Enlightenment: Praise of the Mastery of Nature in Eighteenth-Century Historical Literature*. Farnham: Ashgate, 2011.

———. 'Rousseau and the Love of Animals.' *Philosophy and Literature* 32 (2008): 293-302.

———. *Subjugated Animals: Animals and Anthropocentrism in Early Modern European Culture*. Amherst: Humanity Books, 2006.

Part III

DECODINGS

Visceral Pleasures and Pains

Otniel E. Dror

Abstract
The chapter deals with the nineteenth-century scientific view of the direct connection between affect and visceral-physiological processes. At the point in the history of science when the visceral basis for emotions attracted sustained attention of the medical community, the borderline between physical and emotional pain practically collapsed. The discourse on the physiology of emotions not only contributed to the expansion of the field of emotions beyond its existing vocabulary but also transformed the concept of the viscera: numerous processes on the visceral level were henceforth re-interpreted in terms of emotions. One of the consequences of this development was the physiologists' marginalisation of the spoken word, the overt gesture, and other exteriorisations of feeling.

Key Words: Viscera, pleasure, physiology, emotions, gestures, history of pain, nineteenth-century science.

*****

1. Visceral Emotions

> We have seen that the physical embodiment of feelings varies, in all probability, to as great an extent as their proper mental tone varies; so that if the diffusive action were on all occasions capable of being traced by an observer, the states of an individual mind would express themselves as variously as they are felt. No such power of tracing the physical outgoing of an emotional wave is possessed by us.[1]

> all our emotions we express by physiological processes . . . fear by heart palpitation; anger by increased heart activity and elevation of blood pressure and a change in carbohydrate metabolism. ... [These] processes belong to our normal life and have no ill effects.[2]

In the 'Test and Questions' section of chapter IX, 'Feeling and Emotion,' of *Business Psychology*, Hugo Münsterberg, a Harvard psychologist, posed a series of questions regarding the relationships between 'pleasure feeling' and 'work.' One subset of queries interrogated the relationships between the body proper and emotions: 'How does the body itself respond to feelings?' What are 'the bodily reactions of a businessman who has just received joyful news'?[3] These particular questions, which focused on the businessman and his body, shifted the reader's attention from the more traditional concerns of hedonism with agency, the springs of action, motivation, and conation, to the internal-*visceral* workings of the physiology of pleasure.

Traditionally, hedonistic theories—of a Jeremy Bentham (Utilitarianism) or a W. Stanley Jevons (Neoclassical economics)—approached pleasure and pain not from the visceral perspective but in the context of agency and (the springs of) action. Physiologists and psychophysiologists, in contrast, studied hedonism on the visceral plane and in the *milieu intérieur*.[4] Though their motivations and their theories of visceral hedonism differed, they all shared in this innards-looking perspective on pleasure and pain, and they all provided a variety of mechanistic, dynamogenic, teleological or Darwinian interpretations of the relationships between visceral processes and the experiences of pleasure and pain.

Here I interrogate this shift to the viscera and to the internal *habitus* of the body during the late nineteenth and early twentieth century.[5] The shift to the viscera presented and signified a fundamental transformation in the identity, possibilities and realms of the emotions. Physiologists of emotions construed a realm of emotions which were invisible to the naked eye and unperceived by the feeling subject, but were evident in visceral response. These sometimes unperceived but ubiquitous emotions—i.e., visceral actions that *were* emotions—greatly expanded the realms, presence and reach of the emotions. The new visceral emotions sometimes overlapped with, sometimes opposed and sometimes simply marginalised psychological-experiential notions and conceptions of emotions.

I begin with a brief overview of the multiple meanings and possibilities of the shift to the viscera and the embodiment of emotions. I then indicate that the turn to the viscera in the study of emotions drew on the history of the study of pain. In the remainder of the chapter, I examine three salient aspects of the turn to the viscera in the study of emotions—the scientification of emotions, the logic of visceral affect and exteriorisation. Since my major objective is to present an overview of the shift to the viscera, my approach is analytical rather than contextual.

2. Visceralisation: Embodiment

Physiological study of emotions during the late nineteenth and early twentieth centuries was one of embodied-visceral reactions.[6] Though physiologists of emotions were centrally concerned with experience, experience was not the material that they directly worked with on a day-today basis. They worked with blood flows, contracting and dilating viscera, urine, sweat, saliva, blood—with the body and its materiality. Visceral substrata were the materials that they observed, touched, measured, recorded and ultimately wrote about.

Physiologists observed a variety of embodied patterns that were written in the language of the material elements of the body and interpreted them in terms of emotions. A particular blood pressure curve, a unique pattern of gastric or rectal contractions, or a specific change in metabolic rate or cardiac function was read in terms of an emotion. Visceral emotions were no longer defined or identified in terms of subjective experience, overt gesture, facial expression or verbal report, but were recognised in and through the viscera. These visceral emotions were not un-conscious or sub-conscious; they were expressions of emerging visceral-*physiological* identities for emotions.

The visceralisation-embodiment of emotions introduced new possibilities for theorizing, arranging and studying the emotions. One novel discussion, which emerged from and drew on the shift to the body, pertained to the historicity of emotions. Were emotions universal and 'timeless,' or was 'the form they take at any time … historical, restricted and limited in specific ways,' as Bertolt Brecht believed.[7] Did the experience of emotions change over historical time, as their physiological-visceral substratum and embodiment shifted or evolved?

Alexander Bain (1859) had presented the historicising implications of embodiment for a true history of feelings. Since 'the conventions of civilised man' inflected the natural biological expressions of the instincts, they changed the 'allocation of the members that receive the recoil of the state of mental exhilaration' and altered 'the character of the consciousness.'[8] The history of human conventions and manners—or, to borrow Marcel Mauss's term, the history of 'body techniques'—necessarily implicated and created a history of feelings. Other nineteenth-century theorists, like Charles Darwin and William James, adopted similar approaches. Mental experience and bodily expressions of emotions were mutually constitutive and had evolved over phylogenetic and/or social time.

The shift to the viscera also signified a shift from a focus on coarser emotions, which were favoured by observers of emotions from Aristotle to Darwin—since they were clearly and overtly observable—to a focus on subtle emotions, which were devoid of overt and unmistakable expressions. It signified an expansion of the purview of science to encompass all those emotions which had no outlet in action or expression.

This expansion of the realm of emotions by the new physiology implicitly presented an image of science as the epitome of 'sensibility.' The scientific men of the laboratory detected 'microscopic changes' that signified the presence of heretofore invisible and unrecognised emotions.[9] These microscopic changes included infinitesimal changes in second-order heart rate, ephemeral shifts in blood flow to the viscera or brain, minute fluctuations in the production of sweat and more. The most ardent representatives and the most radical instantiations of the culture of sensibility were not to be found in sensitive women or men of feelings, but in the new science of emotions.

Hand-in-hand with this expansion in emotions, the visceralisation-embodiment of emotions also signalled a contraction in studied emotions. Many emotions were excluded from the purview of the new science of emotions, since they lacked a visceral identity. One such emotion was love. In contrast to the rich and varied physiologies of love in tales, myths, and archaic knowledge—going back to Erisistratus and Boccaccio—modern *experimental* physiology of the emotions did not study love in any significant sense of the term.

Charles Darwin had already argued in *The Expression of the Emotions* (1872) that love had no 'proper or peculiar means of expression' and was therefore an unsuitable object for his study on the expressions of the emotions: 'Love, though one of the strongest emotions of which the mind is capable, can hardly be said to have any proper or peculiar means of expression; and this is intelligible, as it has not habitually led to any special line of action.'[10] There was no real 'expression' of love that paralleled the numerous expressions of the varied emotions that Darwin studied in *The Expression of the Emotions*.

This absence did not signify that love was left out of nineteenth-century discussions, but it was not studied inside the laboratory as blush, erection, tears, jealousy, fear or anger, i.e., as a physiological object of knowledge.[11] What was the fate of such emotions from the perspective of a science that strove to physiologise and naturalise human experience? Darwin did not offer an alternative solution or strategy.

3. The Visceral Physiology of Pain

The turn to the viscera in the study of emotions and the construction of visceral emotions partly drew on and grew out of the physiology of pain. Nineteenth-century physiologists studying pain presented a visceral model of pain, which functioned as a template that framed visceral emotions. During the mid-1850s, the French physiologists François Magendie and Claude Bernard had already observed that imperceptible excitations of *sensory* nerves influenced the actions of the heart, though the animal itself did not manifest any sign of experiencing pain.[12] Their observations and those of numerous other physiologists constituted and framed a realm of 'pain' phenomena that was defined by and visible only in terms of the viscera. These pains were not felt or experienced by the subject or animal. They were physiological pains, defined and identified in terms of physiological reactions to sensory stimulation.

Physiological pain introduced a category of non-felt and non-perceived pain that was registered physiologically in response to the stimulation of sensory nerves. This physiological reflex reaction of the body to potentially damaging stimuli was clearly distinct and distinguished from the psychologically felt experience of *physical* pain. The former was independent of and could take place without the latter.

The genealogy and history of this physiology-type pain harked back to the eighteenth century. In the early nineteenth century Xavier Bichat, the renowned French physiologist, presented a discrete physiology of pain, which was visible in terms of visceral response. For Bichat, the viscera and their physiology of pain defined, identified and authenticated pain. The truth and reality of pain was visceral. 'Voulez-vous savoir si une douleur est feinte?' Bichat observed, 'explorez le pouls.'[13]

For Bichat, true pain was visible in visceral response. If pain had originally been the quintessential technology of extracting truth from bodies, Bichat's concerns focused on the authentication of the authenticator. The truth of pain, of its presence, Bichat suggested, resided in visceral response. Rather than identifying and defining the truth of pain in verbal locution or in overt bodily expressions or gestures of pain, Bichat presented a visceral-physiological response as the ultimate indication that pain was indeed present and not feigned.[14]

These preliminary distinctions in the study of pain would be explicitly conceptualised and articulated in terms of Charles Scott Sherrington's notion of the 'nociceptive.'[15] This was the *physiological* dimension of the reaction to potentially damaging stimuli. It presented a pain that was distinct from felt pain.[16]

4. Scientifying Emotions

Physiologists who studied visceral emotions drew on the templates and practises of the physiology of pain. Like physiologists of pain, they changed overtly observable and naturally readable experiences into unobservables, in order to remake them observable only in terms of the viscera and through the mediation of new scientific technologies and practices. In introducing their new emotions, physiologists of the emotions critiqued a variety of alternative modes of speaking, seeing and knowing emotions. They critiqued the innate and natural—i.e., lay—ability to recognise emotions. They rejected language, facial expressions and gestures as indicators or media for conveying and knowing emotions. And they argued that only non-emotionally affected scientists could properly observe disturbing emotions; only trained and self-composed scientists could register emotions.

In rejecting non-visceral modes of knowing emotions, investigators emphasised the limitations and drawbacks of studying only 'superficial' facial expressions. Even Charles Darwin, whose analysis of emotions depended on facial expressions, explained that subjects tended to inhibit the natural and overt expressions of emotions and thereby skewed his observations on the expressions of emotions. Darwin also lamented his failure to capture certain expressions of emotions—'I have been trying to get a London Photographer to make me one of a young baby screaming or crying badly; but I fear he will not succeed. ... I presume it will be hopeless, from constant movement, to get an insane person photographed, whilst crying bitterly'; he also mentioned the 'difficulty' of photographing 'shaky subjects.'[17] Angelo Mosso, the Italian physiologist of emotions, also complained that (civilised) subjects deliberately 'subdue[d] the reflex movements' and skewed his observations on facial expressions of pain.[18]

Physiologists also criticised the approach which assumed that everyone had a natural and innate ability to study expressions of emotions. They made emotions unobservable to all but the expert scientific investigator. Charles Darwin, for example, modelled the study of facial expressions on the study of natural history. The study of facial expressions, like the study of natural history, demanded expert observers. In his study, Darwin appealed to the special observational skills of the botanist J. Scott of Calcutta, whose 'habit of accurate observation, gained by his botanical studies, has been brought to bear' on Darwin's interest in the expressions of the emotions.[19] Darwin also mobilised the expert observational skills of clinicians, who noted a variety of facial expressions of emotions in their correspondence with Darwin.[20] Darwin's science of emotions depended on 'experts' in order to study the seemingly mundane and natural expressions of emotions.[21]

Duchenne de Boulogne, the renowned French clinician, also targeted non-scientific observers of emotions. In *Mécanisme de la physionomie humaine* (1862), Duchenne faulted some of the great classical artists and sculptors for misrepresenting numerous expressions of emotions. His scientific observations purported to correct these misrepresentations.

In addition to criticising the aptitude and reliability of lay observers, physiologists implicitly indicated that the observation of embodied emotions demanded singular scientific traits. In 1806 Charles Bell, the British physiologist, drew a distinction between the anatomist and the artist in terms of their distinct personalities. 'The mere conviction in the mind of the painter, that anatomy is necessary to the perfection of his science,' Bell explained, 'will seldom be sufficient to insure his application to a very difficult and somewhat of a disgusting study.'[22]

Duchenne de Boulogne presented a parallel argument in respect to emotions. In *Mécanisme de la physionomie humaine* he deliberately omitted his most convincing empirical evidence in respect to emotions, since he feared that his lay readers would be 'disgust[ed]' by his observations on fresh cadavers.[23] The observation of emotions demanded not only a keen scientific eye, but also the professional traits of emotional control and imperturbability. A second and major focus of the criticisms of physiologists who studied visceral emotions was language. In presenting alternative physiological media and technologies for the scientific study of emotions, investigators of emotions criticised diverse aspects of language.

One recurring critique of language targeted the relationships between words and psychological entities. The relationship between actual emotions and words that denoted emotions was regarded as flawed. Thus Alfred Lehmann, the late nineteenth-century Leipzig psychophysiologist rejected the structure that language imposed on the relationships between affects and moods. He pondered whether he should bend language to fit affective entities, or whether he should change the meaning of words to reflect the interrelationships between emotions, affects and moods.[24] Other researchers voiced the same general argument, but instead of asserting that language introduced fictitious distinctions, as Lehmann had argued, they asserted that necessary distinctions were collapsed in language.

Carl Georg Lange presented this latter type of criticism in arguing for his 'vasomotor' theory of emotions, as did William James. There were, Lange explained in referring to the vasomotor apparatus, 'innumerable shades of transition [of emotions], which so far have no name in speech.'[25] Lange criticised common-sense ideas of emotions, and proposed a new classificatory system, which he based on 'natural' physiological patterns.

William James was also critical of the poverty of language. In *The Principles of Psychology* (1890), he presented a general critique of the 'absence of a special vocabulary for subjective facts,' which 'hinders the study of all but the very coarsest of them.' 'Empiricist writers,' he explained,

> are very fond of emphasizing one great set of delusions which language inflicts on the mind. Whenever we have made a word, they say, to denote a certain group of phenomena, we are prone to suppose a substantive entity existing beyond the phenomena, of which the word shall be the name. But the *lack* of a word quite as often leads to the directly opposite error. We are then prone to suppose that no entity can be there; and so we come to overlook phenomena whose existence would be patent to us all, had we only grown up to hear it familiarly recognized in speech. It is hard to focus our attention on the nameless.[26]

Four decades later, John B. Watson practically repeated James' criticism almost verbatim. 'Owing to their concealed nature,' Watson argued in referring to *visceral* actions,

> society cannot get hold of visceral behaviour to lay down rules and regulations for its integration. It follows as a corollary from this that we have no names, no words with which to describe these reactions. They remain unverbalized. ... Because, then, of the fact that we have never verbalized these responses, a good many things happen to us *that we cannot talk about. We have never learned how to talk about them. There are no words for them.*[27]

Despite these critiques, physiologists did not enumerate new emotions, which the viscera and the body revealed to them, but for which they could not find a pre-existent linguistic term. On the one hand, they were critical of the poverty and ineptitude of language to represent emotions; on the other, they refrained from introducing new terms for them.[28]

Duchenne de Boulogne's famous study of facial expressions exemplifies this pervasive tension. His *Mécanisme de la physionomie humaine* explored the mental possibilities of the emotions by studying their possibilities of expression.[29] Duchenne produced a myriad of expressions by irritating the muscles of the face with an electric current. Each and every artificially produced expression was recognised, labelled and categorised by Duchenne in one of three terms: the 'normal,' the 'pathological' and the 'grimace.' The 'grimace' stood for all those expressions that did not immediately call forth a pre-existent emotional term. These expressions were meaningless for him.

Duchenne's system did not leave conceptual space for expressions which might have been manifestations of as yet unnamed emotions. Rather than presenting his science as an opportunity to extend language and/or discover new emotions in the body, Duchenne's study of embodied emotions was circumscribed by pre-existing linguistic referents.[30]

Hand-in-hand with the rejection of existing modes of studying emotions physiologists construed a new genealogy for the new science of emotions. Investigators appealed to a history of great figures who served as sources of inspiration for their own physical-material approach to emotions. Carl Georg Lange (1884) and Duchenne de Boulogne (1862) invoked Newton's colour theory as a model for their own transition from 'subjective' modes of observing emotions, which relied on the experiences of observers, to objective modes, which depended on the physiological attributes of the emotions. Alfred Lehmann (1892) proposed organic chemistry as a template for his new and 'natural' system. Other investigators invoked René Descartes's 1649 *Les Passions de l'âme* as the primary and direct source for their own physical approach. Still others, like the renowned late nineteenth- and early twentieth-century British physiologist Charles Scott Sherrington, regarded the James-Lange-Sergi theory of emotions as presenting 'the extreme antithesis to the spiritualistic conception of emotion.'[31] And still others, like the early twentieth-century psychologist Carney Landis, observed that Charles Bell's 1806 treatise *Anatomy and Philosophy of Expression* was the direct forerunner of Darwin's and James's physiological approach, since Bell had insisted that bodily expression was a basic fact of emotion.

5. The Logic of Visceral Affect

The turn to the viscera presented both continuities and fractures in the logic of affect. On the one hand, investigators often extended the logic of external expressions and gestures of emotions to the innards of the body. On the other hand, the turn to the viscera presented numerous possibilities, which were unavailable, inconceivable or paradoxical from the perspective of the externally observed and studied body or from a psychological perspective.

One major conundrum which preoccupied and baffled investigators and clinicians who studied visceral emotions was the logic of visceral emotions. What were the reasons for the particular effects of specific emotions on specific visceral processes and organs? Or, why did particular visceral processes occur during particular emotional states? Sherrington had expressed this general difficulty and the perplexing logic that undergirded the viscera:

> The instinctive bodily expressions of emotion arose … as attitudes and movements useful to the animal for defence, escape, seizure, embrace, etc. These as survivals have become symbolic for states of mind. Hence an intelligible nexus between the muscular attitude, the pose of feature, etc., and the emotional state of mind. But between action of the viscera and the psychical state the nexus is less obvious.[32]

In making sense of and rationalizing visceral emotions, prominent late nineteenth-century physiologists interpreted the viscera in terms of Darwin's study of the exterior expressions of emotions.[33] Physiologists like Sherrington proposed a variety of evolutionary schemes and models that gave meaning and purpose to visceral functions during emotions. This extension of the logic of 'expression' into the viscera explained the universal and shared patterns of visceral action during emotions. The Darwinian framework was not essential, however, since physiologists who objected to emerging Darwinism, such as the French physiologist Elie de Cyon (1873), also rationalised visceral expressions of emotions by identifying universal patterns of visceral emotions and reading emotions in the viscera.[34]

The extension of the dominant logic of the external body into the viscera was also apparent in the logic of representation. This extension was clearest in the basic representation of pleasure and displeasure. In the physiology of emotions, pleasure and displeasure—i.e., *visceral* pleasure and displeasure—were represented in terms of the opposition between an ascending pleasure curve versus a descending displeasure curve. This basic visceral logic of pleasure and displeasure continued a logic of representation, which, as Oksana Bulgakova has argued in *Factory of Gestures*, can be traced back to Quintilian's *De institutione oratoria*, and appeared in a variety of historical texts, including those of the Munich Jesuit Franziskus Lang, the Berlin pedagogue Johann Jakob Engel, and the method of François Delsarte (up versus down is happy versus sad is pleasure versus displeasure).[35]

In parallel with the continuity in the dominant logic, its extension into the viscera, and its adoption in the representation of visceral feelings, the turn to the viscera presented breaks and significant transformations. Physiologists rearranged the topology of emotions, collapsing what other disciplines and approaches perceived as ostensibly antagonistic emotions. They presented confluence where other perspectives presented antagonisms and vice versa.

Darwin had already noted in passing in his study of the external expressions of the emotions that the heart accelerated in both fear and anger. Late nineteenth-century French scientists A. Binet and J. Courtier dismissed the long-standing identification between fear and pain. The visceral physiology of fear, they asserted in explicitly challenging the dominant view, was discontinuous with the physiology of pain.[36] The intimate associations between pain and fear disappeared on the visceral plane.

Twentieth-century physiologists greatly extended these early visceral possibilities. In contrast to Darwin's passing allusion to fear and anger, they reframed the logic of these two basic emotions. Fear and anger, which were often positioned and sited in opposition to each other—as observed in bodily gesture, in terms of their opposite effects on the behaviour of organisms, and in terms of their mental relationships (anger often eliminated fear)—were strikingly similar, perhaps identical, when observed in terms of their visceral-physiological manifestations. Both fear and anger/rage elicited the same physiological processes inside the body. Their *visceral* logic was identical.

A second major challenge of visceral emotions pertained to the relationships and distinctions between the substantive and affective valence and effect of objects in the world. Charles Féré, the late nineteenth-century

French psychophysiologist, introduced this distinction in discussing the effects of 'bouillon' on the convalescing patient. As Féré explained, it was well known that the administration of bouillon to patients contributed to a speedy convalescence. Since chemical analysis had demonstrated that bouillon contained insignificant amounts of nutritious elements, Féré explained that the positive effects of bouillon reflected the physiology of the pleasure value of bouillon.[37] The healing effect of bouillon was not a matter of an experienced mental pleasure but that of a concrete visceral physiology of pleasure. It was the visceral physiology of pleasure that aided the patient.

Alfred Lehmann, a contemporary of Féré, made these distinctions in terms of laboratory praxis. In *Die Hauptgesetze des menschlichen Gefühlslebens* (1892), Lehmann published a series of experiments on feelings. One of his experiments studied the feelings that were aroused by smoking a cigarette inside the laboratory.

As Lehman explained, the cigarette was the ideal stimulus for resolving a major difficulty in the study of feeling states. It was well known that every laboratory stimulus worked on two different planes: a direct physiological-substantive effect on the body and a physiological-affective effect that depended on its affective quality. The laboratory that studied the psychophysiology of affective states had to distinguish between the physiological changes that were due to the direct physical or toxicological effects of the stimulus and the physiological effects that were due to the affective—pleasure or displeasure—effects of the same stimulus. Smoking a cigarette was an *experimentum crucis*, since the same physical stimulus, the cigarette, evoked contradictory affective responses in different individuals—either an acute pleasure or an acute displeasure. By comparing the physiological response of subjects who savoured cigarettes to the physiological response of subjects who were disgusted by them, Lehmann isolated the physiology of the affective experiences of pleasantness and unpleasantness. The cigarette was a perfect stimulus for a science that construed a distinction between the substantive and the experiential-affective physiologies of a given stimulus, i.e., between the physiology of the pleasure of tobacco and the physiological-chemical effects of the tobacco itself.[38]

Féré's and Lehman's studies underlined and exemplified the continuous tensions and paradoxes of the new visceral emotions. On the one hand, investigators turned their attention from mental experience to visceral emotions. On the other hand, these same investigators conceived the physiological actions of the body in terms of psychological categories, like pleasure and displeasure, and they privileged these psychological categories over mechanistic-biological-chemical forces in explaining observed physiological processes. Thus, the pleasure in food was privileged over the nutritional value of this same food in explaining the physiological effects of 'food' inside the body.

6. Exteriorisation

The turn to the viscera created new venues through which the body came into contact with or opened to the world. It was no longer only the bowels, mouth and genitalia—'the sites of evacuation, consumption and its sites of pleasure'—that were thresholds to the world, but the entire body was now a threshold.[39] Physiologists collected and archived these visceral patterns and functions and interpreted them in terms of emotions.

The conspicuous presence of the viscera on the surface of the body became a source of critical tensions. Various late nineteenth- and early twentieth-century investigators of emotions, among them E. W. Scripture, A. Mosso, C. H. Sherringon, W. B. Cannon, C. Darrow, and C. Ruckmick, expressed the tensions that inhered in a science that depicted emotions—even the most sublime and subtle ones—in terms of the body's innards and/or its pollutions. As E. W. Scripture explained in 1908, 'some people have objected to the sweat glands being dignified into organs of the emotions. But dignity does not exist for science.'[40] Chester Darrow, future head of the Society for Psychophysiological Research and member of the Institute of Juvenile Research in Chicago, diffused these tensions during the interwar years when he discovered that the more ideational emotions did not perturb the body as much as the sensory ones. Or as reported by Christian Ruckmick of the University of Iowa (1930), the 'higher emotions or sentiments' had different galvanic behaviours and rules when compared to 'primitive emotions.'[41]

This exteriorisation can be read in terms of a rigidly Foucauldian framework. The registration and study of visceral emotions would then be seen 'as an instrument by which the body is enlisted in the production of legibility in order to serve at surveillance's creation of domesticable bodies.'[42] The increased legibility of the body worked to augment demands for self-discipline. No longer limited to external gestures, the new subject disciplined the interior body. Increased legibility led inexorably to new modes of visceral self-discipline, which went hand-in-hand with the increased demand for interior self-control.[43]

Were the new demands for and new practices of visceral self-control akin to the etiquette literature of the period, which prescribed increased bodily control of overt gestures and manners? Was attention to the manners of the viscera, i.e., putting on a visceral mask and controlling one's viscera, simply an extension of 'manners' into the interiority of the body? Was it akin to putting on a disguise in the post-Rousseau moral and political meaning of inauthenticity? Or was it a return to the ancient notion of masks as transformative—'as makers, not destroyers of true identities,'[44] or an amalgamation of both?

A clear exemplification of the cultural resonance of visceral emotions and of the preoccupation with visceral control and visceral dissimulation emerged with the advent of the lie-detector test during the 1920s. In the lie-detector, the focus on visceral emotions and on the dissimulation of emotions shifted from the external body to the interiority of the viscera. Beating the lie-detector required visceral dissimulation. Feigned and faked emotion was no longer a product of the manipulation of one's overt gesticulations or pose; it was now constituted in terms of the manipulation of one's visceral patterns.

As the *Capital Time* for Dec. 4, 1931, reported, when Mr Stephens 'beat' the lie-detector he explained that the production of 'faked' emotions worked not by dissimulation and mimicry but by changing one's visceral functions and patterns.[45] With the shift of emotions to the viscera, the very meaning of creating, mimicking and dissimulating shifted to the viscera.

John B. Watson's early twentieth-century science of behaviourism offers a similar case in point. Watson's behaviourism was a manifesto for the education of the viscera. Conditioning was a theory and a praxis that introduced manners into the viscera and promoted and projected a reality in which the viscera, like external gestures, would be totally controlled:

> The 'cold sweat' of fear . . . the 'palpitating heart' of the swain or maiden, are more than merely literary expressions; they are bits of genuine observation. I want to develop the thesis later on that society has never been able to get hold of these implicit concealed visceral and glandular reactions of ours, or else it would have schooled them in us, for society has a great propensity for regulating all of our reactions.[46]

Watson's behaviourism and conditioning offered society a totalising technique for 'school[ing]' the viscera qua emotions and the emotions qua viscera.

7. Concluding Remarks

> The viscera are the voice and vocabulary of the emotions.[47]

Visceral emotions and the visceral logic of emotions presented an alternative cosmology of emotions. The visceral perspective challenged externally observed and psychologically felt emotions, in proposing new possibilities for emotions and their inter-relationships.

Rather than reducing the physiology of emotions to the minor role of challenging a supposedly pre-eminent and existing set of categories and distinctions, which privileges literary, medical or psychological conceptions of emotions, we can suggest that physiologists of emotions provided an alternative reading of emotions and of their possibilities. Their physiological emotions broadened the possibilities and presence of emotions.

The history of the physiology of emotions contributed to a history of the viscera. By identifying emotions in the viscera, physiologists not only changed the concept of emotions but they also transformed the viscera. Numerous processes on the visceral level were henceforth re-interpreted in terms of emotions. Visceral emotions reconceived the viscera and indicated an important shift in the modern history of the viscera. Our study of the history of physiological-visceral emotions during the nineteenth century endows the viscera with a true history and provides an initial periodisation for their modern history.

The study of visceral emotions offers two contending interpretations. On the one hand, physiologists marginalised the spoken word, overt gestures and expression of emotions, and the psychologically felt. On the other hand, they greatly expanded the realms and possibilities of emotions by identifying and bringing to light numerous invisible emotions lurking under the skin.

Notes

[1] Alexander Bain, *The Emotions and the Will*, ed. Daniel N. Robinson (London: John W. Parker, 1859), 28.
[2] Franz Alexander, 'Psychological Aspects of Medicine,' (March 10, 1938). F. Alexander to A. Gregg, 3.9.38, folder 46, box 4, Institute for Psychoanalysis, Reports (6), 1938 -1941, 216 A, Series 216, Record Group: 1.1, Projects, Rockefeller Archive Center, Sleepy Hollow, NY.
[3] See Hugo Münsterberg, *Business Psychology* (Chicago: La Salle Extension University, 1924), 134. In this chapter Münsterberg argues that the economic sphere of modern society—manufacture and consumption of goods—depends on the productions of pleasantness in the producer and the customer.
[4] Literally in the internal organs and internal environment of the body.
[5] In theorising the pre-modern body, Gail Kern Paster has proposed 'an internal division within the conception of the bodily habitus.' She distinguishes between 'the ensemble of techniques Mauss writes about as the body's external habitus, its socially and self-perceptible details of address, bearing gesture, bodily behavior' and between an 'equally formable, if not equally visible, internal habitus. This is the enshrouded domain of the body's internal workings.' (Gail Kern Paster, *The Body Embarrassed* [Ithaca: Cornell University Press, 1993], 2-4).
[6] We should thus avoid the penchant of telling the history of the physiology of emotions in terms of our contemporary preoccupations with the *neuro*physiology of emotions and the history of the brain.

[7] Bertolt Brecht, *Brecht on Theater*, trans. John Willett (New York: Hill and Wang, 1964), 145.
[8] Bain, *Emotions and Will*, 14-15.
[9] For 'microscopic changes,' see Hugo Münsterberg, *On the Witness Stand: Essays on Psychology and Crime* (New York: McClure, 1908), 118-19.
[10] Charles Darwin, *The Expression of the Emotions in Man and Animals* (New York: Appleton, 1872), 212-213. Despite Darwin, later Darwinians, like the famous clinician George W. Crile, approached love's physiological expressions from an evolutionary—Spencerian—perspective.
[11] Despite this physiological absence, love did not elude the commentaries of Darwin, Whewell, Mosso, James, Maudsley, and Duchenne, who referred to love in the context of their preoccupations with motherly love, sexual love, and instinctual love, and the distinctions or similarities between them. Darwin, for one, was careful to state that the physiology of motherly love and love between 'opposite sexes' was different. Others begged to differ. Their transgression impoverished the repertoire of emotions. They combined and collapsed what society had defined and experienced as different types of love into the same 'love.' This process of fusing 'different' emotions gained momentum in physiology, as the twentieth century approached. There was also a literature on the maladies of love—which is not the focus of my present study. See *JAMA* 93, no. 17 (1929): 1323, Foreign Letters: 'A Medical Study of Love' which summarises Paul Voivenel's book, *La maladie de l'amour*.
[12] Claude Bernard, 'Sur la physiologie du coeur et ses rapports avec le cerveau,' *Leçons sur les propriétés des tissus vivants*, coll. and ed. M. Émile Alglave (Paris: Germer Baillière, 1866), 458-60.
[13] 'If you wish to know whether a pain is feigned, examine the pulse.' Cited in Théodule Ribot, *Psychologie des sentiments* (Paris: Alcan, 1896), 30.
[14] One cultural context for Bichat's concern with the authenticity of pain was the emerging practice of mesmerism. The absence of pain in the body of the mesmerised subject (woman) was often advanced as proof of the authenticity of mesmerism. Yet how could one authenticate the authenticator and assure that the mesmerised subject was not simply feigning her indifference to pain. Bichat offered one solution—examine the pulse. On this problem during the early nineteenth century, see Thomas Burgess, *The Physiology or Mechanism of Blushing* (London: John Churchill, 1839), 51-52. On mesmerism, see Alison Winter, *Mesmerized: Powers of Mind in Victorian Britain* (Chicago: University of Chicago Press, 1998).
[15] Charles S. Sherrington, *The Integrative Action of the Nervous System* (New Haven: Yale University Press, 1906).

[16] The long history and genealogy of physiological pain harked back to earlier developments. For a comprehensive history of pain, see Roselyne Rey, *The History of Pain*, trans. Louise Elliott Wallace, J. A. Cadden and S. W. Cadden (Cambridge, MA: Harvard University Press, 1995).
[17] Darwin to Crichton-Browne, June 8, 1870, *Evolution: Selected Letters of Charles Darwin, 1860-1870*, ed. Frederick Burkhardt, Samantha Evans and Alison Pearn (Cambridge: Cambridge University Press, 2008), 245; Crichton-Brown to Darwin, April 3, 1871, letter 7658, ibid.; Correspondence Project, Cambridge. In fact, Darwin's book on *The Expression of Emotions* contains various photographs of mimicked facial expressions rather than 'natural' ones.
[18] Angelo Mosso, *Fear*, 5th edition, trans. E. Lough and Frederich Kiesow (London: Longmans and Green, 1896), 201.
[19] Darwin, *The Expression*, 21.
[20] Darwin's appeal to expert observers was only partial: he also relied on the non-expert observations of mothers who observed the expressions of their young children.
[21] There is a tension in Darwin's approach. On the one hand, he argued and demonstrated that various facial expressions were universal; on the other hand, he often appealed to expert witnesses. Thus Darwin distinguished between the innate and natural ability to recognise certain emotions and the expert ability to accurately describe the features of the expression of the emotions.
[22] Charles Bell, *Essays on the Anatomy of Expression in Painting* (London: Murray, 1806), 19.
[23] G. B. Duchenne (de Boulogne), *Mécanisme de la physionomie humaine ou analyse électro-physiologique de l'expression des passions applicable à la pratique des arts plastiques* (Paris: Jules Renouard, 1862), 131-32.
See also Mosso, *Fear*, 201; Lorraine Daston, 'Fear and Loathing of the Imagination in Science,' *Daedalus* 127 (1998): 73-95.
[24] Alfred Lehmann, *Die Hauptgesetze des menschlichen Gefühlslebens* (Leipzig: O. R. Reisland, 1892), 61.
[25] Carl Georg Lange, 'The Emotions: A Psychophysiological Study,' in *The Emotions*, by Carl Georg Lange and William James (Baltimore: Williams & Wilkins, 1922), 80.
[26] William James, *The Principles of Psychology* (New York: Henry Holt, 1890), 195.
[27] John Watson, *Behaviorism* (New York: W. W. Norton, 1930), 166.
[28] Nevertheless, a few did suggest sub-types of existing emotions. In studying physiological parameters, G. Dumas discovered two different types of joy and three different types of sadness; and Binet discovered two different types

of fear. See A. Binet and J. Courtier, 'Influence de la vie émotionnelle sur le coeur, la respiration et la circulation capillaire,' *L'Année psychologique* 3 (1896): 65-126.
[29] The legitimacy of the biology of facial expressions and of their combinations reflected the regularities of combinations and appearances of the experiences of emotions.
[30] Duchenne did argue, however, for the discovery of novel *combinations* of emotions.
[31] Charles S. Sherrington, 'Experiments on the Value of Vascular and Visceral Factors for the Genesis of Emotion,' *Proceedings of the Royal Society of London* 64 (1900): 391; Harvey W. Wiley, 'Pepsin, Pep, and Patience,' *Good House-keeping* 61 (1915): 805-809.
[32] Ibid.
[33] This concern is evident in the research of Angelo Mosso, Michael Foster, Paolo Mantegazza, Charles Scott Sherrington, George W. Crile, and Walter B. Cannon.
[34] See M. E. Cyon, 'Le coeur et le cerveau,' *Revue scientifique de la France et de l'étranger* 21 (1873): 481-89. The rationalisation of visceral emotions often worked by interpreting visceral behaviour in terms of comparable overt gestures. For Cyon's passionate hatred of Darwinism, see Gerald L. Geison, *Michael Foster and the Cambridge School of Physiology: The Scientific Enterprise in Late Victorian Society* (Princeton: Princeton University Press, 1978), 351. This Darwinian-teleological interpretation of visceral 'expressions' was for the most part absent from Darwin's own study of *The Expression of the Emotions*.
[35] Oksana Bulgakova, personal communication.
[36] Binet and Courtier, 'Influence de la vie émotionnelle sur le coeur.'
[37] Ch. Féré, *Sensation et mouvement: Études expérimentales de Psycho-Mécanique* (Paris: Felix Alcan, 1887), 48.
[38] Lehmann, *Hauptgesetze*, 98.
[39] Gail Kern Paster, *Body Embarrassed*, 16.
[40] E. W. Scripture, 'Detection of the Emotions by the Galvanometer,' *Journal of the American Medical Association* 50 (1908): 1164. This was part of a larger shift from Victorian to Modern representations of the body. See Otniel E. Dror, 'Creating the Emotional Body: Confusion, Possibilities and Knowledge,' in *An Emotional History of the United States*, ed. Peter N. Stearns and Jan Lewis (New York: New York University Press, 1998), 174-93; Stephen Kern, *The Culture of Love: Victorians to Moderns* (Cambridge, MA: Harvard University Press, 1992), 92-93; Peter N. Stearns, *American Cool: Constructing a Twentieth-Century Emotional Style* (New York: New York University Press, 1994), 66-67.

[41] Christian A. Ruckmick, 'Emotions in Terms of the Galvanometric Technique,' *British Journal of Psychology* 21 (1930): 149-59.
[42] Mary Ann O'Farrell, *Telling Complexions: The Nineteenth-Century English Novel and the Blush* (Durham: Duke University Press, 1997), 6.
[43] The increased demand for visceral self-control was already apparent during the early twentieth century. During the post-WW II period it became visible in terms of various 'biofeedback' techniques and technologies.
[44] Lorraine Daston and H. Otto Sibum, 'Introduction: Scientific Personae and Their Histories,' *Science in Context* 16 (2003): 3.
[45] Leonarde Keeler, Newspaper clipping: 'Test 3 with lie detector; results are kept secret,' *Capital Time*, 4 December 1931. Notebook, titled: 'Lie Detector Scrap Book, 1932, Property of Leonarde Keeler,' Unmarked Box, Leonarde Keeler Papers, Department of Defense Polygraph Institute, Fort Jackson, SC.
[46] Watson, *Behaviorism*, 165.
[47] J. L. Fetterman, 'The Correlation of Psychic and Somatic Disorders,' *JAMA* 106 (1936): 30.

Bibliography

Alexander, Franz. 'Psychological Aspects of Medicine.' (March 10, 1938). F. Alexander to A. Gregg, 3.9.38, folder 46, box 4, Institute for Psychoanalysis, Reports (6), 1938-1941, 216 A, Series 216, Record Group: 1.1, Projects, Rockefeller Archive Center, Sleepy Hollow, N. Y.

Bain, Alexander. *The Emotions and the Will.* Edited by Daniel N. Robinson. London: John W. Parker, 1859.

Bell, Charles. *Essays on the Anatomy of Expression in Painting.* London: Murray, 1806.

Bernard, Claude. 'Sur la physiologie du coeur et ses rapports avec le cerveau.' In *Leçons sur les propriétés des tissus vivants*, by Claude Bernard. Collated, edited and arranged by M. Émile Alglave, 421-471. Paris: Germer Baillière, 1866.

Binet, A., and J. Courtier. 'Influence de la vie émotionnelle sur le coeur, la respiration et la circulation capillaire.' *L'année psychologique* 3 (1896): 65-126.

Brecht, Bertolt. *Brecht on Theater.* Translated by John Willett. New York: Hill and Wang, 1964.

Burgess, Thomas. *The Physiology or Mechanism of Blushing*. London: John Churchill, 1839.

Cannon, Walter B. *Bodily Changes in Pain, Hunger, Fear, and Rage: An Account of Recent Researches into the Function of Emotional Excitement*. 2nd Edition. New York: Appleton, 1929.

Crichton-Browne, James, to Charles Darwin. 3 April 1871, letter 7658, Darwin Correspondence Project, Cambridge.

Cyon, M. E. 'Le coeur et le cerveau.' *Revue scientifique de la France et de l'étranger* 21 (1873): 481-89.

Darwin, Charles. *Evolution: Selected Letters of Charles Darwin, 1860-1870*. Edited by Frederick Burkhardt, Samantha Evans and Alison Pearn. Cambridge: Cambridge University Press, 2008.

———. *The Expression of the Emotions in Man and Animals*. New York: Appleton, 1872.

Daston, Lorraine. 'Fear and Loathing of the Imagination in Science.' *Daedalus* 127 (1998): 73-95.

Daston, Lorraine and H. Otto Sibum. 'Introduction: Scientific Personae and Their Histories.' *Science in Context* 16 (2003): 1-8.

Dror, Otniel E. 'Creating the Emotional Body: Confusion, Possibilities, and Knowledge.' In *An Emotional History of the United States*, edited by Peter N. Stearns and Jan Lewis, 173-194. New York: New York University Press, 1998.

Duchenne (de Boulogne), G. B. *Mécanisme de la physionomie humaine ou analyse électro-physiologique de l'expression des passions applicable à la pratique des arts plastiques*. Paris: Jules Renouard, 1862.

Féré, Ch. *Sensation et Mouvement: études expérimentales de Psycho-Mécanique*. Paris: Felix Alcan, 1887.

Fetterman, J. L. 'The Correlation of Psychic and Somatic Disorders.' *JAMA* 106 (1936): 26-31.

Geison, Gerald L. *Michael Foster and the Cambridge School of Physiology: The Scientific Enterprise in Late Victorian Society*. Princeton: Princeton University Press, 1978.

JAMA 93 (1929): 1323. Foreign Letters: 'A Medical Study of Love.'

James, William. *The Principles of Psychology*. New York: Henry Holt, 1890.

Keeler, Leonarde. Newspaper clipping: 'Test 3 with lie detector; results are kept secret,' *Capital Time*, 4 December 1931. Notebook, titled: 'Lie Detector Scrap Book, 1932, Property of Leonarde Keeler,' Unmarked Box, Leonarde Keeler Papers, Department of Defense Polygraph Institute, Fort Jackson, SC.

Kern, Stephen. *The Culture of Love: Victorians to Moderns*. Cambridge, MA: Harvard University Press, 1992.

Lange, Carl Georg. 'The Emotions: A Psychophysiological Study.' In *The Emotions*, by Carl Georg Lange and William James, 33-90. Baltimore: Williams & Wilkins, 1922.

Lehmann, Alfred. *Die Hauptgesetze des menschlichen Gefühlslebens*. Leipzig: O. R. Reisland, 1892.

Mosso, Angelo. *Fear*. 5th Edition. Translated by E. Lough and Frederich Kiesow. London: Longmans and Green, 1896.

Münsterberg, Hugo. *Business Psychology*. Chicago: La Salle Extension University, 1924.

———. *On the Witness Stand: Essays on Psychology and Crime*. New York: McClure, 1908.

O'Farrell, Mary Ann. *Telling Complexions: The Nineteenth-Century English Novel and the Blush*. Durham: Duke University Press, 1997.

Paster, Gail Kern. *The Body Embarrassed*. Ithaca: Cornell University Press, 1993.

Rey, Roselyne. *The History of Pain*. Translated by Louise Elliott Wallace, J. A. Cadden and S. W. Cadden. Cambridge, MA: Harvard University Press, 1995.

Ribot, Théodule. *Psychologie des sentiments*. Paris: Alcan, 1896.

Ruckmick, Christian A. 'Emotions in Terms of the Galvanometric Technique.' *British Journal of Psychology* 21 (1930): 149-59.

Scripture, E. W. 'Detection of the Emotions by the Galvanometer.' *Journal of the American Medical Association* 50 (1908): 1164-65.

Sherrington, Charles S. 'Experiments on the Value of Vascular and Visceral Factors for the Genesis of Emotion.' *Proceedings of the Royal Society of London* 64 (1900): 390-403.

———. *The Integrative Action of the Nervous System*. New Haven: Yale University Press, 1906.

Stearns, Peter N. *American Cool: Constructing a Twentieth-Century Emotional Style*. New York: New York University Press, 1994.

Stearns, Peter N., and Jan Lewis, editors. *An Emotional History of the United States*. New York: New York University Press, 1998.

Watson, John. *Behaviorism*. New York: W. W. Norton, 1930.

Wiley, Harvey W. 'Pepsin, Pep, and Patience.' *Good Housekeeping* 61 (1915): 805-09.

Winter, Alison. *Mesmerized: Powers of Mind in Victorian Britain*. Chicago: University of Chicago Press, 1998.

The Code of Pain in Chekhov

Natalia Pervukhina-Kamyshnikova

Abstract
Chekhov's works exhibit a distinctive pattern of references to human suffering that corresponds to his reserve in matters concerning his personal life. Signals of the pain and suffering of his characters represent an understated but identifiable code that allows the audience to interpret the meaning of the characters' muted emotions. Chekhov was especially sensitive to inconspicuous human pain, hushed despair and humiliation of those who were unable to express their grief due to a lack of confidence and of a sense of their own worth. The code emerges as a strand of literary devices, often perceived as incongruities, which signal that we are confronted with the unutterable. This article offers an inventory of discursive elements that occur in disturbing situations and convey unease without naming its reasons.

Key Words: Chekhov, *The Cherry Orchard*, 'St Peter's Day,' discursive incongruities, psychological pain, signals of pain, mistreatment of elderly and dependents, the unutterable.

*****

Anton Chekhov (1860-1904) died of tuberculosis, an illness that ran in his family. It had carried away his cousin when she was twenty-six and his brother Nikolai in 1889, at the age of thirty-one. Chekhov, a trained physician, had diagnosed the disease in the case of his brother, who had moved in with him three years earlier.

The writer himself had had numerous intestinal symptoms since the age of fifteen, and the diagnosis of gastrointestinal tuberculosis was on his medical history. He spat blood for the first time in 1884, and more serious bleeding happened twice a year thereafter. He was undoubtedly aware of the significance of such symptoms but avoided the fatal word in reference to himself even after a massive haemorrhage in 1887, when he was finally diagnosed with advanced lung tuberculosis. Yet he refrained from open discussion of his disease, whether because he knew that it was practically incurable at the time, or because he did not want to trouble his family and friends. Most importantly, however, he wished to protect his privacy (a remarkably general trait of his personality). However, Chekhov's grave illness and his professional understanding of it strongly affected his view of the human condition and consequently his writings.

Chekhov's knowledge about illnesses and suffering, both physical and mental, informed everything that he wrote. 'My knowledge of medicine,' he often said, 'saved me from many mistakes, mistakes that even Tolstoy himself could not avoid.'[1] Here I shall demonstrate that Chekhov's references to physical and emotional pain in his writings are coded - in keeping, as it were, with his muting the signs of his own suffering in his life. Furthermore, he was especially sensitive to understated human pain, hushed despair and humiliation of those who were unable to express their grief due to a lack of confidence and to a damaged sense of their own worth. Financially dependent elderly and single women in a hopeless search for love were among the less articulate characters whose pain Chekhov communicated through a subtle code developed in his writings.

1.

In the twentieth century, Chekhov's achievement as an artist was dismissed by almost all of the best Russian poets, including Anna Akhmatova, Marina Tsvetaeva, Osip Mandelstam and later Joseph Brodsky. The harshly critical comments of these writers, scattered throughout their letters and essays, are based on their perception of Chekhov's works and even of his personality as the ultimate expression of the prosaic world disconnected from, and hostile to, the Romantic and heroic ideals they cherished. Even more importantly, they saw Chekhov's writings as detached from the realm of poetry. There is a kind of ironic injustice in the fact that Chekhov's inconspicuous stylistic innovation in presenting human suffering was not recognized by the very artists who considered their aesthetic sensitivity as at one with their ethical position.[2]

In 1880-1886, the first six years after his move to Moscow from provincial Taganrog, Chekhov combined medical studies with literary work to support his parents and siblings. During that period he wrote more than four hundred short stories and vignettes, which were published in popular humorous journals in Moscow and St. Petersburg. In early 1886, Alexei Suvorin offered him double pay and triple space in the influential conservative newspaper *Novoe Vremia* (*New Times*), which he published. For several years, Chekhov tried to divide his time between medicine, his 'legitimate wife,' and literary fiction, his 'paramour,'[3] as he wrote to Suvorin, who kept trying to persuade him to devote himself entirely to literature. Chekhov could refer to his literary work as of lesser importance because the light subject matter of his short stories and their brevity failed to bring him renown as a first-rate author. When Dmitry Grigorovich, a highly regarded writer of the period, wrote him a letter in which he expressed his admiration for Chekhov's talent, the young author responded with astonished gratitude, partially exaggerated, yet with an important confession:

> If I do have a gift that warrants respect, I must confess . . . that until now I have failed to respect it. I felt I had one, but would consider it insignificant. Purely external factors suffice to cause an organism to treat itself with excessive mistrust and suspicion. . . . In the five years I have spent hanging around newspaper offices, the common view of my literary insignificance has taken hold of me; it has not taken me long to take up the same view of my work, and so it went! . . . I have so far treated my literary work extremely frivolously, casually, to no purpose. I cannot recollect working on a *single* story for more than a day. . . . I wrote my stories the way reporters write up fires: mechanically, only half-consciously, without the least concern for the reader or myself... While writing, I would do my best not to waste on the story at hand images and scenes that I cherished, that Heaven knows why, would put them away and carefully conceal.'[4]

This famous letter is partially responsible for the usual distinction between Chekhov's early short stories and his mature works. This distinction does not take into account that, before Chekhov turned to writing for income, he, still a student in Taganrog, already authored a full-length play *Platonov* (*Bezottsovshchina*, 1878-1980), the manuscript of which was discovered long after his death and which already had many of his trademark themes and characters. The direct evidence that Chekhov was not 'nonchalant' in his early writings is provided by the reminiscences of Dr. Rossolimo, his fellow student at Moscow University: 'When completing a paragraph or a chapter he painstakingly selected words for their sound, as if looking for a way to complete the sentence musically.'[5] The ability to weave his ethical message into the very fabric of his works is also evident in all of his writings.

Literature prevailed over medicine in Chekhov's life by the end of the 1880s. His concern for the calibre of his art had grown. The public and critics wanted him to produce a 'great Russian novel,' which would grant him a place in the hierarchy of talents next to Turgenev or Tolstoy. Chekhov never wrote a classical Russian novel. He was striving for different genre experiments, yet his stories became longer, and his 'painstaking selection of words' to produce a desired effect became even more careful.

The worsening state of his health slowed him down. In the last five years of his life Chekhov wrote only fourteen short stories, among which are such renowned gems as 'About Love' ('O liubvi,' 1898), 'The Lady with a Little Dog' (Dama s sobachkoi,' 1899), 'In the Ravine' ('V ovrage,'1900), and 'The Bishop' ('Arkhierei,' 1902). It was his dramatic works, however, that established his place in the literary canon. His five major plays were written in the same period - *Ivanov* (1887), *The Seagull* (*Chaika*, 1895), *Uncle Vanya* (*Diadia Vania*, 1897), *The Three Sisters* (*Tri sestry*, 1900), and *The Cherry Orchard* (*Vishnevyi sad*, 1904).

Chekhov's works exhibit a distinctive pattern of references to human suffering, similar to his reserve in matters concerning his personal life. In his earlier short stories strange comical details that sometimes accompany the characters' calamities might seem incongruous and excessive, yet in his plays the same pattern appears as a defining element of the idiosyncratic 'Chekhovian mood,' the vague but troubling sense of the profound significance of the ordinary. Chekhov found ways to present the experience of abuse, loneliness, humiliation and other kinds of suffering without directly naming them. Oblique ways of exposing his characters' suffering, perfected in Chekhov's mature works, are recognisable even in his earliest stories. In his later dramatic works the web of minimalistic signals of emotional neglect expands, spreading throughout the plays and creating a distinctive Chekhovian atmosphere.

Chekhov's dramatic method was so unusual that most of his contemporaries drew a determined distinction between his plays and his prose. Leo Tolstoy concluded a long friendly conversation with Chekhov with a provocative statement: he confessed that he hated Chekhov's plays because they were even worse than Shakespeare's, who in Tolstoy's opinion, also wrote badly.[6] Yet the very fact of ranking Chekhov alongside Shakespeare testifies to Tolstoy's understanding of the calibre of Chekhov's dramatic works.

2.

Chekhov's art anticipates Wittgenstein's statement that 'what we cannot speak about we must pass over in silence.'[7] Conversely, Wittgenstein's remark, 'There are, indeed, things that cannot be put into words. *They make themselves manifest.* They are what is mystical,'[8] can be read as an indirect comment on Chekhov's writing.

Indeed, most of Chekhov's works leave the audience disconcerted and bewildered,[9] with a lingering troubling indefinable feeling. The difficulty of defining the source of this hurt gives his art a mystical attraction. Why do slapstick short stories often leave the reader with a certain aftertaste? And why is *The Cherry Orchard*, in which a child drowns, a family nest is ruined, and an old servant is abandoned in a locked up house, full of empty babbling, comic mishaps, and intentionally meaningless discourse, packaged as a comedy?

For Chekhov, pain, like other fundamentally private kinds of experience, should be respected and kept concealed.[10] His characters discover the need for secrecy when they have to hide their deepest and most authentic feelings under the carapace of socially accepted lies and therefore come to believe that other people also hide the most significant truth. In 'The Lady with a Little Dog,' on the way to a tryst with Anna, Gurov takes his little daughter to school and explains to her the weather phenomena while thinking, 'The real inner life of every individual is based on mystery, and perhaps it is partly for that reason that civilized man is so nervously anxious that personal privacy should be respected?'[11] The same thought occurs to the character Peter in an earlier story 'Difficult People' ('Tiazhelye liudi,' 1886): he rushed out of his father's house after an ugly family scene and is walking away with depressing thoughts; however, on seeing a neighbour he bows to her with a broad smile, which is answered in kind. The young man then remembers that this lady is very unhappy in her marriage and that her sons have gone the wrong way: she might have shed many tears over her life, but 'it is probably Nature itself that gave people that capacity to lie, so that they could keep the secrets of their nest even at the most difficult moments of intense stress.'[12] The task of an artist is to register the unseen tears.

3.

In a letter to Olga Knipper, the leading actress in the Moscow Art Theatre and his future wife, Chekhov instructed her on playing Masha (*The Three Sisters*) who is trapped in an unhappy marriage and destined to a doomed love affair:

> Are you acting well, my sweet? And mind now! Don't put on a doleful face, not in any single act. Angry yes, sorrowful no. People who have borne grief in their heart for a long time and are used to it just whistle absentmindedly and often sink into thought. So, on the stage, you get pensive from time to time while people are talking.[13]

Indeed, a prominent feature of Chekhov's work is the nuanced discrepancy between his characters' psychological state and their actions. This striking discrepancy produces the effect of a breakdown of communication. The effects of miscommunication are disastrous in terms of human suffering, and yet they are consistently underplayed. The apparently improbable mannerisms and anecdotic locutions in Chekhov's work were often perceived as a flaw. Even Petr Bitsilli, one of the earliest and most discerning interpreters of Chekhov's art, believed that Chekhov's drama was a regrettable lapse from the artistic standards of his short stories, mainly because of the 'many incongruities which Chekhov let slip in':

> The characters in his plays indulge in melodramatic outpouring of feelings; they argue emotionally about topics from 'progressive articles' using a 'literary' language full

> of complex sentences, which people would ordinarily never use in conversations. The lack of verisimilitude is even more striking and shocking when the characters suddenly switch to everyday, conversational language.[14]

However, Bitsilli insightfully pointed out that 'the mere fact of these inconsistencies' was extremely important.[15] The discursive incongruities resulted, he thought, from the author's miscalculation of the impression such elements would produce on stage.

Nevertheless, it was sensitive readers like Bitsilli who were the first to notice and be disturbed by the inane dialogues of Chekhov's characters and the incongruous elements in his plays, elements that pointed to the essence of Chekhov's genius. Indeed, such 'striking and shocking' incongruities of discourse are often engraved in the readers' and theatre audiences' memory more deeply even than the plot line. The reason for this is that the incongruities signal the specific significance of a situation, or a particularly sensitive moment in a characters' presence on the stage.

In short stories, incongruous details and the distorted speech of the characters play the same role. In his groundbreaking *Chekhov's Poetics*, A. P. Chudakov wrote that details 'presented in their incidental qualities and combinations' have 'an ultimate purpose and reveal the dogma or system of dogmas.'[16] They form an oblique reference to the issues critical to a character. Such a strategy is part and parcel of the elaborate system of concealing the author's personal beliefs and attitudes. The boundary between his inner and outer life that Chekhov so carefully protected found its analogue in the development of a Chekhovian psychological code for presenting the conditions of torment, conflicts and pain.

When Chekhov's works are read in their entirety, the code emerges as a strand of literary devices which signal that we are confronted with the unutterable. For example, a sensitised reader would not be deceived when a Chekhovian character (or, for that matter, the writer himself in his letters) complains of boredom ('in fact, it is boring,' 'let's leave it, it's boring'). Such asides as complaints of boredom, references to pauses, whistling and humming of the characters are part of the code, and as such usually frame and disguise a central compositional feature of the text. For example, in a letter to A. N. Pleshcheev, a fellow writer, Chekhov describes his literary plans, and attempts to discuss some of his most personal and private convictions about life:

> my aim is to kill two birds with one stone: to depict life truthfully and, at the same time, to show how far this life diverges from the norm. I don't know what the norm is, just as none of us knows what it is. We all know what a

> dishonourable action is, but what honour is we don't know. I shall keep myself within the limits which are closest to my heart and which have been tested by people who are stronger and cleverer than I am. These limits are - the absolute freedom of man, freedom from violence, from prejudice, from ignorance, from the Devil, freedom from passions, etc.
> Actually, this is boring. Where are you going this summer?[17]

One can actually construct an inventory of incongruous elements in Chekhov's stories and plays, elements that occur in disturbing situations and that convey unease without naming its cause. Incongruities often signal pain on both sides: the ones who suffer from the mistreatment and aggressive misconduct but also the mindless perpetrators of pain, unable to realise themselves in a more productive and harmless way. Below are some of the most obvious examples.

a. *Funny, 'nonsensical' words*, such as 'tara-ra … bumbia,' 'merlekhlundiia,' and the mock-Latin 'renyxa,' (in Russian it reads as '*chepukha,*' 'nonsense'), all found in the play *The Three Sisters*, prolong the conversation that is troubling for one of the participants. Often, a character who is mostly a commentator on the main characters' monologues or complaints repeats such interjections obsessively. In *The Three Sisters* it is the hapless doctor Chebutykin who responds with 'tara-ra … bumbia' to Irina's emotional monologue: 'But just yesterday something happened, as if some dark mystery now looming over me.'[18] The nonsense of 'Tara-ra … bumbia' not only deflates Irina's pathos but also attracts attention to Chebutykin's failure in life, to his despair. His 'Tara-ra … bumbia' may be considered a trademark of characteristically Chekhovian incongruities.

b. *Malapropisms, would-be 'learned' words*, tend to be used by the characters who emerge as agents of oppression and humiliation. For example, when in the slapstick comical story 'St. Peter's Day' (1882) a pretentious dunce uses the word 'sceptic' instead of the implied 'misanthrope,' his incoherent babbling masks cruelty.

c. *Distorted grammar* enhances the effect of meaninglessness. There are numerous examples of infelicities of speech, from the early short stories to the last play, *The Cherry Orchard*, where the absurd Epikhodov, nicknamed 'Two-and-Twenty Troubles,' declares: 'Abroad everything is in full complexity' or 'I cannot say I approve our climate. I cannot. Our climate cannot promote just right.' Such apparently comical absurdities uttered by a marginal character add to our sense of the loss of meaning in the lives of the protagonists. In one of Chekhov's last stories, 'At Christmas Time' ('Na sviatkakh,' 1900), a letter written for the illiterate old peasants by a village scribe in irrelevant disconnected formulas of a military-service regulation is included in its entirety. The senselessness of such correspondence, produced by an arrogant 'well-fed, lusty fellow, with a coarse snout and a red nape,' is a key to understanding the unutterable feelings of the helpless old parents and their daughter.

d. *Shop-talk and obscure terminology* comically camouflage heart-rending situations. For example, in the story 'A Wedding with a General' ('Svadba s generalom,' 1884), a retired general, unaware of being 'rented' as a guest of honour for a wedding party, entertains the company with his jargon-laden monologue until he learns about his humiliating role. In 'Polinka' (1887), the growth of emotional tension between the haberdashery-shop clerk and the girl with whom he is in love is accompanied by the ever-increasing number of professional terms.

e. *Catch-words and clichés* ('oh, well', 'and all such things', 'yes, well') are used even by articulate people such as Sorin in *The Sea-Gull* or Vershinin in *The Three Sisters* when they are embarrassed and at a loss for words.

f. *Uncontrolled loquacity*, which the protagonist of *Ivanov* calls 'catarrh,' fits of verbal incontinence, afflict the characters when they are uncomfortably over-conscious of their inappropriate behaviour - in, for instance, 'The Duel' ('Duel', 1891) or 'The Story without an Ending' ('Rasskaz bez kontsa,' 1886) .

g. *Inane or insipid language* is usually attributed to vulgar petty tyrants who enjoy their control over dependent people, most often family members, children, or subordinates.

h. *Coarse jokes and vulgar imitation of an accent* foreshadow a gloomy outcome of a conflict. The most famous examples are the so-called humour of Solenyi in *The Three Sisters*: 'homemade wine enhanced with cockroaches,' 'my hands smell like a corpse.' In *Ivanov* Count Shabelsky crudely mimics the Yiddish accent of the ill-fated heroine.

i. *Formulaic platitudes*, the would-be 'noble' verbiage, mask an indifference to the essence of the matter or to the plight of family members. Tyranny in a family is one of the most common scenes of suffering in Chekhov's writings: 'Paterfamilias' ('Otets semeistva,' 1885); 'Good people' ('Khoroshie liudi,' 1886); 'The Duel' (1891); 'At Home' ('V rodnom uglu,' 1897).

j. *Tired and sometimes inaccurate quotations* from familiar texts by Pushkin, Lermontov, Krylov, Turgenev and even Shakespeare (*Hamlet, The Merchant of Venice*) fill in the blanks of conversations and usually signal the falsity and discomfort of the situation for the participants. One of the most poignant examples is in *The Seagull* - Masha's obsessive repetition, at moments of sadness and despair, of a folklore based line '*U lukomorjia dub zelenyj*' ('A green oak by the sea') from Pushkin's poem 'Ruslan and Ludmila' that had become a staple of children's poetry.[19] A similar effect is produced when the characters compulsively quote lines from popular songs and period sayings.

k. *Vapid irrelevancies mark tormenting emotional situations*: the old news reported by Chebutykin, the helpless provider of non-sequiturs, that 'Balzac got married in Berdichev,' is needlessly repeated by Irina in *The Three Sisters*; the same Chebutykin strangely informs the audience about 'Tsytsykar. Here the small-pox is rampant';[20] in *Uncle Vanya,* Astrov notes, *à propos de rien*, that 'It must be bitterly hot in that Africa now.'[21] At the least appropriate moments Gaev of *The Cherry Orchard* resorts to pool-table terminology, e.g., 'Off the white on the right, into the corner pocket! Red ball goes into the middle pocket!' When 'Deeply moved, nearly crying' (according to a stage direction), he mutters, 'The train... The station... Cross in the middle, a white double in the corner...'[22]

l. *Disparaging comments* on one's own just uttered confession of despair and grief deflate its significance. Thus, in *The Seagull* after saying 'I have a feeling as if I were born very long ago; I am dragging my existence with an effort like an endless train... Often I have no wish to live at all,' Masha adds 'It certainly does not matter,' almost replicating Chekhov's abrupt conclusions of self-revealing passages in his letters ('This is boring').[23]

m. *Complaints of boredom* in response to poignant confessions by other characters reveal an acute sense of loneliness and helpless compassion as a background of this exchange. For example, in *Ivanov*, an aging hanger-on, Shabelsky, dreams of a miraculous jackpot which would allow him to go to Paris and spend the rest of his life at his wife's grave, 'thinking and praying.' His words 'My wife is buried in Paris' are followed by a pause and by Anna's line: 'It is terribly boring. Let's play a duet?'

n. *Gestures indicated by stage directions* such as 'whistling,' 'laughing,' 'waving her hands,' are sometimes at odds with the utterances that they accompany. Sorin's words to his self-absorbed and stingy sister, the actress Arkadina, 'you are a generous, noble woman,' are accompanied with the direction 'whistling'; his reference to his own scarcity of means is followed by the stage remark 'laughing.' Painful feeling is swallowed by the gap between the meaning of the words and the semiotics of the gestures. The stage directions are the only clue to the painful feeling underlying Sorin's timorous attempts of appeal to Arkadina's 'generosity.'

o. *Similar to the stage directions,* in the short stories *there are recurrent references to the eating, smoking, or drinking habits* of a character. They may signify a muting of budding emotionality. The most evident examples are that of Masha's snuff-taking in *The Seagull* and Gurov's eating

> water-melon right after the first love scene in 'The Lady with a Little Dog.' In both instances, those characters are destined for powerful love, unrequited in Masha's case and life-transforming in Gurov's.

The inventory of such ostensibly non-functional details could be continued.[24] The most striking among them in Chekhov's plays are the different forms of reticence: pauses, unfinished sentences, disconnected utterances. In the short stories, the narrator often conveys a state of anguish and suffering when he registers the meaningful silence of the characters. If, as a commentator observes, in Wittgenstein's *Philosophical Investigation* 'meaning emerges in blank spaces between paragraphs,'[25] in Chekhov, the mystery of the ineffable looms through a theatrical equivalent of blank spaces.

Chekhov broadened the framework of silence by including in it such apparently uninformative speech gestures as pleonasms, recurring asides, out-of-place giggling, awkward, confused smiles and nonsensical rants. All of those are code signals of the characters' distress, embarrassment, humiliation and anguish. Such signals often indicate the impossibility for a character to find an adequate form of expression for their feelings, yet the reader may learn to recognize these feelings and perhaps more perceptibly than the personages on the stage.

4.

To the confusion of theatre directors, Chekhov subtitled his first and his last stage works, *The Seagull* and *The Cherry Orchard*, 'comedy.' While these plays, along with *The Three Sisters*, have by now taken their place on Parnassus alongside Balzac's *The Human Comedy* and Dante's *Divine Comedy*, theatre-goers and scholars have long attempted to understand the hidden implications of such a puzzling genre attribution for these gloomy works. Yet existential anguish is combined throughout Chekhov's writings with elements of the comedy of manners

In his early medley of short stories, ostensibly humorous, Chekhov plants the same signals of pain, abandonment, discomfort or embarrassment that will develop into a ubiquitous system of conveying the suffering of the characters in his mature plays. From among numerous examples, I shall focus on the motif of the misery of neglected and abused elderly, found in one of Chekhov's earliest stories and in his last play.

Thus the 1881 'St Peter's Day' is a hilarious account of a hunting-trip by a party of rather ineffective hunters. Saint Peter's Day, June 29, was the opening day of the hunting season. The following year, 1882, Chekhov wrote yet another story, in which the same theme is stated explicitly in the title: 'June 29. A Tale of a Hunter Who Never Hits His Target.' In both stories the narrator focuses on various silly mishaps that spoil a hunting trip. The hunters' grotesquely comic behaviour is, however, a thin disguise for their very real cruelty. The combination of the tragic and the comic often manifests itself in an almost macabre way.

In 'St. Peter's Day' a retired captain kills a ground squirrel (*suslik*) with a stone, and a mathematics teacher shoots a skylark. Neither squirrels nor skylarks are useful prey; moreover, the skylark is a bird renowned for the beauty of its song. These killings are brutal and senseless. They are followed by a gross scene of an autopsy performed by the hunters on the dead squirrel:

> The retired captain killed a ground squirrel with a stone.
>
> 'Gentlemen, let's dissect this squirrel!' suggested the clerk for Marshal of the Nobility, Nekrichikhvostov [a name in a Gogolian tradition, meaning 'Mr. Do-Not-Shout-Tail' – N. P.].
>
> The hunters sat down on the grass, got out their pocket-knives, and busied themselves with anatomy.
>
> 'I can't find anything in this squirrel ('ia v etom suslike nichego ne nakhozhu' - There is nothing worthwhile I can find'),' said Nekrichkhvostov, once the squirrel had been cut up into tiny pieces. 'There's not even a heart. But intestines - there's plenty of those. You know what, gentlemen? Let's go to the swamp. What can we kill there?'[26]

'The heart' (*serdtse*) can also mean 'soul' or 'essence.' The 'soul' or 'essence' of nature is what eludes those hunters; they find only a channel for excrement.

All the components of the story, including incongruity between the characters' comical *anti-aptonyms*, converge in a portrait of mankind as a destructive force at odds with the harmony and beauty of nature. Over half of the text of 'Saint Peter's Day' is a record of inane squabbles among the hunters. There is only one participant, Kuzma Bolva, who remains silent throughout the story but whose role is crucial. His age and appearance mirror his name's implied meaning. 'Bolva' derives from the Latin *boletus*, a type of mushroom called in Russian *borovik* or *mokhovik*. In Russian folklore an old man is frequently referred to by the expressions *starik-borovik* (old boletus), *sushenyi grib* (a dry mushroom) , *starichok-mokhovichok* (little old boletus).[27] Chekhov highlights Bolva's old age and physical resemblance to an old mushroom:

> There crept Kuzma Bolva, a commoner from Arkhangelsk, an old man in boots without heels, in *a ginger top-hat*, with a twenty-five pound double-barrel shotgun and *yellowish-green spots on his neck.* … a plebeian, but the gentlemen, out of respect for his advanced years (he was born at the end of the last century) and his ability to hit a twenty-kopeck coin thrown in the air, are not squeamish when it comes to his plebeian origins and take him along on their hunts.[28]

Bolva's fate, at the end of this would-be comical story, is mysterious and terrible. The other hunters, absorbed in their petty quarrels and the excitement of the hunt, forget about the old man and abandon him in the forest:

> 'Gentlemen, where is Bolva?'- exclaimed Mangé. The hunters looked at each other. 'Where is Bolva?' - he repeated.
> 'He must be on that troika. Gentlemen,' cried Egor Egorych. 'Is Bolva with you?'
> 'Not here, not here,' shouted Kardamonov.
> The hunters were perplexed.
> 'Well, to hell with him,' decided the general. 'We can't go back for him.'
> 'We've got to go back, your Excellency. He is awfully weak. He'll die without water. He won't make it.'
> 'If he wants to, he'll make it.'
> 'But the old man will die, he is ninety!'
> 'Nonsense.'[29]

Ultimately, in all of Chekhov's writings the other, more prominent characters reveal their best and worst traits through their treatment of marginal figures. Kuzma Bolva is the first in a series of memorable old men and women in Chekhov's works. Among the others are Firs, the loyal serf in *The Cherry Orchard*, the old nanny Anfisa and the old watchman Ferapont in *The Three Sisters*. In the list of *dramatis personae*, Chekhov provides an age designation 'old man, old woman' only in reference to them; the other characters' ages are not indicated. As if this were not enough, Chekhov is careful to indicate the precise age of those elders: Bolva is ninety years old, Firs is eighty-seven, Anfisa is eighty.

The 'comedy' *Cherry Orchard* ends with Firs, the old and feeble servant, left behind by his masters in the boarded-up house they have sold. He is abandoned not because of anyone's intentional cruelty but due to a chain of blunders:

> *Ania.* Has Firs been taken to the hospital?
> *Iasha.* I told them to this morning. I suppose they've sent him.
> *Anya* (*To Epikhodov, who is passing through the hall).* Semyon Panteleevich, please, check if Firs has been taken to the hospital.
> *Iasha (offended).* I told Egor this morning. What is the use of asking ten times?
> *Epikhodov.* The aged Firs, in my conclusive opinion, is beyond repair. It is time he joined his forefathers. I only envy him. *(Puts a trunk on a hat-box and squashes it.)* Well, of course. I thought so! *(Exit.)*
> *Iasha. (Grinning).* Two-and-twenty troubles.
> *Varia (behind the door).* Has Firs been taken to the hospital?
> *Ania.* Yes.
> *Varia.* Then why didn't they take the letter to the doctor?
> *Ania.* So it should be send later on. *(leaves)*[30]

It is difficult to understand from this conversation who in fact was originally responsible for taking Firs to the hospital. They all *want* to believe that the unpleasant task of placing a faithful family servant in a hospital has already been carried out; they cannot accept their own responsibility for depriving Firs of the only home he has ever known. Firs's words at the conclusion of the play have a particularly tragic ring because a loyal servant and in fact a member of the family blames nobody but himself. His final colloquialism *nedotiopa*, a Russian equivalent of 'a good-for-nothing, worthless, bungler' is a feature of a slapstick comedy, which he addresses to himself; the word, however, sums up all the wasted life of the play's characters and the lost Eden of the Cherry Orchard that its inhabitants let slip away.

> *Firs (goes to the door and touches the handle).* Locked. They've gone. *(Sits on the sofa).* They forgot about me... Never mind... I'll sit here a while. And I reckon Leonid Andreevich didn't put on his fur coat, I'll bet he went off in the light one. *(A worried sigh).* I should have seen to it, these young folk have no sense *(mutters something which cannot be understood).* Life's slipped by somehow, as if I never lived it *(Lies down.)* I'll lie down a while... You've got no strength left, nothing at all, nothing... Yes, you bungler... *(lies motionless).*[31]

It is typical of Chekhov to make a marginal figure convey the most poignant idea of the play.

Characteristically, the outcome of Bolva's predicament is not clarified; we do not know for certain that Bolva will perish in the forest just as we do not know whether Firs is actually supposed to die in the abandoned house. It is the author's silence about further possibilities that leaves us with a sense of the cruel consequences of neglect. The examples of the extreme loneliness of neglected old people may be read as an emblem of the essential loneliness of all: we all ultimately remain alone in face of pain and death.

Thus in Chekhov's 'comedies' the leading characters may wear their hearts on their sleeves and pronounce the most heart-wrenching (ultimately deflated) monologues on their wasted lives, but it is the marginal characters who raise our awareness of the omnipresence of the genuine and unarticulated pain of the human condition.

Notes

[1] Ivan Bunin, *About Chekhov: The Unfinished Symphony* (Evanston: Northwestern University Press, 2007), 5; Richard Carter, 'Anton P. Chekhov, MD (1860-1904): Dual Medical and Literary Careers,' *The Annals of Thoracic Surgery* 61 (1996): 1557-63; Jefferson J. A. G. Gatrall, 'The Paradox of Melancholy Insight: Reading the Medical Subtext in Chekhov's 'A Boring Story,'' in *Bloom's Modern Critical Views: Anton Chekhov* (New York: Chelsea House, 2009), 55-76.

[2] Cf. D. S. Mirsky: 'the self-conscious intellectual elite was always conspicuously cool to him. The highbrows of the beginning of the century even affected to (or sincerely did) despise him.' *A History of Russian Literature from its Beginning to 1900* (New York: Vintage, 1958), 383. See also Lidia Chukovskaia, *Zapiski ob Anne Akhmatovoi* (Paris: YMCA Press), 1: 182-83; 2: 486-87; Osip Mandelstam, 'O piese A. Chekova *Diadia Vania*,' *Sobranie sochinenii* (Ann Arbor: Ardis, 1981), 4: 107-09; Marina Tsvetaeva, 'Pis'ma Mariny Tsvetaevoi,' *Novyi Mir* 4 (1969): 194.

[3] Letter to A. S. Suvorin, September 11, 1888, *Letters* 2: 326. All references are to Anton Chekhov, *Polnoe sobranie sochinenii i pisem* [*Complete Works in 30 vols.*] (Moscow: Nauka, 1973-1988). This publication includes 12 volumes of *Letters*; henceforth abbreviated as *PSSP* and as *Letters*.

[4] March 28, 1886. Letters 1: 216-18.

[5] G. I. Rossolimo, *Chekhov v vospomimnaniiakh sovremennikov* (Moscow: Goslit-izdat, 1952), 499.

[6] George Orwell explains Tolstoy's attack on Shakespeare ('O Sheskpire i o drame,' 1903) by his religious rejection of humanistic values and the aim of his later years 'to narrow the range of human consciousness. One's interests,

one's points of attachment to the physical world and the day-to-day struggle, must be as few and not as many as possible.' 'Lear, Tolstoy and the Fool,' in *All Art is Propaganda* (Orlando: Harcourt: 2008), 325. In the nuanced complexity of Chekhov's plays, Tolstoy probably perceived the similar abundance of life and denial of the simplification (*oproshchenie*) which he sought at that point in his life.

[7] Ludwig Wittgenstein, *Tractatus Logico-Philosophicus* (London: Routledge and Kegan Paul, 1961), 74.

[8] Ibid., 522, 73.

[9] Virginia Woolf wrote about the bewilderment that Chekhov provoked in his readers in 1925 in her essay 'The Russian Point of View,' *Collected Essays* (New York: Harcourt, Brace and World, 1967), 1: 240.

[10] Chekov married Olga Knipper after she agreed to keep the place and the date of their marriage a secret from all friends and family.

[11] Chekhov, *PSSP* 10: 142.

[12] Chekhov, *PSSP* 5: 328.

[13] 2 January 1901. *Letters* 9: 173.

[14] Peter M. Bitsilli, *Chekhov's Art: A Stylistic Analysis* (Ann Arbor: Ardis, 1983), 118.

[15] Ibid., 119-20.

[16] A. P. Chudakov, *Chekhov's Poetics* (Ann Arbor: Ardis, 1983), 205. James Wood expresses a similar understanding: 'Chekhov thinks of detail as a story, and thinks of story as an enigma.' *The Broken Estate: Essays on Literature and Belief* (New York: Random House, 1999), 65.

[17] 9 April 1889, *Letters* 3:186. Interestingly, in many selections from Chekhov's letters, those telling digressions from direct ideological statements are omitted by translators as conventional and insignificant. See *Letters of Anton Chekhov*, ed. Avrahm Yarmolinsky, trans. Bernard G. Guerney and Lynn Solotaroff (New York: Viking, 1973), 114; S. S. Koteliansky and P. Tomlinson, *The Life and Letters of Anton Tchekhov* (New York: Benjamin Bloom, 1965), 154.

[18] Chekhov, *Three Sisters*, act IV. *PSSP* 13: 176.

[19] *PSSP* 13-14: 124, 185.

[20] *PSSP* 13-14: 147-48 (Act II). Cf. a strikingly similar use of the word 'Madagaskar' by Natasha Rostova at a moment of intense anguish in Tolstoy's *War and Peace* (Vol. 2, Part 4, Chapter 9).

[21] *PSSP* 13-14: 114 (Act IV).

[22] *PSSP* 13-14: 252 (Act IV).

[23] Cf. Chekhov's letter to Pleshcheev, note 17 above.

[24] See Natalia Pervukhina, *Anton Chekhov: The Sense and the Nonsense* (New York: Legas, 1993).

[25] Matt Greenfield, 'The Valve. A Literary Organ.' Internet blog posting on 08/16/05. Primitive Language Games, http://www.thevalve.org/go/search/results/ 8b7bca15d832adec05b5c412bee7fe7c/, Viewed on March 5, 2012.
[26] *PSSP* 1: 74.
[27] Cf. in Chekhov's *Notebooks*: 'Only old women live on that street, that's why it's called Mushroom street,' *PSSP* 17: 95. In his discussion of the etymological link between the roots *grib* and *greb* in Russian, Roman Jakobson mentions an 'age-old connection of the whole onomatopoetic set with chthonic imagery, which is quite typical of the Slavic name for a mushroom, *grib*.' Roman Jakobson, 'The Etymology of Grib (E. Sl. fungus, W. Sl. Boletus),' *Selected Writings* 7 (The Hague: Mouton, 1985): 336-37.
[28] *PSSP* 1: 68.
[29] Ibid., 74-75.
[30] *PSSP* 13-14: 246.
[31] Ibid., 253-54.

Bibliography

Bitsilli, Peter M. *Chekhov's Art: A Stylistic Analysis*. Ann Arbor: Ardis, 1983.

Bunin, Ivan. *About Chekhov: The Unfinished Symphony*. Translated by Thomas G. Marullo. Evanston: Northwestern University Press, 2007.

Carter, Richard. 'Anton P. Chekhov, MD (1860-1904): Dual Medical and Literary Careers.' *The Annals of Thoracic Surgery* 61 (1996): 1557-63.

Chekhov, Anton. *Letters of Anton Chekhov*. Selected and edited by Avrahm Yarmolinsky. Translated by Bernard G. Guerney and Lynn Solotaroff. New York: Viking, 1973.

———. *Polnoe sobranie sochinenii i pisem, PSSP* (*Complete Works* in 30 vols; Sochineniia18 vols, Pisma 12vols). Moscow: Nauka, 1973-1988.

Chudakov A. P. *Chekhov's Poetics*. Ann Arbor: Ardis, 1983.

Chukovskaia, Lidia. *Zapiski ob Anne Akhmatovoi*. Paris: YMCA Press, 1976.

Gatrall, Jefferson J. A. 'The Paradox of Melancholy Insight: Reading the Medical Subtext in Chekhov's 'A Boring Story.'' In *Bloom's Modern Critical Reviews: Anton Chekhov*. Edited by Harold Bloom, 55-76. New York: Chelsea House, 2009.

Greenfield, Matt. *The Valve*. A Literary Organ. Internet blog posting on 08/16/05. Primitive Language Games, http://www.thevalve.org/go/search/results/ 8b7bca15d832adec05b5c412bee7fe7c/. Viewed on March 5, 2012.

Jakobson, Roman. 'The Etymology of Grib (E.Sl. fungus, W.Sl. Boletus).' In *Selected Writings*, 7: 336-37. The Hague: Mouton, 1985.

Koteliansky, S. S. and P. Tomlinson. *The Life and Letters of Anton Tchekhov*. New York: Benjamin Bloom, 1965.

Mandelstam, Osip. *Sobranie sochinenii* (*Collected Works*). Ann Arbor: Ardis, 1981.

Mirsky, D. S. *A History of Russian Literature from its Beginning to 1900*. New York: Vintage, 1958.

Orwell, George. 'Lear, Tolstoy and the Fool.' In *All Art is Propaganda*, 316-36. Orlando: Harcourt, 2008.

Pervukhina, Natalia. *Anton Chekhov: The Sense and the Nonsense*. New York: Legas, 1993.

Rossolimo, G. I. *Chekhov v vospominaniiakh sovremennikov*. Moscow: Goslit-izdat, 1952.

Tsvetaeva, Marina. 'Pisma.' *Novyi Mir* 4 (1969): 184-214.

Wittgenstein, Ludwig. *Tractatus Logico-Philosophicus*. London: Routledge and Kegan Paul, 1961.

Wood, James. 'What Chekhov Meant by Life.' *The Broken Estate: Essays on Literature and Belief*. New York: Random House: 1999.

Woolf, Virginia. 'The Russian Point of View.' *The Common Reader*, 243-56. New York: Harcourt, Brace and Company, 1925.

After the Camps: Semantic Shift and the Experience of Pain

Manuela Consonni

Abstract
The Shoah as an historical event transformed the interrogation of the meaning of existence, raising radical questions about pain, death and individual finitude. If hermeneutics aims to define the space of expression, i.e., the semantic field which enables things to exist according to a determinate meaning, it must also open up to possibilities of semantic changes under the influence of new types of experience. In order to trace the changes in the structure of separate members in a semantic field and to map the progression of such changes one must have a critical mass, a number of meaningful events and of recurrences of the word in its new usage. If a word appears in a specific meaning only once, as a kind of *hapax legomenon*, it does not suffice for such a linguistic development. The Being as being towards death in the camps has led to paramount semantic shifts. Such semantic shifts are at the centre of this study and their object is pain. Death is lived through the presence of pain which becomes locus for its articulation. This pain is the multiple experience of an actual physical wound, of the disruption of the harmony of being and of the being's unfitness for the world. It is also a metaphysical anguish that leads one to anticipate one's own death. It is not a philosophical pain of death, nor a cosmic pain in regards to the mortality of the being but the ineffable essence of camp experience. In this experience, the sense of life as being in the world, the Heideggerian *Dasein*, is 'being towards death' in both the figurative and the literal sense. Movement towards death is the shared experience of people in the camps, their shared identity.

Key Words: Auschwitz, death, testimony, epistemology, hermeneutics, language, historical semantics, Primo Levi, Charlotte Delbo, Robert Antelme.

*****

> During the terrible years of the Yezhov terror I spent seventeen months in the prison queues in Leningrad. One day someone 'identified' me. Then a woman with lips blue with cold who was standing behind me, and of course had never heard of my name, came out of the numbness which affected us all and whispered in my ear (we all spoke in whispers there):
>
> 'Could you describe this?'
>
> I said, 'I can!'

> Then something resembling a smile slipped over what had once been her *face*.
> -Anna Akhmatova, 'In Place of an Introduction,' *Poem without a Hero* (1957).

Those among us who deal with the reconstruction of the past regard memory as a central theme and an instrument of analysis for their work. Since the middle of the twentieth century, the importance of memory has gained enhanced emphasis in projects devoted to the memory of the Holocaust and of the Gulag as well as to the memory of post-colonial countries, largely owing to the recognized need of historical-symbolic compensation for the victims.[1] The present paper is motivated by this need, though it is also part of the on-going debate about the limits of representation after Auschwitz.[2]

The knowledge produced by the victims, *pace* Hilberg's 1961 monumental work based on archive and official documents mostly composed by the perpetrators,[3] generates a narrative of their existential experience. This complements the historical narrative by giving us a sense of the Final Solution from inside, at the stages when its implementation was gradual rather than swift. In other words, the content of this knowledge encompasses the enormity of intense protracted personal suffering, suffering that transformed the interrogation of the meaning of existence, of individual finitude, of death; suffering whose records are still impacting this interrogation. [4]A major component of this knowledge, as this paper shows, is the ability to decode shifts in the semantic field of pain.

The texts, 'linguistically charged and humanly meaningful,'[5] written by survivors of concentration and death camps have forged a new language, seeking to improve the narrative model approximating camp experience. The meaning of the event, lived and reconstructed *a posteriori* by the survivors, active agents in producing a critical mass of knowledge and reweaving the threads of history from the standpoint of the victims, demands an investment also from readers, because readers too find themselves implicated, though at a distance in space and time, and are called upon to examine their own attitudes to the realities represented.

Nor do survivors themselves avoid being implicated, at least in a kind of imaginative failure, or be it self-protection, that blinds one to the pain of the degraded body of another. Thus Robert Antelme tells of the first witnessed death of a Buchenwald companion:

> Someone lifted up one side of the tent, and two men holding a blanket by either end came out and placed it on the ground. Something on the blanket came into view. Grey-black skin clinging to bones: his face. Two purple

> sticks protruding from the nightshirt: his legs. He didn't say anything. Two hands rose from the blanket, and the two men each grabbed a hand and pulled; the two sticks were now standing. His back was towards us. He bent forward, and we saw a wide black crack between two bones. A stream of liquid shit shot in our direction. A thousand guys standing there had seen that black crack, the curve of that stream. ... Then he fell. ... The guy lay outside on the blanket. He wasn't moving. His round eyes were open. ... Those who had brought him out of the tent returned. They leaned over him, but they couldn't tell whether he was dead. They pulled gently on the sleeve of the nightshirt; he didn't move. They didn't dare to touch his skin. There was no telling whether he was dead. ... It was from the shit that we'd known he was alive.[6]

The description of this humiliating gratuitous death is similar in substance to that of 'the Somogy thing' in Primo Levi's *If This Is a Man*: a depleted Hungarian Jew is seen as a dummy that crashes on the floor of the barrack with the noisy sound of the 'shameful wreck of skin and bones.'[7]

Yet survivor memoirs also tell us of what it felt like to be thus dehumanized, or driven towards the extreme, whether by deprivation or by active violence. Pain was often caused by 'useless violence,' violence as an end in itself, 'always redundant, always disproportionate,' whose sole purpose was creating pain.[8] Useless violence transformed sealed trains from means of transportation to ambulatory prisons and instruments of death. Useless violence - or perhaps covertly calculated violence - reigned in the ceremony of the spoliation of the body at the arrival and at the periodical selections: standing naked before the SS was already an anticipation of death, 'a naked and barefoot man feels that all his nerves and tendons are severed: he is a helpless prey'; without clothes, he no longer 'perceives himself as a human being. ... He knows that he can be crushed at any moment.'[9] One was condemned not only to die but to die in pain.

Camp experience is one of the causes of what Dan Diner describes as the onset of the 'historical crisis.'[10] With compelling universality, this crisis challenges the assertion of purpose and meaning in the historical process, along with the complacent belief in the intelligent design (the philosophical idea which Alexander Pope captured in the line 'whatever is, is right'). After Primo Levi's *If This Is a Man*, Pope's *Essay on Man* can hardly be quoted without irony.

The Holocaust is the historical event that changed the concept of death as 'the millionfold death has acquired a form never feared before and has taken on a very different nuance.'[11] But the radical semantic shifts in the perception of death have been caused not by the event itself but by the discourse of survivors who could bear witness to this new modality of dying. Death in Auschwitz lacked features of conventional representations of death: it was not odourless, decorated, and ceremonial. It was massive, collective, ugly, and, as Levi said, trivial, bureaucratic, and mundane - unexplained and not relieved by tears. True, there has never been a time in which human death has been understood, considered 'natural,' serenely accepted without fear or apprehension, whatever place it occupied in the social imagination.[12] Yet death is not a phenomenological invariant. As Ariès notes, in the twentieth century the fear of death inflated, and the new collective sensibility that has grown around death has now become the characterizing trait of our epoch.[13] The fear of death has not slackened; death has resisted subjection: it is as if death changed its nature, or another death has been added to the natural one. The kind of dying that took place in the camp destroyed the social and cultural systems in which death was earlier comprehended and dealt with, leaving the individual naked before it. If death is eschewed, extreme experience that may obliterate mnemonic registration does not alter the content of the memory, which, when resurfacing, brings with it the pain of the offence, 'denying the peace to the tormented.'[14]

I shall not enter the debate on the historical uniqueness of the Holocaust, or raise the Holocaust to the rank of metaphysical category with a 'superhistorical' meaning,[15] or resort to functionalist historicisation, that 'methodological retreat into the description of structures.'[16] I see Auschwitz as a paradigm of the kind of death that can be (because it has been) inflicted, and I believe that one should try to approximate an understanding of the human experiential aspect of this paradigm in all its specificity, without objectifying the victims and without allowing 'the banality of the implementation' to spill over to their experience.[17]

Key cultural concepts, such as death, are not fixed and timeless; they are moulded and remoulded by their political and social contexts. The political, social and even geographical contexts of the genocidal extermination help to explain the changes that such contexts have undergone; the narratives of the victims help to decode these changes. The experience of the concentration camps was characterized by constant 'fearful anticipation.'[18] Hannah Arendt emphasises the hopeful uncertainty involved in this state of mind, 'a remarkable and very characteristic uncertainty which impedes both rebellion and any clear articulated understanding of the thing feared.'[19] By contrast, what I discuss in this paper is the content of the anticipation, the knowledge of how details of current deprivation, still part of camp life, signify the beginning of camp death.

According to Reinhart Koselleck, language and the concrete socio-political situation do not coincide with the way they are 'available or comprehensible' to the speaking subjects themselves.[20] If a group is empirically formed on the basis of

> command or consent, of contract or propaganda, of necessity or kinship, concepts are needed in order for the group to recognize and define itself. Through the shared experience and its linguistic recognition, the group can present itself and rewrite itself as a functioning and active agency in creating a 'new discourse' on the epistemic level of the event and on the ethical one. Therefore the concept is not merely a sign for, but also a factor in political or social groupings.[21]

Despite developments in the inner structure of concepts, in each historical period the semantic area covered by a lexical unit is in tension with the repetition of this unit, and the latter lags behind change.[22] The grids of experience are replicable and recyclable but spaces of experience move and open new semantic horizons. Linguistic possibilities are developed or disappear, old meanings become fuzzier or are 'enriched.' Kosseleck notes the 'methodological antinomy' that prevails between the linguistic figures of historical singularity and structural iterability: history is

> never identical with its linguistic registration and formulated experience, whether this is expressed orally or in writing, but at the same time, it is not independent of these linguistic articulations. Our counterconcepts then prove the iterability, as well as the novelty, of the situations they refer to.[23]

The perspective of the victims, the linguistic self-registration of their experience, reveals both the structural iterability of their suffering and its language and the novelty of its concrete forms.

Holocaust concentration camps have added words to dictionaries. They have built a new semantic field that includes such words as *Selektia*, *Rampa*, *Muselmann*, *Capo*, *Stuck*, *Prominenten*, etc., and, with the help of survivor texts, idioms like 'Hier ist kein warum.' But they have also expanded the semantic structure of separate words - semantic structure as a combination of the denotation and the multiple connotations of a word. The shift in question is the way in which the semantic structure of apparently neutral words or concepts, words that are widely used in our everyday life, was changed in the camps, so that their connotations were modified even after the camps. Most of the words that underwent such sematic shifts are words pertaining to the inroads of death into the *Haftling's* body.[24]

If hermeneutics aims to define the space of expression, i.e. the semantic field which enables things to exist according to a determinate meaning, it must also be open to possibilities of semantic changes under the influence of new kinds of experience. In order to trace the changes in the structure of separate members of a semantic field and to follow the progression of such changes, one has to have a 'critical mass,' a number of events of meaning, a number of recurrences of the word in its new use. If a word appears in a specific meaning only once, as a kind of *hapax legomenon*, its case does not suffice for registering a semantic shift.

The Jewish genocide pursued by the Nazis, a drive conceived not as a means to an end but as an end in itself, placed its victims in the position of 'being for death.' In their experience, 'the sense of life as being in the world, the Heideggerian *Dasein*, is being towards death in both the figurative and the literal meanings. Movement towards death is the shared experience of the people in the camps, in a sense, their shared identity.'[25] The being towards death in the camps is testified to by more than one surviving witness, and so are semantic shifts in the field of pain to which it gave rise. Death is lived through the presence of suffering that becomes the site of its articulation.

The knowledge of this pain is *pàthei màthos,* a knowledge that mediates suffering, a knowledge that comes only after suffering that unfolds at the very edge of the unknowable.[26] Here, as throughout Holocaust sites, the experience of the limit is tested. The limit in question is death - a boundary which consciousness can approach but not cross.

The pain of the victims is both the experience of an actual physical wound, of the disruption of the harmony of the being and an experience of the being's unfitness for the world. It is also a metaphysical anguish, the fearful anticipation of one's own death, desperate and usually without solution. Pain is the ineffable essence of camp experience - not philosophical pain or cosmic pain in the face of general mortality, but pain that hooks the individual human being to his or her finitude while casting death as traumatic, setting it in the context of defilement. No 'partial shelter' from this kind of death - in 'sleeping and eating and drinking and laughter,'[27] no screen of willed ignorance was possible: 'The ocean of pain, past and present, surrounded us. ... It was useless to close one's eyes or turn one's back to it, because it was all around, in every direction, all the way to the horizon and beyond.'[28]

In 1965, the Auschwitz survivor Charlotte Delbo still remembers her experience and uses bodily imagery to express it:

> I see myself, my own self as I know I was: hardly able to stand on my feet, my throat tight, my heart beating wildly, frozen to the marrow, filthy, skin and bones; the suffering I feel is so unbearable, so identical to the pain endured there,

> that I feel it physically, I feel it through my own body which becomes a mass of suffering; and I feel death fasten on me, I feel that I am dying.[29]

Pain in the concentration camps is not compensated by any emotional relief of the kind granted and available to individuals sentenced to death.[30]

In concentration-camp experience, pain is proof and judgment of the meaning of one's existence. It is experienced as part of one's own self-individuation, which enables the human being to constitute him- or herself integrally as individual. In pain, as in death, the individual is not replaceable. The experience of happiness is sharable, even if diverse, but in pain, at its meaningful moments, individuals are alone. They are non-interchangeable in the experience of pain because the pain of each is an anticipation of *his or her own death*, because pain reduces one's self, one's life, until they are diminished to nothing. In pain one experiences the intensity of the loss, the deprivation of the self; one also experiences the external power that dispossesses the subject of itself in regard to the 'I before.' Pain is the experience that we have of death, inscribed in the body. It is the objectivity of the physical, of the natural mortal vulnerability of the form (the Aristotelian soul) and the matter of the individual. The experience/knowledge nexus is configured in a remarkable way: if pain is known through experience, experience leads to a new kind of knowledge - the radical nature of the experience does not cancel knowledge but redeploys and sharpens it. Along with Salvatore Natoli, I believe that the radical nature of the Holocaust experience can be ascribed to precisely this: it repositions experience and knowledge, giving rise to a new way of perceiving the world and comprehending the events that take place in it.[31] Concentration camp experience unveils a typology of knowledge that is incommensurable with other forms of epistemology because of the shift that the experience produces in regard to the connotations of the words, affecting, as we have seen in Delbo, not only perception but also memory.

It is precisely because the semantic shift affects neutral and frequently used words that the world at large, beyond the boundaries of the camp, seems to have changed entirely. Camp experience shatters the ordinary rhythm of existence forever and produces enough discontinuity to cause the world to be seen as it had never been seen before. The camp draws its survivors towards an existential tension that, when not totally destructive, widens the limits of perception. Natoli describes pain as a vector of knowledge,[32] but in the camp pain was the test, the proof and the dominant mode of each individual's existence.

Words such as 'thirst,' 'cold,' 'hunger,' 'winter,' 'summer,' 'mud' or 'shoes' are redefined in the context of pain. For example, Primo Levi makes the following now famous statement (echoed in Paul Auster's 1987 *In the Country of Last Things*) about shoes:

> Death begins with the shoes; for most of us, they show themselves to be instruments of torture, which after few hours of marching cause painful sores which become fatally infected. Whoever has them is forced to walk as if he was dragging a convict's chain, . . . he arrives last everywhere, and everywhere he receives blows. He cannot escape if they run after him; his feet swell and the more they swell, the more the friction with the wood and the cloth of the shoes become insupportable. Only the hospital is left: but to enter the hospital with a diagnosis of 'dicke Füsse' (swollen feet) is extremely dangerous, because it is well known to all, especially to the SS, that here there is no cure for that complaint.[33]

Auschwitz survivor Charlotte Delbo gives us this example:

> someone who has been tortured by thirst for weeks on end, could never again say, 'I am thirsty. How about a cup of tea?' This word has also been split into two. *Thirst has turned back into a word for commonplace use.* But if I dream of the 'thirst' I suffered in Birkenau, I once again see the person I was, haggard, half-crazed, near to collapse; I feel physically that 'real thirst' and it is an atrocious nightmare.[34]

The chronic hunger of *Lager* inmates was likewise of a kind unknown to free people, as was the tormenting cold, another pathway to death. Robert Antelme recollects:

> We put paper between our shirts and jackets. We feared for our lungs. It was a collective fear. There was nothing to help you get through pneumonia. The toughest peasants, never bothered by the rain hitherto, now felt menaced by it. All of a sudden they sensed the fragility of their bodies . . . they knew they could be done in by a sprinkle. ... Anxiously, they would watch the big clouds, watch the sky darken. ... No longer did they have confidence in their bodies; they knew that for their bodies there would be no help.[35]

Pain is reflected in the lack of a solid symbolic structure, the lack of a universal common platform for explaining it. Language loses its power as a form of cognitive socialization because words are building blocks that belong to different narrative constructs. For survivors, the act of returning to the liberated word was often more meaningful than the act of going home. The language of civilisation confirmed that they had again become human beings and social creatures. Concurrently, however, this language represented the limit of their ability to return to society because their own words had a countervalue, a surfeit of meaning that undermined the foundations of the existing social discourse. The unspeakable, the unnameable signalled the head-on collision between writing and experience, between the conventionalities of familiar language and the lapidary character of camp experience. Language can represent experience, but cannot express or convey it. Perhaps it cannot even signify it. The difficulty is not the lack of a vocabulary to denote or describe the extreme, not a semantic gap in the testimony, but the inadequacy of any given language for rendering the experience in which language itself is gradually lost. Primo Levi often comments on the mutilation of the language and on the hopelessness of the effort to confer a shareable meaning on something that is not shareable:

> Just as our hunger is not the feeling of missing a meal, so our way of being cold has need of a new word. We say 'hunger,' we say 'tiredness,' 'fear,' 'pain,' we say 'winter' and they are different things. They are free words, created and used by free men who lived in comfort and suffering in their homes. If the Lager had lasted longer a new, harsh language would have been born; and only this language could express what it means to toil the whole day in the wind, with the temperature below freezing, wearing only a shirt, underpants, cloth jacket and trousers, and in one's body nothing but weakness, hunger and knowledge of the end drawing nearer.[36]

One of the reasons for this inadequacy is that writers have at their disposal a vocabulary that no longer reflects their experience, and yet they have no choice but to use this discredited lexicon. The result is a crisis of representation for those who write and for those who read. The sign remains the same but the interpretation of the sign varies between people who shared the experience and those who did not. Each word holds specific connotations for the first group that it does not hold for the second. Thus the linguistic question turns into a social question associated with hegemony and authority. The functioning of the word in social discourse is efficient when the speaker (a writer in our case) and the listener share a cultural code. The experience becomes knowledge when the word and the narrative act are authoritative guarantors of the experience itself. In post-war years, codes were not shared, and if the denotations of words written and read may have been the same, their connotations were widely different. As a result the unintelligibility of survivor texts kept them from joining the hegemonic discourse, and their marginal status was, in its turn, detrimental to their accessibility.[37]

Humankind has always tried to endow pain with meaning. The individual's pain found meaning in grand images sanctified as models. Versions of the pain scenario are also the places where the relationship between the individual's pain experience and its universal meaning is established. As Salvatore Natoli observes, this interweaving of individual and universal, indivisible from the experience of pain, allows the experience to become a language: the reflection of the universal in the individual is what allows the sufferer to communicate experience[38]. Though the pain of the other is considered unknowable, it can be imagined and recognized *a posteriori*: suffered pain can be universalised as possible pain that, in turn, finds its ordinary confirmation in the suffered pain. Thanks to this recourse, the presence of pain is familiarised to the imagination, sometimes distant but always re-emerging. Personal reflection on pain then becomes a projection of the self onto general suffering. The possible is, thus, the middle term between the individual and the universal: all are candidates for the unexpected and unpredictable blows. Images of pain are scenarios in which an individual casts him- or herself as a suffering person, in quest of a vocabulary and ideas that would help one come to terms with pain and interpret it. Shareable myths fuse with the reality of pain; they shape the individual's pain as they interpret it. Pain experience is familiarised and formalised in faiths, theologies, ceremonies and rituals - frameworks for the representation of pain that give it legitimacy and meaning, creating the ritual space in which pain can be communicated. Faiths and cultures, along with their ceremonies and rituals, have a lexicon for pain. In a sense, ceremonies and rituals exist to give meaning to human suffering and pain, to fill the gap of silence that falls on man when pain strikes and stays. In the absence of ceremonies and rituals surrounding pain and death in the concentration camps, their place is taken by narrative, which ceremonies and rituals can dispense with. The survivors' words become meaningful to the extent of becoming, or replacing, ceremonies and rituals. The semantic structure of the items in such vocabularies accommodates the concentration camps' semantic fields of pain, creating a new social mask for it.

The kind of pain bred in the concentration camp belongs to the category of 'the monstrous, perhaps unrepeatable' in human history; when an attempt is made to tell it, 'friends, children, readers, or even strangers sense this, beyond their indignation and commiseration; they understand the uniqueness of our experience, or at least make an effort to understand it.'[39]

And yet the survivors who know this experience also tend to assume guilt, or feel shame, for their own share, as it were, in a general human responsibility for inflicting suffering. In the essay 'Shame,' echoing John Donne's prose poem 'No man is an island,' Primo Levi represents the survivor's shame as a consequence of ordinary omission:

> It was not possible for us, nor did we want, to become islands, the just among us, neither more nor less numerous than in any other human group, felt remorse, shame and pain for the misdeed that others and not they had committed, and in which they felt involved, because they sensed that what had happened around them in their presence, and in them, was irrevocable. It would never again be able to be cleansed; it would prove that man, the human species - we, in short - were potentially to construct an infinite enormity of pain; and that pain the only force that is created from nothing, without cost and without effort. It is enough not to see, nor to listen, nor to act.[40]

In order to reach some level of understanding of camp pain, one has to stage the following experiment: accept the anaesthetising social mediation of the discourse of pain in order to prevent silence about it, and then try to transcend it through exertions of the imagination.

The Holocaust constitutes, intellectually, an *archè,* that is, a chronological beginning, even though it is popularly associated with the possibility of the end, an apocalypse. Lyotard suggests that Auschwitz is a model rather than an example. While an example has the function of illustrating an idea, it does not stand in a necessary relation with what it has to illustrate and so remains indifferent to it. A model, by contrast, is what initiates the idea. According to Lyotard, Auschwitz is a kind of 'para-experience' in which the dialectic meets an undeniable negative, initiating what cannot be continued because of the absence of an appropriate precise language able to contain the experience.[41] In a sense, Lyotard seems to take at face value Sigmund Freud's assertion that death 'is an abstract concept with a negative content for which no unconscious correlative can be found. It would seem that the mechanism of the fear of death can only be that the ego relinquishes its narcissistic libidinal cathexis in a very large measure, that is, gives up itself.'[42] Freud concludes, 'I believe that the fear of death concerns an interplay between the ego and the super-ego.'[43] In this sense, then, the unconscious cannot have an experience of death; untouched by it, it appears to itself immortal, eternal and timeless. Yet in the camps the fear of death became a concrete encounter with the real, as if the unconscious had been touched by death itself, not only by the fear of death. A special language was born out of this encounter, a language that bears the mark and the awareness of one's having been, once, a being towards death. This language opens the way for self-reflexive discourse, as well as for efforts of imagination. It is a language in which the idea of death and the experience of dying coincide, removing the gap between the signified and the signifier. Dying in the camp is the literal materialisation of death; the black hole to which one is pulled. Being in the camp is none other than being towards death: life is moving towards the horizon which does not recede apace.[44]

To rebuild the semantic field of the camps means to build an awareness of the language in which connotations of words interact in ways different from the links between their denotations. That might go a long way towards rejecting the axiom that the camp experience is untranslatable. Along with Lyotard, I would say that camp experience marks the borders 'wherein historical knowledge sees its competence impugned,'[45] but borders that we can cross. Our choice is not between claiming scientific knowledge of every detail or disowning knowledge because we lack first-hand experience. We also have the option of decoding, and of leaps of imagination that confront the need for decoding. The word 'theft' may serve as an example. In Auschwitz, as Levi recollects, theft was punished by the civil directors of Buna, but authorised and encouraged by the SS in the main camp; by civilians it was considered a normal exchange operation; among *Häftlinge* theft from outside was heroism; theft from fellow prisoners was generally punished (but the punishment fell both on the thief and the victim). 'We invite the reader to contemplate the possible meaning of "good" and "evil"; "just" and "unjust"; let everybody judge . . . how much of our ordinary moral world could survive on this side of the barbed wire.'[46] Understanding the complicated load carried by the word 'theft' not in the framework of the ten commandments but in the context of camp logistics reduces the distance between ordinary language and the cognitive aspects of camp experience.[47]

In his invitation to the reader to rethink the connotations of words, Primo Levi more than others has posed the challenge to learn a new language, to understand and compensate for the inability of customary linguistic forms to convey the experience of the 'other' death. Though the goal of imaginative capturing of that ultimate experience is not attainable, one can at least come closer to it by learning to recognise the changes that the semantic structures of familiar words have undergone in the camps. Camp testimonies are 'inconvenient' texts,[48] not only because of the information they contain, but also because they affect the semantic structure of the words in our own use, expanding and shifting their connotations and thus affecting the way in which we see our own world. The expansion of the semantic field of words pertaining to bodily suffering also compensates for the limited success of the attempts to give an innovative account of the intellectual content of camp experience - that content was reduced by suffering and the quest for alleviation.

Knowledge that emerges from the texts of the victims is not useless. One must, of course, beware of endowing its source with the kind of meaning which, as Hannah Arendt noted in regards to Eugen Kogon's and David Rousset's books, might allow any kind of 'positive interpretation'[49] for the sake of psychological consolation. The usefulness of the knowledge of the camp experience lies in that it enhances and complicates the awareness that we are living in the world in which Auschwitz was possible, and this awareness brings along visible changes 'in the secularly grounded and rationally organized structures of civilization,'[50] including language. The *novum* that emerges from the victims' narratives allows us to make a cognitive use of their experience for theoretical and interpretative purposes, to decode the universal historical, ethical and epistemological meaning of the extermination with the help of the hermeneutic force of their language, of the shifts that take place in the content and the outlines of their concepts.

When the memoirs were first published, their target audience included many fellow survivors and people who had undergone much suffering, though of other kinds, during the war. This audience largely shared the camp memoirists' cultural code, therefore they may have remained unaware, except subconsciously, of the semantic shift in which their own vocabulary participated. Half a century after the event, readers no longer automatically share that cultural code. It was quite prophetic on the part of Charlotte Delbo, Robert Antelme, Primo Levi and others to foresee this 'normalisation' of language and insert in their narrative explanations of the semantic expansion which they experienced, for the benefit of the new generation of readers who do not share their cultural code and must be guided in deciphering the special import of seemingly ordinary words.

Notes

[1] Cf. also Carlo Ginzburg, 'Memoria e globalizzazione,' *Quaderni Storici* 120 (2005): 665.

[2] It is also a part of a broader project on the history of death after the Shoah based on philosophical and historiographical writings and memoire literature sources.

[3] See Raoul Hilberg, *The Destruction of European Jews* (New Haven: Yale University Press, 2003 [1961]). Hilberg's was 'the first clear description of (the) incredibly complicated machinery of destruction' (Hannah Arendt, *Eichmann in Jerusalem* [New York: The Viking Press, 1964], 71). His empirical descriptive methodology was used to process the huge archives of Nazism in order to delineate the history of the political, legal, administrative and organizational mechanisms of perpetrating the Final Solution, as seen

through German eyes, often those of anonymous clerks whose unquestioning dedication to their duties was central to the efficacy of the industrial project of genocide. In keeping with this aim, Hilberg refrained from emphasis on the suffering of Jews, the victims.

[4] Valiant attempts to re-read individual testimony and to integrate it within Holocaust historiography have been made in Shaul Friedländer, *Nazi Germany and the Jews: The Years of Persecution, 1933-1939* (New York: HarperCollins, 1997); *The Years of Extermination* (New York: HarperCollins, 2007); as well as Christopher Browning, *Remembering Survival: Inside a Nazi Slave-Labor Camp* (New York: Norton, 2010).

[5] Martin Jay, 'Of Plot, Witnesses, and Judgments,' in *Probing the Limits of Re-presentation: Nazism and the Final Solution*, ed. Shaul Friedländer (Cambridge: Harvard University Press, 1992), 98-99.

[6] Robert Antelme, *The Human Race*, trans. Jeffrey Haight and Annie Mahler (Marlboro: Marlboro Press, 1992 [1957]), 29.

[7] Primo Levi, *If This Is a Man: The Truce*, trans. Stuart Woolf (London: Abacus, 1987 [1947, 1963]), 178.

[8] Primo Levi, *The Drowned and the Saved*, trans. Raymond Rosenthal (London: Abacus, 1989 [1986]), 83.

[9] Ibid., 90.

[10] Dan Diner, *Beyond the Conceivable: Studies on Germany, Nazism and the Holocaust* (Berkeley: University of California Press, 2000), 160-70.

[11] Theodor Adorno, 'Selection from Metaphysics: Concepts and Problems: The Liquidation of the Self': 430.

[12] Cf. Levi, *The Drowned and the Saved*, 83: 'Death, even when not provoked, even the most clement, is a violence, but it is sadly useful: a world of immortals (Swift's Struldbruggs) would be neither conceivable, nor liveable, would be more violent than the present life, violent though it is.'

[13] For a discussion of changes in the perception of death through the centuries see the monumental works of Philippe Ariès, *L'Homme devant la mort* (Paris: Seuil, 1977), 641-730. See also Michel Vovelle, *La mort et l'Occident de 1300 à nos jours* (Paris: Gallimard, 1983), 700-93. Both authors maintain that in order to speak about death after WWII we should build new parameters of analysis.

[14] Levi, *The Drowned and the Saved*, 12.

[15] See Enzo Traverso, *La violenza nazista: Una genealogia* (Bologna: Il Mulino, 2002), 10.

[16] Diner, *Beyond the Conceivable*, 165.

[17] '[I]n the historiographical realm, the obvious dichotomy between banality in implementation and monstrosity in individually experienced victimization

reflects the fundamental divide between two different approaches to, and presentations of, the Final Solution' (Ibid., 166).

[18] Hannah Arendt, 'The Concentration Camps,' *Partisan Review* 15 (1948): 744.

[19] Ibid.

[20] Reinhart Koselleck, *Futures Past: On the Semantics of Historical Time* (New York: Columbia University Press, 2004), 157ff.

[21] Ibid., 156.

[22] Useful for our discussion is Koselleck's definition of binary concepts which contain not only claims of universality but the possibility of their translation into political language: 'The historical world . . . operates for the most part asymmetri-cal concepts that are unequally antithetical,' such as the contrast between a Hellene and a Barbarian, a Christian and a Heathen, as well as 'between the human and non human, superhuman and subhuman' (Ibid., 157).

[23] Ibid., 159-60.

[24] Hannah Arendt's description of 'fearful anticipation' and Michel Foucault's discussion of 'the threshold of biological modernity' (*Histoire de la sexualité.* 1: *La volonté de savoir* [Paris: Gallimard, 1976]) have anticipated Giorgio Agamben's discussion of a camp inmate as *homo sacer*, a person who, according to ancient Roman law, can be killed without that action being considered murder; see Agamben, *Homo Sacer: Il potere sovrano e la nuda vita* (Torino: Einaudi, 1995), 80-81; as well as *Quel che resta di Auschwitz: L'archivio e il testimone (Homo Sacer III)* (Torino: Bollati Boringhieri, 1998); *Stato di eccezione* (Torino: Bollati Boringhieri, 2003), *passim*.

[25] Manuela Consonni, 'Primo Levi, Robert Antelme, and the Body of the Muselmann,' *Partial Answers: Journal of Literature and the History of Ideas* 7 (2009): 253-56. On the Muselmann debate, in terms of the Heideggerian *Dasein* and the concentration camps, see Agamben, *Quel che resta di Auschwitz*, 37-80.

[26] See Giorgio Agamben, *Infanzia e storia: Distruzione dell'esperienza e origine della storia* (Torino: Einaudi, 1978), 10-11.

[27] 'And meanwhile we have gone on living, / Living and partly living, / Picking together the pieces, / Gathering faggots at nightfall, / Building a partial shelter, / For sleeping and eating and drinking and laughter.' T. S. Elliot, *Murder in the Cathedral* (New York: Harcourt Brace, 1935), 43.

[28] Levi, *The Drowned and the Saved*, 65-66.

[29] Charlotte Delbo, *Days and Memory* (Marlboro: Marlboro Press, 1990), 3.

[30] 'For people condemned to death, tradition prescribes an austere ceremony,

calculated to emphasize that all passions and anger have died down, and that the act of justice represents only a sad duty towards society which moves even the executioner to pity for the victim. Thus the condemned man is shielded from all external cares, he is granted solitude and, should he want it, spiritual comfort; in short, care is taken that he should feel around him neither hatred nor arbitrariness, only necessity and justice, and by means of punishment, forgiveness' (Levi, *If This Is a Man*, 20-21).

[31] Salvatore Natoli, *L'esperienza del dolore: Le forme del patire nella cultura occidentale* (Milano: Feltrinelli, 2001), 8.

[32] Ibid., 9-12.

[33] Levi, *If This Is a Man*, 40-41.

[34] Delbo, *Days and Memory*, 4. Semantic shifts are suggested throughout Delbo's trilogy *Auschwitz and After* which includes 'None of Us Will Return,' 'Useless Knowledge,' and 'The Measure of Our Days' (*Auschwitz and After,* trans. Rosette C. Lamont, introduction by Lawrence L. Langer [New Haven: Yale University Press, 1995]).

[35] Antelme, *Human Race*, 47-48.

[36] Levi, *If This Is a Man*, 129.

[37] On the epistemological and social 'situatedness' of knowledge in autoethno-graphy and its hermeneutics associated with some of the issues raised in the essay, Clifford Geertz writes: 'This issue, negotiating the passage from what one has been through "out there" to what one says "back here," is not psychological in character. It is literary. It arises for anyone who adopts what one may call, in a serious pun, the I-witnessing approach to the construction of cultural descriptions. ... [It] is to pose for yourself a distinctive sort of text-building problem: rendering your account credible through rendering your person so. ... To become a convincing "I-witness," one must, so it seems, first become a convincing "I"' (Clifford Geertz, *Works and Lives: The Anthropologist as Author* [Stanford: Stanford University Press, 1988], 78-79).

[38] Salvatore Natoli, *L'esperienza del dolore,* 14.

[39] Levi, *The Drowned and the Saved*, 122.

[40] Ibid., 66.

[41] On the discussion of Auschwitz as a model or/and an example, see: Theodor W. Adorno, *Negative Dialectics* (New York: Continuum Publishing Company, 1973), 361-73; and Jean-François Lyotard, *Le differend* (Paris: Minuit, 1983), 32-58, 86-106. Lyotard, however, notes, at the end of his chapter devoted to the referent and the name, that 'there would be no history with a differend, that a differend is born from a wrong and is signalled by a silence indicating that phrases are in abeyance of their becoming event [*en souffrance de leur évenement*], that the feeling is the suffering of this

abeyance [*cette souffrance*].' I concur in his recommendation that the historian should 'break with the monopoly over history granted to the cognitive regime of phrases, and he or she must venture forth by lending his or her ear to what is not presentable under the rules of knowledge. Every reality entails this exigency insofar as it entails possible unknown senses' (57-58). Auschwitz is indeed the most real of realities, 'its name marks the confines wherein the historical knowledge sees its competence impugned. It does not follow that one falls into a non-sense. The alternative is not: either the signification that learning [*science*] establishes, or absurdity be it of the mystical kind'.

[42] Sigmund Freud, 'The Subordinate Relationships of the Ego,' in *The Ego and the Id* (London: Hogarth Press, 1957), 85-86.

[43] Ibid., 86.

[44] On the question of the new language born out of the experience see the appendix 'Auschwitz Terms' in Janusz Nel Siedlecki et al., *We Were in Auschwitz* (New York: Welcome Rain Publishers, 2000 [1946]). There, the list of the neologisms is preceded by the epitaph-like sentence: 'The isolation and extraordinariness of the surroundings, the mix of many languages, and the official German language all combined to produce a distinctive camp language, which like the language of conspiracy, still needs to be codified' (188).

[45] Lyotard, *Differend*, 58.

[46] Levi, *If This Is a Man*, 92.

[47] The Gulag survivor Varlam Shalamov wrote on the same issue: 'Values shift here, in Kolyma, and any one of our concepts - even though its name may be pronounced in the usual way and spelled with the usual letters - may contain some new element or meaning, something for which there is no equivalent on the mainland. Here everything is judged by different standards: customs and habits are unique, and the meaning of every word has changed. Semantic metamorphoses touch not only such concepts as Love, Family, Honor, Work, Virtue, Vice, Crime, but even words that are quite specific to the world of the Far North, and that have been born within its bowels - for example *ESCAPE*' (Varlam Shalamov, *Kolyma Tales*, trans. John Glad [London: Penguin, 1994], 343). Shalamov writes about the adoption by the inmates of the criminal language that affects ordinary language: 'When it is impossible to describe a new event, feeling, or concept for which ordinary human language has no word, a new term is created, borrowed from the language of the legislator of taste in the Far North - the criminal world' (Ibid.). The striking phenomenon in the prisoners' language that this paper focuses on is the semantic shift that occurs within the units of the language already at the disposal of the prisoners.

[48] See Bernard Harrison, *Inconvenient Fictions: Literature and the Limits of Theory* (New Haven: Yale University Press, 1991).
[49] Hannah Arendt, 'The Concentration Camps,' 744.
[50] Diner, *Beyond the Conceivable*, 160.

Bibliography

Adorno, Theodor W. *Negative Dialectics*. New York: Continuum, 1973. Original: *Negative Dialektik.* Frankfurt: Suhrkamp, 1966.

———. 'Selection from *Metaphysics: Concepts and Problems:* The Liquidation of the Self.' In *Can One Live after Auschwitz? A Philosophical Reader*, edited by Rolf Tiedeman, 427-36. Stanford: Stanford University Press, 1978.

Agamben, Giorgio. *Homo Sacer. Il potere sovrano e la nuda vita*. Torino: Einaudi, 1995.

———. *Infanzia e Storia. Distruzione dell'esperienza e origine della storia.* Torino: Einaudi, 1978.

———. *Quel che resta di Auschwitz. L'archivio e il testimone (Homo Sacer III)*. Torino: Bollati Boringhieri, 1998.

———. *Stato di eccezione*. Torino: Bollati Boringhieri, 2003.

Akhmatova, Anna. *Poems of Akhmatova*. Selected, translated and introduced by Stanley Kunitz with Max Hayward. Boston: Little and Brown, 1973.

Améry, Jean. *At the Mind's Limit: Contemplations by a Survivor on Auschwitz and its Realities*. Translated by Sidney Rosenfeld and Stella P. Rosenfeld. Indiana: Indiana University Press, 1980. Original: *Jenseits von Schuld und Sühne. Bewältigunversuche eines Überwältigten.* Stuttgart: Klett-Cotta, 1977.

Antelme, Robert. *The Human Race*. Translated by Jeffrey Haight and Ann Mahler. Marlboro: Marlboro Press, 1992. Original: *L'Espèce humaine,* Paris: Gallimard, 1957.

Arendt, Hannah. 'The Concentration Camps.' *Partisan Review* 15.2 (1948): 743-62.

———. *Eichmann in Jerusalem*. New York: The Viking Press, 1964 (revised edition).

Ariès, Philippe. *Essais sur l'histoire de la mort en Occident: du moyen âge à nos jours*. Paris: Seuil, 1975.

———. *L'Homme devant la mort*. Paris: Seuil, 1977.

Browning, Christopher. *Remembering Survival: Inside a Nazi Slave-Labor Camp*. New York: Norton, 2010.

Consonni, Manuela. 'Primo Levi, Robert Antelme, and the Body of the *Muselmann*,' *Partial Answers: Journal of Literature and the History of Ideas*, 7 (2009): 243-59.

Delbo, Charlotte. *Days and Memory*. Translated by Rosette C. Lamont. Marlboro: Marlboro Press, 1990.

———. *Auschwitz and After*. Translated by Rosette C. Lamont, with an introduction by Lawrence L. Langer. New Haven: Yale University Press 1995.

Diner, Dan. *Beyond the Conceivable: Studies on Germany, Nazism and the Holocaust.* Berkeley: University of California Press, 2000.

Elliot, T. S. *Murder in the Cathedral.* New York: Harcourt Brace, 1935.

Foucault, Michel. *Histoire de la sexualité.* 1. *La volonté de savoir*. Paris: Gallimard, 1976.

Freud, Sigmund. 'The Subordinate Relationships of the Ego.' In *The Ego and the Id*, 68-88. London: Hogarth Press, 1957.

Friedländer, Saul. *Nazi Germany and the Jews: The Years of Persecution, 1933-1939*. New York: HarperCollins, 1997.

———. *Nazi Germany and the Jews: The Years of Extermination.* New York: HarperCollins, 2007.

Geertz, Clifford. *Works and Lives: The Anthropologist as Author*. Stanford: Stanford University Press, 1988.

Ginzburg, Carlo. 'Memoria e globalizzazione.' *Quaderni Storici* 120 (2005): 657-70.

Harrison, Bernard. *Inconvenient Fictions: Literature and the Limits of Theory*. New Haven: Yale University Press, 1991.

Hilberg, Raoul. *The Destruction of European Jews*. New Haven: Yale University Press, 2003 [1961].

Jay, Martin. 'Of Plot, Witnesses, and Judgments.' In *Probing the Limits of Representation: Nazism and the Final Solution*, edited by Shaul Friedländer, 97-107. Cambridge, MA: Harvard University Press, 1992.

Koselleck, Reinhart. *Futures Past: On the Semantics of Historical Time*. Translated by Keith Tribe. New York: Columbia University Press, 2004. Original: *Vergangene Zukunft. Zur Semantik geschichtlicher Zeiten*. Frankfurt: Suhrkamp, 1979.

Levi, Primo. *If This Is a Man. The Truce*. Translated by Stuart Woolf. London: Abacus, 1987. Originals: *Se questo è un uomo*. Torino: Da Silva, 1947. *La Tregua*. Torino: Einaudi, 1963.

———. *The Drowned and the Saved*. Translated by Raymond Rosenthal. London: Abacus, 1989. Original: *I sommersi e i salvati*. Torino: Einaudi, 1986.

Lyotard, Jean-François. *Le differend*. Paris: Minuit, 1983.

Natoli, Salvatore. *L'esperienza del dolore: Le forme del patire nella cultura occidentale*. Milano: Feltrinelli, 2001.

Shalamov, Varlam. *Kolyma Tales*. Translated by John Glad. London: Penguin, 1994.

Siedlecki, Janusz Nel, Krystyn Olszewski and Tadeusz Borowski. *We Were in Auschwitz*. New York: Welcome Rain Publishers, 2000 [1946].

Traverso, Enzo. *La violenza nazista: Una genealogia*. Bologna: Il Mulino, 2002.

Vovelle, Michel. *La mort et l'Occident de 1300 à nos jours*. Paris: Gallimard, 1983.

Part IV

EPIPHENOMENA

Folk Theodicy in Concentration Camps: Literary Representations

Leona Toker

Abstract
Literary works, whether memoiristic or fictional, written by survivors of concentration camps frequently represent attempts by prisoners to explain the metaphysical meaning of their suffering in order to preserve their religious beliefs or their religiously held social ideology. This 'folk theodicy' (a term coined by analogy with 'folk etymology' and 'folk psychology') is an epiphenomenon of suffering and a strategy for orientation in the midst of a religious or ideological crisis. Its traditional forms, such as belief in punitive justice or in service of remote goals, break down when the suffering to which it responds is particularly prolonged and acute. Folk theology is then either relinquished along with faith itself or else reversed: the God that failed is imagined as helpless and suffering. While the literary records of the folk theology of Holocaust victims can provide a conceptual framework for redescribing the conduct of communist true believers in the Gulag, Gulag literature can shed light on the mechanics of *deconversion*, that is on the factors that led up to the loss of faith. Whereas neither counterarguments nor their own unjustly inflicted suffering could shake religiously held communist beliefs, such beliefs were, apparently, irreparably damaged by the almost visceral experience of moral disgust. It stands to reason that a similar sense of disgust with the world in which the Nazi atrocities could unfold was the cause of the loss of religious beliefs among some of the victims or at least the cause of the renunciation of the practices associated with religious beliefs.

Key Words: Concentration camps, Gulag, Auschwitz, theodicy, folk theodicy, Varlam Shalamov, Primo Levi, Solzhenitsyn, Iurii Dombrovskii, deconversion.

*****

Pain, physical or moral, individual or collective, has always raised the issue of evil. In the shape of theodicy this issue has been explored by philosophers, theologians and writers. But attempts to justify God also take place at the grass-roots level, among the less learned, and in close connection with conventional morality. These grass-root attempts to vindicate the ways of God is what I propose to call *folk theodicy*.

Folk theodicy is a Phoenix that keeps rising from its ashes. For Voltaire, the Lisbon earthquake meant the end of standard theodicy, yet we find the call for theodicy periodically renewed. In his elegiac poem 'In Memoriam' Alfred Tennyson writes:

> Be near me when this sensuous frame
> Is racked with pangs that conquer trust;
> And Time, a maniac scattering dust,
> And Life, a Fury slinging flame. (50: 1-4)

The addressee of these lines is not, as might be expected, God, but the dead friend, Arthur Hallam, whom the poem mourns. The pain of bereavement merges with physical pain, with which the 'sensuous frame,' the body, is 'racked,' and the two threaten to prevail against 'trust' - the faith-based world view. The loss of belief further exacerbates the pain: 'Time' becomes a madman scattering the dust of the archaeological and geological digs which to a mid-Victorian intellectual suggests that, as a species, mankind can also be reduced to ashes. 'Life, a Fury slinging flame,' is an actively evil avenger, more cruel than life in Macbeth's nihilistic vision, where it is but a tale 'told by an idiot, full of sound and fury, signifying nothing' (*Macbeth*, Act V, scene 5).

The key parts of the poem defenestrate the deistic perspective on the notion of 'the intelligent design' - Alexander Pope's '[w]hatever is, is right.' In the prologue Tennyson expresses a longing for a sense of a more personal agency that might subjugate partial evil to ultimate good; in the end he does reach some plateau of theodicy and testifies to a return of emotive religiosity. Yet a few generations later, and on other meridians, this kind of emotive theodicy received new and more crushing blows. As to rational theodicy, 'from Augustine to Leibnitz and beyond,' it remains fascinating and 'impressive in some of its detailed arguments, but few theologians and no philosophers would want to claim nowadays that its achievement runs much beyond that of giving us a clearer view of the problem' of suffering.[1] Folk theodicy, by contrast, allows a better understanding of individuals' ways of coping with the kind of pain that is perceived as unprecedented and disorienting.

I shall here discuss the directions and the fate of folk theodicy in concentration camps - the Nazi Lagers and the Soviet Archipelago - as represented in memoirs and fiction by intellectuals such as Primo Levi, Varlam Shalamov, Evgenia Ginzburg and Yurii Dombrovskii. These works thematise what I here call *folk theodicy* as one of the main ways (complete with impasses) in which people attempted to resist the assault of continuous acute pain on their religious beliefs. This mainly applies to people for whom the loss of faith was not liberation but a disaster in itself. The authors of the memoirs tend to explore folk theodicy not as their own way of coping with disorientation but as that of others, whom they observe. In ghettoes and concentration camps there was usually just about enough time for folk theodicy to be formed and deployed. By contrast, in places like Babi Yar, Treblinka or Katyn, death came too fast for that to happen.

Here the Lagers will be discussed in so far as they overlapped with the Nazi drive towards the annihilation of the Jews, forming a kind of Holocaust by instalments. In Isaac Bashevis Singer's *The Penitent*, echoing Judges 6:12-14, a Holocaust survivor asks, 'Where was God when they burned His Torah and ordered those who had studied it to dig their own graves?' or 'Where was His love when the Nazis tortured Jewish children?'[2] In Soviet camps, religious Christians, Jews or Muslims tended to be, paradoxically, sustained by their faith, which was most often further enhanced; this is especially clear from representations of the behaviour of various sectarians in the works of Solzhenitsyn, Shalamov, Margolin and other Gulag survivors. But a religious crisis experienced by the Jews as an epiphenomenon of the Holocaust was, in the Gulag, partly replicated by the crisis of faith in the specifically Soviet sense. The Gulag 'true believers' were those who refused to give up their religiously held *communist* convictions despite being victimised by the very system that they had struggled to create and maintain; some of them are scathingly discussed in the chapter entitled 'The Loyalists' (*blagonamerennye*) in Solzhenitsyn's *The Gulag Archipelago*[3]; recollected in most Gulag memoirs, they are represented with the harshest criticism by former members of other parties.[4] The similarity between communist commitments and religion, especially 'religion' in the Durkheimian sense, is by now a matter of common knowledge[5]; I shall treat it as a given. The ideological challenge for these true believers was to find ways to justify the party and the communist state not only in respect to the injustice of sending *them* rather than others down what Solzhenitsyn called 'the sewer' but also for the lack of the proverbial divine omniscience ('How come they don't know?'). Their plight, and their outcry, was like Job's 'I will say to God, 'Do not condemn me, show me wherefore thou contendest with me'' (10:2). The interrogators frequently did show them documents, false or true depositions, sometimes of the people closest to them, that subverted that demand.

For concentration-camp inmates pain was not sporadic; it formed the 'medium' of existence.[6] Folk theodicy in concentration camps is an epiphenomenon of this acute and constant suffering against the background of a cognitive dissonance. This essay attempts to sketch its dominant shapes, the reasons for its breakdown, and the results of this breakdown. It ends by considering the ways in which the literature of the Gulag and the literature of the Holocaust may shed light on each other's processing of folk theodicy and of its reversals.

1. Folk Theodicy: The Concept

Folk theodicy, by contrast with philosophical or theological theodicy, is practise rather than theory. It amounts to popular strategies for staving off the loss of religious faith by finding a justification for suffering; these popular strategies have little connection to scholarly endeavours, such as Rabbi Kalonymus's attempts to work out the problem of evil and a justification of God in the Warsaw ghetto, or even with the standard Jewish notion of God hiding His face (which, I believe, explains much of the pathos in the works of Ka-Tzetnik). The term 'folk theodicy' is coined by analogy with such notions as 'folk etymology' and 'folk psychology': all the three are ways of maintaining one's bearings under conditions in which the precise information that one craves is inaccessible.

'Folk etymology' is popularly held beliefs (mostly false) about the origins of specific words, as well as changes in the pronunciation, meaning or spelling of words under the influence of such beliefs. The English word 'shamefaced,' for instance, gained its current form through the association of shame and the wish to hide one's face, though its true etymology is 'shamefast,' that is, held in the grip of shame. Folk etymology thus subverts the archaeology of language but can produce insights into cultural history.

The no more patrician phenomenon of 'folk psychology,' isolated by Jerome Bruner,[7] refers to the tendency we all share to attribute the behaviour of others to beliefs or desires with which we are familiar, usually from our own experience. 'Folk psychology' is a tool for orientation in the social world; its inventory changes from culture to culture. One of the main uses of 'folk psychology' is the processing of the exceptional and extraordinary with the view to reducing it to a combination of ordinary folk-psychological patterns; this is a common procedure for domesticating otherness both in the reading of literature and in attempts to cope with a fast-changing 'real' world in which what once seemed unthinkable has degenerated into the merely unwieldy.

Folk theodicy likewise seeks to tame the extraordinary. It fails when the extraordinary turns into the extreme, when the suffering is massive and unbearable. Concentration camps constitute extraordinary and extreme conditions, though their exceptional status is relative in view of the huge numbers of inmates. The Holocaust, in particular, combined the intentionality of moral evil with the dimensions of natural disasters, so-called 'acts of God.' The challenge of genocides to theodicy in general is, indeed, double: prior to the twentieth century moral evil and natural disasters tended to present separate problems for the vindication of God, even though history-book accounts of the sacking of cities would tell us otherwise; in the twentieth century they were drastically conflated, for instance when the Stalinist terror in the Soviet Union, betraying a version of the genocidal agenda, starved millions of Ukrainian peasants by the artificial famine of the early 1930s, or had whole nations deported to Siberia under conditions of at least partly deliberate deadly neglect. The forms of faith that survived in concentration camps, e.g. the faith of sectarians in the Gulag, or the faith of fervent Hasidic scholars during the Holocaust (e.g., as represented in the novels by Ka-Tzetnik and Hasidic tales[8]) rejected a preoccupation with theodicy *a priori* instead of risking its breakdown.

Folk theodicy is mainly based on two patterns of thought - punitive justice and teleology. Both collapsed in the two systems of concentration camps.

2. Punitive Justice and Teleology

The popular idea of *retributive justice*: God is punishing us for our sins, or for the sins of the fathers. Most communist true believers in the Gulag had, however, been sentenced on charges that had little or no relationship to reality, whatever other crimes, unregistered in the official indictment, they may have been guilty of. In interrogation rooms great numbers of them had confessed to crimes they had not committed, succumbing to blackmail, torture, pharmacology, or manoeuvring. Their suggestibility enhanced by hunger and sleeplessness, some may have been sufficiently confused to *accept* the criminal view of themselves created by the investigation protocols.[9] Most did not retain that state of mind afterwards, when serving their sentences in the camps. As to the real crimes in which they may have taken part, such as organising the famine in the Ukraine or victimising earlier 'enemies of the people,' arrays of ideological arguments were available for explaining them away. The idea of the sins of the fathers was trumped by prioritising nurture over nature: communist upbringing could overcome the ideological heritage of non-proletarian antecedents, leaving one morally and ideologically pure - unless one had concealed one's non-proletarian class origins. Yet even in the latter case the punishment was felt to be incommensurable with the crime.

A sense of monstrous incongruity in the relationship between crime and punishment was more intense in Auschwitz. Whatever the sins of the individual or of the whole Jewish community (godlessness, for example), the retribution was excessive. In a 1967 symposium on Jewish values after the Holocaust, Elie Wiesel compared the victory celebrated on Purim and that celebrated on Hanukkah:

> Hanukkah: The Greeks sought to absorb Judea spiritually; some Jews responded favorably . . . but then the Macabees rose up in arms in the battle against Hellenism. ... When Haman planned to exterminate the Jews, the Jews, led by Mordecai, proclaimed three days of prayer and fasting. The question is asked: Why did Jews oppose spiritual resistance

> to physical threat and physical resistance to spiritual threat? The Midrash explains this paradox in the following way: the Jewish people entered a covenant with God. We are to protect His Torah, and He, in turn, assumes responsibility for Israel's presence in the world. ... [I]t seems that for the first time in our history, this very covenant was broken. This is why the Holocaust has terrifying theological implications.[10]

Among those less profoundly steeped in Jewish learning, the religious crisis was couched in other terms. In a television interview Chief Justice Haim Cohen (1911-2002), whose brother and other family members perished at the hands of the Nazis, accounted for his rebellious deconversion by saying that what he learned about the Holocaust made him think that if God exists, he is not the God of law or the God of justice. 'I don't want such a God,' concluded Haim Cohen.[11] If the Nazis were blind instruments of the vengeful God, then God's only justification could indeed be that he does not exist.

The other pattern in folk theodicy is *teleological* - partial evil as a way to universal good. We may wish to believe, with Tennyson's *In Memoriam*, that 'not a worm is cloven in vain, / That not a moth with vain desire / Is shrivell'd in a fruitless fire, / or but subserves another's gain.' But if we do so, we place ourselves in bad company - in his 'Poem on the Lisbon Disaster' Voltaire is understandably outraged by the philosophers who explain away the horror of the earthquake: 'This misery, you say, is anothers' good' ('Ce malheur, dites-vous, est le bien d'un autre être,' l. 97). Purged of mystical overtones such consequentialism was an article of faith among communist true believers, who easily resorted to slogans like 'it is better that ninety-nine innocent people should suffer than that one guilty person should escape,' 'You cannot make an omelette without breaking eggs' (or, to use the exact calque, 'Chips fly when trees are cut' - a version of the Machiavellian 'the-end-justifies-the-means' principle), and 'Revolution is not made in white gloves.' For their own suffering they could account by the margin-of-error statistics; moreover, having devoted their lives to what they regarded as self-denying service to the party, they could accept the possibility that the new service which they were challenged to render lay in accepting individual injustice for the sake of the great goal of the construction of communism. It was more difficult when what was required of them in this service was to resign not only to losing their lives but also to giving up their honour. In Arthur Koestler's novel *Darkness at Noon*, the interrogator reminds the protagonist Rubashov that honour is 'to serve without vanity, and unto the last consequence.'[12] If at the current juncture the party needs to discredit opposition, perhaps the scapegoat true believer's insistence on his honourable innocence is just moral squeamishness, a wish to emulate the condemned Danton's grand stand; if so, that too must also be sacrificed on the altar of the struggle for a better future. Koestler's view of the matter comes close to the kind of scholarly fantasy that we also find in Borges's 'Three Versions of Judas': 'The ascetic, for the greater glory of God, vilifies and mortifies his flesh; Judas did the same with the spirit.'[13] In a sequel to this train of thought, God is imagined as incarnating himself not just in man but 'in a man to the point of infamy, a man to the point of reprobation and the abyss' - Judas; and the true believer seeks 'the grace of joining his Redeemer in Hell.'[14]

Teleological theodicy cannot withstand the onslaught of emotion in the face of the suffering of children. What Voltaire's 'Poem on the Lisbon Disaster' cannot even try to justify is the sight of '[t]his child and mother heaped in common wreck.' What Dostoevsky in *The Brothers Karamazov* pits against secular teleology is a *Gedankenexperiment*: would we accept a perfect Utopia at the price of continual torture inflicted on one child?[15] Camus's *The Plague* gives a secular version of this topos: at the point of crisis the newly produced and still untested serum only prolongs the suffering of the child to whom it is given. Folk theodicy is doomed if such events can be expected to bring about any sort of redemption since the goal - redemption itself - is contaminated by the means. The corruption, the suffering and the death of children are among the most insistent recurrent subjects of both the literature of the Holocaust and that of the Gulag.

When these two standard forms of folk theodicy, punitive justice and teleology, break down, there are still two other options for those who wish to retain their faith. One, as noted above, is to relinquish the problem; the other is to reverse it.

3. Relinquishing the Problem

In the midst of the Holocaust, *relinquishing* the problem of theodicy was often tantamount to inscribing oneself and one's community into the tradition of regarding any Jewish death during a mass crisis, even though not heroic or a matter of choice, as martyrdom, *Kiddush Hashem* (literally, sanctifying God's name). A redefinition of *Kiddush Hashem* under the circumstances of mass extermination was theorised by Rabbi Shimon Huberband in the Warsaw ghetto before he was killed in an extermination camp:

> *Kiddush Hashem* is performed in three ways: (a) a Jew sacrifices his life when others attempt to make him abandon his Jewish faith, (b) a Jew gives his life to save a fellow Jew, and even more so - to save a group of Jews, (c) a Jew dies while fighting to defend other Jews. Maimonides rules that if a Jew is killed, even without any

> overt attempt to make him abandon his Jewish faith, but because he is a Jew, he is considered a martyr.[16]

Yet Huberband tends implicitly to exclude *Judenrat* members from this category, along with, likewise implicitly, other Jews who collaborated with the Nazis for any reason. Not totally denying that if eventually killed they too might be regarded as cases of 'passive *Kiddush Hashem*,'[17] Huberband prefers to emphasise the stories of those who suffered for active individual resistance to the perpetrators or 'refused to issue lists' or cause other hardship for their brethren:

> The latter Jews acted in accordance with the ruling of the *Shulchan Arukh*, which states: 'If Gentiles say to Jews, 'Give us one of yours and we shall kill him, otherwise we shall kill all of you'; the Jews should not give them one of their own, unless the Gentiles specified him and said, 'Give us so-and-so.' And there are those who say that even in such a case one should not hand him over, unless he is guilty of a capital offense.[18]

What Huberband is here writing about is what after Primo Levi's *The Drowned and the Saved* has been referred to as 'the gray zone.' Leaving the question of martyrdom aside, in 1970 Elie Wiesel, not yet in possession of that term, was inclined to include even people who compromised themselves in the 'gray zone' in the ranks of the victims, rather than traitors:

> I cannot condemn anyone who failed to withstand trials and temptations. Guilty or not, the ghetto police, the *kapos*, may plead extenuating circumstances. They arouse pity more than contempt. The weak, the cowardly, all those who sold their souls to live another day, another anxious night, I prefer to include them in the category of the victims. More than the others, they need forgiveness. More and in other ways than their companions, they deserve compassion and charity. Their guilt reflects on their tormentors.[19]

Fourteen years later Wiesel pleaded with Ronald Reagan to cancel his visit to Bitburg, attempting, as it were, to forestall the extension of his own tolerant attitude to the morally weak and so to view even the perpetrators as the victims of the regime.

The term 'gray zone' is not widely used in the discourse on the Gulag, but the phenomenon itself is much discussed. Shalamov's Gulag fiction is populated by people whom he considered martyrs who were not heroes, or at least not heroes of active resistance. Some of them were, indeed, as Wiesel put it, 'the weak, the cowardly, all those who sold their soul to live another day, another anxious night,' but the best refused not only to collaborate with the authorities by becoming informers but also to bend the will of fellow-prisoners in the camps by serving as team leaders whose task was to force others to work and thus drive them to lethal depletion. In Shimon Huberband's terms, their suffering was tantamount to 'passive' *Kiddush Hashem.* In fact, the term 'passive' is a mistranslation of the principle of *shev ve-al taaseh* ('remain seated and do nothing'): it applies to outward passivity alone: in the Gulag the choice may have meant a deliberate ethical decision, a refusal to cooperate, which elsewhere I discuss as a Lenten principle, the principle of conscious self-denial.[20] The former communists' opting for such martyrdom instead of seeking positions of prominence in the Gulag was likewise tantamount to relinquishing folk theodicy as irrelevant.

Such a new internal commitment went hand-in-hand with choices of outer conduct - mainly the choice *not* to collaborate with the authorities. All too often, however, a Gulag prisoner was not even offered an opportunity to make such a choice. Among the victims of the Holocaust herded to their deaths, there was no choice except an internal one - to interpret their fate as part of the long history of Jewish martyrdom.[21] Yet, as Primo Levi notes in *The Drowned and the Saved*, the true witnesses are dead: one would like to believe that those who chose to see their deaths as martyrdom could maintain the exaltation or else the serenity of the spirit to their terrible last moments. No certainty is available, and in the very wish to think in such terms one risks becoming sentimentally self-protective. *Kiddush Hashem* was, rather, a way of thinking about the death of another at the hands of 'the evil ones,' as Huberband consistently called the SS and their local associates.

4. Reversing the Problem

By contrast, the *reversal* of folk theodicy meant thinking not about God hiding his face even from the innocent and the meek but about the need to extend a spiritual protection to God - putting God on the receiving end, offering solidarity to a God whose attributes no longer include omnipotence. In the famous episode in Elie Wiesel's *Night* (the one that Mauriac chooses to read as crucifixion), a column of prisoners is marched past the gallows on which three resistance fighters have been hanged. The youngest of the three is a boy, a so-called *pipel*, whose agony is protracted because his body is too light to press on the loop and lead to a prompt death. 'Where is God now?' asks one of the witnesses. Wiesel writes: 'I heard a voice within me answer him: 'Where is He?' Here He is - He is hanging here on this gallows...'[22] This does not mean to say 'god is dead' - it means that God is shrunken, helpless, tortured and in agony along with us, though he has attempted resistance.[23] By a reversal of folk theodicy the episode anticipates what Emil

Fackenheim would see as two extremes in post-Holocaust theodicy: 'a 'God-is-dead' kind of despair and a faith which is not radically altered because one has been 'with God in hell.''[24] Wiesel, whose *Night* is sometimes read as a 'theological drama,'[25] leans towards the second option. Significantly, just before staging this exchange, his narrator notes that the boy's horrible agony is not yet over, that he is not yet dead: 'He was still alive when I passed in front of him. His tongue was still red, his eyes were not yet glazed.'[26] God is not dead for Wiesel; he is suffering along with us. Yet this is no consolation. Indeed, in an interchapter entitled 'God's Suffering: A Commentary' in his memoir *All Rivers Run to the Sea*, Wiesel asks, 'How did God manage to bear His suffering added to our own? Are we to imagine the one as justification for the other? Nothing justifies Auschwitz.'[27]

A bitterly carnivalesque version of this attitude, in which the idea of a suffering God combines with resentment against God as self-indulgent, is narrated by an agnostic author, Primo Levi, in the story 'Lilith' in *Moments of Reprieve*. 'Of course, I don't believe this, but I like to tell these stories,' says a fellow prisoner to the authorial persona - the thought is contemplated at a double remove, as too fantastic to be able even to break down:

> You know that God created Adam, and immediately afterwards He realized it wasn't good for man to be alone and He placed a companion at his side. Well, the cabalists said that it wasn't good even for God Himself to be alone, and so from the beginning, He took as His companion the *Shekhina,* which is to say, His own presence in the Creation. Thus the *Shekhina* became the wife of God and therefore the mother of all peoples. When the Temple in Jerusalem was destroyed by the Romans and we were dispersed and enslaved, the *Shekhina* was angered, left God, and came with us into exile. Actually I myself have thought this: that the *Shekhina* also let herself be enslaved and is here around us, in this exile within exile, in this home of mud and sorrow.
>
> So God has remained alone; as happens to many, He has not been able to endure solitude and resist temptation and has taken a mistress. Do you know who? Her, Lilith, the she-devil, and that was an unimaginable scandal. … [T]his obscene tryst has not ended, and won't end soon. In one way it's the cause of the evil that occurs on earth; in another way, it is its effect. As long as God continues to sin with Lilith, there will be blood and trouble on Earth.[28]

'It is inexplicable,' adds Primo Levi 'that fate has chosen an unbeliever to repeat this pious and impious tale, woven of poetry, ignorance, daring acumen, and the unassuageable sadness that grows on the ruins of lost civilisations.'[29] Thus, even an unbeliever is caught in a web of reverse folk theodicy,[30] even the writer who would later say, 'There is Auschwitz, and so there cannot be God. [. . . I don't find a solution to this dilemma. I keep looking, but I don't find it],'[31] thus reversing Dostoevsky's 'If there is no God, then everything is permitted.' In the original 1978 Italian edition *Moments of Reprieve* bore the title *Lilit e altri racconti*, testifying to the importance of this short story in Levi's corpus.

There may be less drama and fascination in the Gulag prisoners' attempts to protect the God that failed. Often, especially during the war with Germany, it took the shape of dedicated work - as dedicated as the prisoner's physical condition would allow. In the case of less admirable forms of service to the regime and its octopus limbs, pragmatic considerations and plain sycophancy usually dwarfed the ideological. A vast paradigm of such attitudes, with their nuances and attendant circumstances, is deployed in Solzhenitsyn's monumental *The Gulag Archipelago*.

5. Deconversion

Can Gulag and Holocaust materials shed light on each other on the issue of folk theodicy and its transformations? Perhaps so.

The fate of folk theodicy in the Lagers may indeed provide an indirect comment on the attitudes of the true believers in the Gulag. True communist believers had to give up their absolute trust in the infallibility of the party and its 'organs' and admit that 'mistakes happen' - though banal, this thought was traumatic. Stalin does not know, many believed; he is kept in ignorance by the careerists who have taken over executive power, by maliciously mischievous lower-rank police officers, the minor devils. Accordingly, many of the true believers kept writing letters and appeals; others deliberately confessed to horrendous treachery in the hope that the absurdity of the accusations would be apparent to all, upon which the evil web of demiurge penal processes would be blown away.[32] This attitude may in some cases have been a post-facto rationalization of having been broken by torture, yet the sense that things have got out of hand, that there is an obscene mess in the system, may also have given individuals the strength to hope that order might still be reinstated and that even under these strange conditions one could still work unsparingly for the Motherland and the Party. This way of thinking was strangely consonant with the mythic pattern of a good ruler reinstated after the fall of a usurper. Not surprisingly, after the death of Stalin, the slogan of his successors was that of *Leninist* 'collective leadership,' the good ruler emerging, as it were, out of an eclipse - no longer hiding his face.

Conversely, Gulag materials can also comment on ideological developments among victims of Nazi camps. They can, in particular, contribute to our understanding of the mechanics of the loss of faith after traditional folk theodicy breaks down and is not compensated by mystical surrogates. In the sketch 'From Zybin's Notes,' a companion piece to his novels *The Keeper of Antiquities* and *The Faculty of Unnecessary Things*, the Gulag survivor Iurii Dombrovskii tells the story of a prisoner who is a true believer, a veteran revolutionary, and a well-trained Marxist. No rational argument can persuade him to blame the regime for his own suffering and for that of others. This Job will not curse God - because his closed system can explain everything, and explain away everything else. Eventually, however, he does lose his faith. What leads to this development is not a logical argument but a gut response to a specific scene that he finds totally disgusting - the sight of two guards, a man and a woman, conducting a vulgar flirtation in the prisoner's bathhouse, amidst scenes that, as Varlam Shalamov also testified, are incompatible with minimal human dignity.[33] Arthur Koestler seems to have understood the process of deconversion in a similar way - it is Rubashov's disgust with the role he is made to play that leads him to doubt his convictions: 'Perhaps it was not suitable for a man to think every thought to its logical conclusion.'[34]

Visceral disgust is, thus, what produces a change tantamount to deconversion, to irrevocable loss of faith.[35] Memoirs of former true believers such as Evgenia Ginzburg, Lev Kopelev and even Aleksandr Solzhenitsyn indeed suggest that their deconversion was caused by recurrent experience of physical or moral disgust on witnessing forms of injustice and depravity that literally turned their stomach - in their cases this was a process, an incremental sequence rather than a single novelistic about-face.[36] It is not impossible that in the Nazi camps the loss of faith, or at least the loss of total commitment to an Orthodox way of life (Wiesel's case) may also have been the result of such accumulating and repetitive gut responses. One might recollect Wiesel's scenes of the moral degradation of starving people - which must, of course, in retrospect be read against the later accumulated awareness of the personality changes that are produced by lethal chronic hunger.

Interestingly, the protagonist of Singer's *The Penitent* returns to faith, or at least to the Orthodox way of life, likewise owing to a strong sense of revulsion against what he comes to categorise as life in modern society. If seventeenth- and eighteenth-century spiritual autobiographies tended to present the conversion to religious life (the born-again experience) as stimulated by acute suffering, the literature that deals with the Holocaust and the Gulag suggests that it is not so much acute or prolonged pain as a strong sense of *disgust* that leads up to abrupt ideological shifts. One may surmise that this deconversion may well be followed by a reconversion, a return to faith (the case of Singer's fictional Shapiro and perhaps of the actual writer

Tadeusz Borowski), if the social conditions, after the long crisis is over, are also nauseating. This may be among the reasons why thousands of Gulag survivors applied for reinstatement in the Communist Party during and after the period of Khrushchev's 'Thaw'; though for the most part this was done for practical reasons.[37]

In any case, in whatever way one's change of beliefs was rationalised, disgust seemed to play a role comparable to pain in the force of its psychological consequences. And it is equally problematic for textual representation though for a reason different from the notorious ineffability of pain: disgust that leads to ideological change is all too often disgust with one's own hardened self, with one's own shame-fast ego.

Reading Holocaust literature with the literature of the Gulag often allows the prominent aspects of one of these two systems to help us understand the veiled aspects of the other, so long as one eschews or at least minimises the danger of obtunding the Holocaust or trivialising the Gulag. The relationship of pain-generated folk theodicy and visceral disgust or its mental counterparts is a case in point; it may improve our understanding of these two concentration-camp worlds which have become ineluctable parts of our current view of the human subject, especially when the tensions between faith, pain and disgust continue to encroach on the comforts of the faith-love-hope triad.

Notes

[1] Bernard Harrison, *Inconvenient Fictions: Literature and the Limits of Theory* (New Haven: Yale University Press, 1991), 182.

[2] Isaac Bashevis Singer, *The Penitent* (Harmondsworth: Penguin, 1983), 20, 100. The narrator of Jonathan Littell's *Les Bienveillantes* (*The Kindly Ones*) connects such a questioning with the idea of the banality of evil: every cog in the machine is to blame for doing his job, 'et Dieu là-haut qui permet tout ça'; he discusses this system as an example of what Marx meant by the product's alienation from the worker. (Paris: Gallimard, 2006), 25, 26.

[3] See, in particular, Aleksandr Solzhenitsyn, *The Gulag Archipelago: An Experi-ment in Literary Investigation*, vol. 2, trans. Thomas P. Whitney (New York: Harper & Row, 1974), 322-52.

[4] The theme of the shameful stance of the communist faithful in the camps runs almost throughout the memoir of, for instance, the SR (Socialist Revolutionary) party member Ekaterina Olitskaia *Moi vospominaniia* (Frankfurt: Possev, 1971).

[5] See, among others, Arthur Jay Klinghoffer, *Red Apocalypse: The Religious Evolution of Soviet Communism* (Lanham: University Press of America, 1996), esp. 1-7 and 9n3-4, and chapter 1 of Nanci Adler's *Keeping Faith with*

the Party: Communist Believers Return from the Gulag (Bloomington: Indiana University Press, 2012).
[6] David B. Morris, *The Culture of Pain* (Berkeley: University of California Press, 1991), 169.
[7] See Jerome Bruner, *Acts of Meaning* (Cambridge, MA: Harvard University Press, 1990), 33-66.
[8] In Yaffa Eliach's *Hasidic Tales from the Holocaust* (Oxford: Oxford University Press, 1982) theodicy seems to be made unnecessary by the supporting presence of a *tsaddik*.
[9] See Igal Halfin, *Stalinist Confessions: Messianism and Terror in the Leningrad Communist University* (Pittsburgh: University of Pittsburgh Press, 2009).
[10] 'Jewish Values in the Post-Holocaust Future: A Symposium,' *Judaism* 16/3 (1967): 281.
[11] See also Tom Segev, *The Seventh Million: The Israelis and the Holocaust*, trans. Haim Watzman (New York: Hill and Wang, 1993), 263-64. For a discussion of a similar story of a loss of faith, told by Ysrael Aviram about his father Yosef, see Daniel Landes, 'Spiritual Responses in the Camps,' in *Genocide: Critical Issues of the Holocaust. A Companion to the film GENOCIDE,* ed. Alex Grobman and Daniel Landes (Los Angeles: The Simon Wiesenthal Center, 1983), 261-78.
[12] Arthur Koestler, *Darkness at Noon* (New York: Macmillan, 1975), 190.
[13] Jorge Luis Borges, 'Three Versions of Judas,' in *Labyrinths: Selected Stories and Other Writings*, trans. James E. Irby (New York: New Directions, 1964), 97.
[14] Ibid., 99, 100.
[15] Ursula Le Guin's 'The Ones Who Walk Away from Omelas,' in *The Wind's Twelve Quarters* (London: Victor Gollancz, 1975) is a *Gedankenexperiment* devoted to precisely this hypothesis. I am grateful to Dalit Assouline for calling my attention to this short story.
[16] Shimon Huberband, *Kiddush Hashem: Jewish Religious and Cultural Life in Poland During the Holocaust*, trans. David E. Fishman, ed. Jeffrey S. Gurock and Robert S. Hirt (Hoboken, NJ: Ktav, 1987), 247.
[17] Ibid.
[18] Ibid., 248. On the contexts of Huberband's analysis of the problem see David Roskies, *Against the Apocalypse: Responses to Catastrophe in Modern Jewish Culture* (Cambridge, MA: Harvard University Press, 1984), 217-18. This injunction from the *Shulchan Arukh*, the code of Jewish law, may be the reason for the particularly pained concern with the Wittenberg affair in the Vilnius ghetto in public and literary discourse (at least eight plays were written about the story of a resistance leader of the ghetto giving himself up

to the Gestapo under the pressure of large parts of the ghetto population in response to the Nazi ultimatum; see Dina Porat, *The Fall of a Sparrow: The Life and Times of Abba Kovner*, trans. Elizabeth Yuval (Stanford: Stanford University Press, 2010), 106-32.

[19] Elie Wiesel, *One Generation After*, trans. Lily Edelman and the author (New York: Random House, 1970), 42.

[20] See Leona Toker, *Return from the Archipelago: Narratives of Gulag Survivors* (Bloomington: Indiana University Press, 2000), 94-100.

[21] See also Landes, 'Spiritual Responses in the Camps,' 200.

[22] Wiesel, *Night*, trans. Stella Rodway (New York: Bantam, 1982), 62.

[23] One of the options for post-Holocaust Jewish thought that Emil Fackenheim rejects - as true (if at all) 'not for our time but all time' - is 'the Whiteheadian God, infinite in goodness but finite in power, unable to destroy evil and hence *this* evil.' *To Mend the World: Foundations of Future Jewish Thought* (New York: Schocken, 1982), 28.

[24] Ibid., 309. Fackenheim cites Richard Rubenstein's *After Auschwitz* as the most influential expression of the former view and Eliezer Berkowitz's *With God in Hell* as that of the latter.

[25] Inga Clendinnen, *Reading the Holocaust* (Cambridge: Cambridge University Press, 1999), 44.

[26] Wiesel, *Night*, 62. On the motif of the suffering Messiah in Wiesel's work, see also Byron L. Sherwin, 'Jewish Messianism and Elie Wiesel,' *Notre Dame English Journal* 11 (1978): 39-40.

[27] Wiesel, *All Rivers Run to the Sea* (New York: Schocken, 1995), 104-105.

[28] Primo Levi, *Moments of Reprieve*, trans. Ruth Feldman (London: Abacus, 1987), 43-44.

[29] Ibid, 45.

[30] I am grateful to Ariela Freedman for this remark.

[31] Ferdinando Camon, *Conversations with Primo Levi*, trans. John Shepley (Marlboro: Marlboro Press, 1989), 68.

[32] Such strategies of communist prisoners' coping with the mystery of their arrest in the Great Purge are catalogued in Alexander Weissberg's account of his Soviet prison experience before he was handed over to the Gestapo after the Molotov-Ribbentrop agreement (*The Accused*, trans. Edward Fitzgerald [New York: Simon and Shuster, 1952]).

[33] See also Toker, *Return from the Archipelago*, 219-20 and 289-90n19.

[34] Koestler, *Darkness at Noon*, 209.

[35] The emotion of disgust is the diametrical opposite of the sense of the sublime

which is an integral part of the religious worldview. Awe, indeed, is replaced by contempt. On the relationship between contempt and disgust see Antonio Damasio, *Looking for Spinoza: Joy, Sorrow, and the Feeling Brain* (Orlando: Harcourt, 2003), 45. For these comments I am indebted to Emily Budick and Na'ama Cohen-Hanegbi.

[36] Nor was this necessarily disgust with camp sexual mores, in particular among the criminal convicts. The contempt with which sexual (and especially homosexual) practises among prisoners are dealt with in some of the literature raises different issues; see Adi Kuntsman, ''With a Shade of Disgust': Affective Politics of Sexuality and Class in Memoirs of the Stalinist Gulag,' *Slavic Review* 68 (2009): 302-28.

[37] These reasons are discussed in detail by Nanci Adler in *The Gulag Survivor: Beyond the Soviet System* (New Brunswick: Transaction, 2002), and, in particular, in *Keeping Faith with the Party*. Further evidence is given throughout Jehanne M. Gheith and Katherine R. Jolluck's collection of interviews and documents, *Gulag Voices: Oral Histories of Soviet Incarceration and Exile* (New York: Palgrave Macmillan, 2011).

Bibliography

Adler, Nanci. *The Gulag Survivor: Beyond the Soviet System.* New Brunswick: Transaction, 2002.

———. *Keeping Faith with the Party: Communist Believers Return from the Gulag.* Bloomington: Indiana University Press, 2012.

Borges, Jorge Luis. 'Three Versions of Judas.' In *Labyrinths: Selected Stories and Other Writings*. Translated by James E. Irby, 95-100. New York: New Directions, 1964.

Bruner, Jerome. *Acts of Meaning.* Cambridge, MA: Harvard University Press, 1990.

Camon, Ferdinando. *Conversations with Primo Levi.* Translated by John Shepley. Marlboro: Marlboro Press, 1989 [1987].

Clendinnen, Inga. *Reading the Holocaust*. Cambridge: Cambridge University Press, 1999.

Damasio, Antonio. *Looking for Spinoza: Joy, Sorrow, and the Feeling Brain.* Orlando: Harcourt, 2003.

Dombrovskii, Iurii. 'Iz zapisok Zybina.' *Vestnik russkogo studencheskogo khristianskogo dvizheniia* 177 (1977): 104-25.

Eliach, Yaffa. *Hasidic Tales of the Holocaust.* Oxford: Oxford University Press, 1982.

Fackenheim, Emil L. *To Mend the World: Foundations of Future Jewish Thought*, New York: Schocken, 1982.

Gheith, Jehanne M. and Katherine R. Jolluck, eds. *Gulag Voices: Oral Histories of Soviet Incarceration and Exile.* New York: Palgrave Macmillan, 2011.

Halfin, Igal. *Stalinist Confessions: Messianism and Terror in the Leningrad Communist University.* Pittsburgh: University of Pittsburgh Press, 2009.

Harrison, Bernard. *Inconvenient Fictions: Literature and the Limits of Theory.* New Haven: Yale University Press, 1991.

Huberband, Shimon. *Kiddush Hashem: Jewish Religious and Cultural Life in Poland During the Holocaust.* Translated by David E. Fishman. Edited by Jeffrey S. Gurock and Robert S. Hirt. Hoboken: Ktav, 1987. Hebrew version, translated from the Yiddish by Joseph Kemish. Edited by Nachman Blumental. Tel Aviv: Zakhor, 1969.

'Jewish Values in the Post-Holocaust Future: A Symposium.' *Judaism* 16 (1967): 266-99.

Klinghoffer, Arthur Jay. *Red Apocalypse: The Religious Evolution of Soviet Communism.* Lanham: University Press of America, 1996.

Koestler, Arthur. *Darkness at Noon.* New York: Macmillan, 1975 [1941].

Kuntsman, Adi. ''With a Shade of Disgust': Affective Politics of Sexuality and Class in Memoirs of the Stalinist Gulag.' *Slavic Review* 68/2 (2009): 302-28.

Landes, Daniel. 1983. 'Spiritual Responses in the Camps.' In *Genocide: Critical Issues of the Holocaust. A Companion to the film GENOCIDE.* Edited by Alex Grobman and Daniel Landes, 261-78. Los Angeles: The Simon Wiesenthal Center, 1983.

Le Guin, Ursula K. 'The Ones Who Walk Away from Omelas.' In *The Wind's Twelve Quarters*, 175-84. London: Victor Gollancz, 1975. Originally published by New Dimensions, 1973.

Levi, Primo. *If This Is a Man / The Truce.* Translated by Stuart Woolf. London: Abacus, 1990. First published in English by Bodley Head, 1965.

———. *Moments of Reprieve.* Translated by Ruth Feldman. London: Abacus, 1987 [1981].

Littell, Jonathan. *Les Bienveillantes.* Paris: Gallimard, 2006. English translation by Charlotte Mandell, *The Kindly Ones.* New York: HarperCollins, 2009.

Morris, David B. *The Culture of Pain.* Berkeley: University of California Press, 1993 [1991].

Olitskaia, Ekaterina. *Moi vospominaniia.* Frankfurt: Possev, 1971.

Porat, Dina. *The Fall of a Sparrow: The Life and Times of Abba Kovner.* Translated by Elizabeth Yuval. Stanford: Stanford University Press, 2010. Originally published in Hebrew under the title *Me'ever le-gishmi.* Jerusalem: Yad Vashem and Am Oved, 2000.

Roskies, David G. *Against the Apocalypse: Responses to Catastrophe in Modern Jewish Culture.* Cambridge: Harvard University Press, 1984.

Segev, Tom. *The Seventh Million: The Israelis and the Holocaust.* Translated by Haim Watzman. New York: Hill and Wang, 1993 [1991].

Sherwin, Byron L. 'Jewish Messianism and Elie Wiesel.' *Notre Dame English Journal* 11 (1978): 33-46.

Singer, Isaac Bashevis. *The Penitent.* Translated by Joseph Singer. Harmondsworth: Penguin, 1983.

Solzhenitsyn, Aleksandr. *The Gulag Archipelago: An Experiment in Literary Investigation.* 3 vols. Translated by Thomas P. Whitney (vols. 1 and 2) and Harry Willetts (vol. 3). New York: Harper & Row, 1978. Original: *Arkhipelag Gulag: Opyt khudozhestvennogo issledovaniia.* Paris: YMCA Press, 1973-1975.

Toker, Leona. *Return from the Archipelago: Narratives of Gulag Survivors*. Bloomington: Indiana University Press, 2000.

Weissberg, Alex. *The Accused*. Translated by Edward Fitzgerald. New York: Simon and Shuster, 1952. Also published as *The Conspiracy of Silence*. London: Hamish Hamilton, 1952.

Wiesel, Elie. *All Rivers Run to the Sea*. New York: Schocken, 1995 [1994].

———. Comments in 'Jewish Values,' 1967: 281-84.

———. *Night*. Translated from the French by Stella Rodway. New York: Bantam, 1982 [1960].

———. *One Generation After*. Translated by Lily Edelman and the author. New York: Random House, 1970.

Pain and Blame: Psychological Approaches to Obstetric Pain, 1950-1980

Paula A. Michaels

Abstract
This chapter[1] reconstructs the recent history of pain in childbirth, a universal physiological phenomenon intertwined with the socio-cultural context in which it unfolds. It focuses on the period from the 1950s through the 1970s, a time of flux in the understanding of childbirth pain within the medical profession and the general public. This era witnessed an emphasis on the role of female psychology in obstetric pain. Two similar psychological approaches to obstetric pain emerged: natural childbirth, promoted by British physician Grantly Dick-Read, and psychoprophylaxis, developed by Soviet neuropsychologist I. Z. Vel'vovskii and popularized in the West by French obstetrician Fernand Lamaze. In an effort to highlight trans-national influences and national idiosyncrasies, I take a comparative approach to the meanings attributed to childbirth pain in France and the United States, viewing them against related relevant developments in the Soviet Union and the United Kingdom and tracing the ways in which the dynamic, dialogic clinical encounter between medical practitioners and their patients inscribed shifting social meanings and values on labour pain.

Key Words: Natural childbirth, labour, obstetrics, psychoprophylaxis, Vel'vovskii, Lamaze, Soviet Union, France, Dick-Read, birth stories.

*****

Elisabeth Bing (b. 1914) has dedicated her life to improving the experience of birth in the United States. For more than six decades she taught childbirth education classes in New York City, and over those many years her underlying perspective on birth and its role in a woman's life as an empowering and transformative experience has remained consistent.[2] 'Giving birth is the most creative thing a woman can do,' she asserts.[3] Her courses promote the idea that childbirth is a normal, natural process and that pregnancy, labour, and birth need not be approached as 'a disease from which women have to be cured.'[4] Through her ability to give birth without resort to pharmacological pain relief, to experience what is colloquially known as 'natural childbirth,' a woman gains new insight into her strengths and abilities. Along with her promotion of non-anesthetized birth, Bing has spent her career advocating the presence and active role of the father during labour and birth; rooming-in, which allows the newborn to stay in the mother's hospital room, rather than in a nursery; and breastfeeding.

Bing's work has helped to transform the American birth into a more 'family-centred' experience. 'We fought to humanize obstetrics and we have been quite successful,' Bing said in a 2000 interview.[5] The presence of fathers and other loved ones is now the norm in American maternity wards. Breastfeeding is strongly encouraged and rooming-in is popular. Only in the realm of obstetric pain management did Bing's aspirations fail to take root in the long term. Bing's belief in the benefits of unanaesthetised birth is today out-of-step with the views of most women in the United States, where 3 out of 4 births involve epidural anaesthesia. In 2001, Bing observed, 'women are not on our side anymore. They are too reliant on machines and want to get childbirth over quickly. They no longer care about achieving anything with their bodies.'[6] Unlike their mothers, relatively few American women of childbearing age today see the point of going through the pain of labour and birth when epidurals allow them to be awake and aware throughout their labour and to participate actively in bringing their child into the world without having to endure discomfort. Bing's judgment of these women is clear, as is her appreciation that her own views have fallen out of favour. 'It isn't just the epidural - it's the attitude toward childbirth. ... Even with regard to pain - there is no satisfaction achieved because the woman does not have to work for anything. We've minimized the sense of achievement one obtains when mastering a difficult experience.'[7] One could certainly challenge Bing's claim that a birth with epidural anaesthesia is an unsatisfying experience, but she is correct that natural childbirth is out of fashion.

Bing's disappointment is understandable. She saw her struggle for natural childbirth as standard for American women rise and fall within one generation. With roots in the 1940s and 1950s, natural childbirth in the United States reached its heyday in the 1970s, after which the number of women seeking to forego the use of anaesthesia began to decline. And the United States was not the only site for opposition to the use of obstetric anaesthesia. For reasons that varied from place to place, the mid-twentieth century witnessed a period of intense debate across Europe, North America and beyond over the origin, meaning and management of labour pain and the role of anaesthesia in birth.

This chapter reconstructs this recent history of pain in childbirth, a universal physiological phenomenon inextricably intertwined with the socio-cultural context in which it unfolds.[8] It deals mainly with the period from the 1950s through the 1970s, an era of acute flux in the understanding of childbirth pain within the medical profession and the general public. Unlike any time before or since, this period witnessed a remarkable emphasis on the role of female psychology in obstetric pain. In an effort to highlight both trans-national influences and national idiosyncrasies, I take a comparative approach to the meanings attributed to childbirth pain. I focus on two distinct national settings, France and the United States, and situate trends there in the context of related, relevant developments in the Soviet Union and the United Kingdom. Two similar psychological approaches to obstetric pain emerged in this era: natural childbirth, promoted by British physician Grantly Dick-Read, and psychoprophylaxis, developed by Soviet psychologist I. Z. Vel'vovskii and popularized in the West through the efforts of French obstetrician Fernand Lamaze. In France, psychoprophylaxis enjoyed far greater popularity than natural childbirth. In the U.S., natural childbirth gained a foothold first, but was then overtaken by and fused with psychoprophylaxis, and the lines between the two became muddy. This chapter aims to expose the ways that the dynamic, dialogic clinical encounter between medical practitioners and their patients inscribed shifting social meanings and values on labour pain in diverse national contexts.

In 1933, Grantly Dick-Read coined the term 'natural childbirth' to describe a satisfying, calm, relaxed birth experience with little or no resort to pharmacological pain relief. Dick-Read's vision of a drug-free birth bucked the trend in obstetric practice at the time. Most British and American urban middle- and upper-class women of the time turned to pharmacological pain relief in labour and birth. The use of nitrous oxide was common among British women, while American women favoured so-called twilight sleep, which combined morphine for pain relief with the amnesic scopolamine. Women drifted in and out of consciousness, frequently needing the aid of forceps to deliver their babies and waking with no memory of having given birth. Dick-Read believed that there was a better, safer, more satisfying way to have babies. Though the phrase 'natural childbirth' came to be a generic way of describing any birth without the use of pharmacological pain relief, for Dick-Read it meant a specific program to prepare a woman for a drug-free labour and birth. Pain management was achieved through deep relaxation and a calm demeanour attained with a proper education in the physiology of pregnancy, labour and delivery. In Dick-Read's estimation, any normal, healthy woman could experience a joyful childbirth without suffering. The mother-to-be had to work hard, certainly, and labour and birth would not necessarily be without some discomfort, but Dick-Read believed that the kind of anguish thought to be an unavoidable part of childbirth was largely the product of women's minds, not their bodies. Modern civilization, in Dick-Read's view, had robbed women of mastery of their own bodies, and of faith in their abilities to endure the rigors of labour. Girls grew up hearing that childbirth was an excruciating, at times fatal experience. Friends and relatives stoked expectant mothers' anxieties with horror stories of their own birth experiences. Anaesthesia denied women the ability to bear witness to and participate in the sacred act of childbirth. Education and training in relaxation fully prepared women for what lay ahead, removing the fear of pain and of the unknown in childbirth. In the first decades of the twentieth century, childbirth education classes were almost non-existent in Dick-Read's Great

Britain and, with the exception of a few urban areas, they were largely unknown in the United States as well.[9] No one routinely taught women what was happening with their pregnant bodies or explained to them what to expect during labour and birth. Dick-Read theorized that childbirth was a naturally painless process, but that fear created muscular tension, which in turn rendered labour and birth painful, a process he described as the fear-tension-pain cycle. 'Tense woman, tense cervix,' he wrote. 'All obstetricians know the effect of a tense cervix: pain, resistance at the outlet and the innumerable complications of a prolonged labor.'[10] Women's minds, not their bodies, made birth painful in his estimation. To return the birth experience to its normal, naturally painless state, it was not anaesthesia they needed, but education and psychological preparation.[11]

For more than a quarter-century after the publication of his first book, until his death in 1959, Dick-Read crusaded to spread his particular approach to unanaesthetised birth. Amid concerns about the effect of anaesthetics on the newborn and women's dissatisfaction with their experience of childbirth, a growing number of expectant mothers and their doctors became partisans of the Dick-Read method in Great Britain and abroad, especially in the United States and, to a lesser extent, elsewhere in the Anglophone world. Dick-Read played a central role in the popularization of childbirth preparation classes in both the U.K. and the U.S. The timing of the 1943 publication of his book *Childbirth without Fear*, an elaboration of the ideas he first articulated in his 1933 *Natural Childbirth*, could not have been more perfect, as World War II wound down and a baby boom took off on both sides of the Atlantic.

Unaware of Dick-Read's work on natural childbirth, medical researchers in the Soviet Union struggled with the same questions about how best to manage the pain of labour and independently came to similar conclusions. In the wake of the catastrophic demographic impact of World War II, the Soviet state sought to raise the birth rate. The USSR enjoyed a post-war baby boom but, unlike its former allies in the West, it suffered from profound shortages of anaesthetics and analgesics. With a pharmaceutical industry unable to meet obstetric demands, it is not surprising that Soviet authorities turned to psychological means of pain relief. Vel'vovskii developed the psychoprophylactic method as a means to ease labour pain without the use of anaesthetics and analgesics. With more than twenty years of research into the application of hypnosis in childbirth, Vel'vovskii sought a more efficient, less time-consuming psychological approach to pain relief. Vel'vovskii's method of psychoprophylaxis attacked the pain of labour in several ways. Like Dick-Read's natural childbirth, a didactic approach to the physiology of pregnancy, labour and birth prepared women by eliminating fear of the unknown. The power of suggestion further eroded negative expectations, as obstetricians emphasised to expectant mothers that they should anticipate a painless labour and birth. Psychoprophylaxis also stressed, far more than in Dick-Read's natural childbirth, the role of conscious relaxation and breathing patterns during labour. Rapid, panting breaths and deep, cleansing breaths were believed to occupy the cerebral cortex and interfere with the transmission of pain signals from the uterus to the brain. Light massage and pressure alleviated residual breakthrough pain. Pavlovian notions of conditional response legitimated psychoprophylaxis, as the method's proponents pointed to the source of its efficacy in the undoing of negative conditioning through education and in the creation of a new set of conditional responses through preparatory work in patterned breathing.[12]

Psychoprophylaxis enjoyed a meteoric rise in the USSR and beyond. Vel'vovskii developed the method in 1948-1949, and it became national policy in the USSR in early 1951, when the Ministry of Public Health launched a campaign for its promotion. Psychoprophylaxis received the state's enthusiastic support because it required relatively little financial investment, had the added appeal of being legitimated on the basis of work by Russia's famous scientist, and supported the regime's pro-natalist agenda. In the summer of 1951, obstetrician Fernand Lamaze travelled to the USSR with a delegation of French communists and their allies to learn about the state of affairs in Soviet medicine and public health. Lamaze witnessed a birth using psychoprophylaxis and returned to France on a mission to spread word of this new gospel. In March 1952, the first French birth using psychoprophylaxis took place at Lamaze's maternity ward at the Pierre Rouquès Metallurgists' Polyclinic. Popularly known as Les Bluets, the polyclinic became a psychoprophylactic training centre where students from all over the world came to learn from Lamaze. At the same time, the USSR promoted the method across Eastern Europe and in the People's Republic of China.

One of Lamaze's patients was American expatriate Marjorie Karmel. So delighted was she with psychoprophylaxis that when she returned to New York City, she wanted to have her second child the same way. Unable to find an American obstetrician willing to support her desires, she was inspired to write *Thank You, Dr. Lamaze*, which appeared in 1959 and helped to catalyse the Lamaze movement in the U.S.[13] In 1960, she joined forces with Elisabeth Bing, who had for more than a decade worked as a childbirth educator and promoter of the Dick-Read method, and obstetrician Benjamin Segal to found the American Society for Psychoprophylaxis in Obstetrics (ASPO), now known as Lamaze International.[14]

Early on ASPO sought to distinguish psychoprophylaxis from the widely known and similar Read method, emphasising the more sophisticated Pavlovian theoretical foundation and more rigorous clinical study of psychoprophylaxis. Lamaze advocates argued that the greater attention to the role of controlled breathing in the mitigation of labour pain and a more conscious, active psychological engagement with the process of labour differentiated psychoprophylaxis from natural childbirth. ASPO leaders also worked to obscure the Soviet origins of psychoprophylaxis, 'given how Americans were feeling about Russians' amid the Cold War.[15] The term 'psychoprophylaxis' faded from use in the U.S., where the method took on the name of the French obstetrician who had brought it across the Iron Curtain.

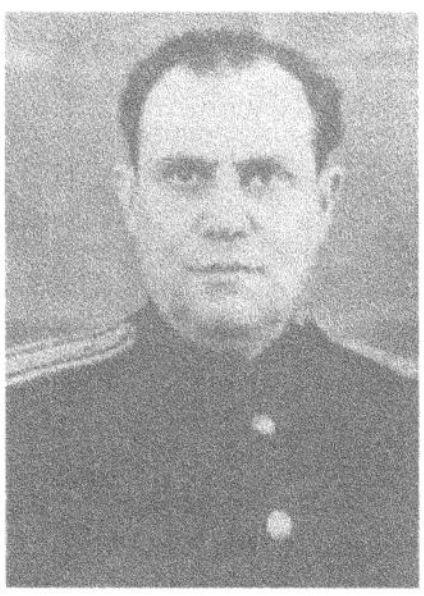

Fig. 1. I. Z. Vel'vovskii, c. 1940s.
Courtesy of Kharkiv Medical Academy of Postgraduate Education

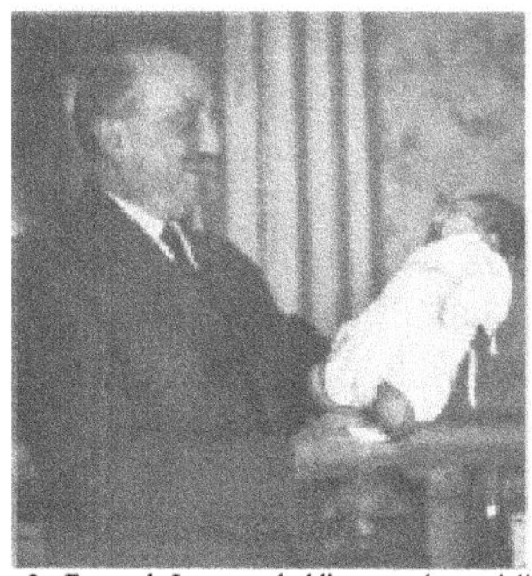

Fig. 2. Fernand Lamaze holding newborn delivered to singer-actress Deanna Durbin, 1951. From Caroline Gutmann, *The Legacy of Doctor Lamaze: The Story of the Man who Changed Childbirth* (New York: St. Martin's Press, 2001). Reproduced with permission

The success of the Lamaze movement in the United States and elsewhere in the Anglophone world to a great extent built and expanded on Dick-Read's effort to promote natural childbirth, even if partisans took pains to draw a bright line between the two approaches. Intense and acrimonious debates over which method was most effective and how precisely they differed marked these rivalries in the 1950s and 1960s. By the 1970s, these arguments receded, dismissed by most childbirth educators, obstetricians and mothers as petty disputes that only detracted from the common goal of promoting birth without the routine use of anaesthesia.[16] 'Natural childbirth' and the 'Lamaze method' became virtually synonymous in the 1970s.

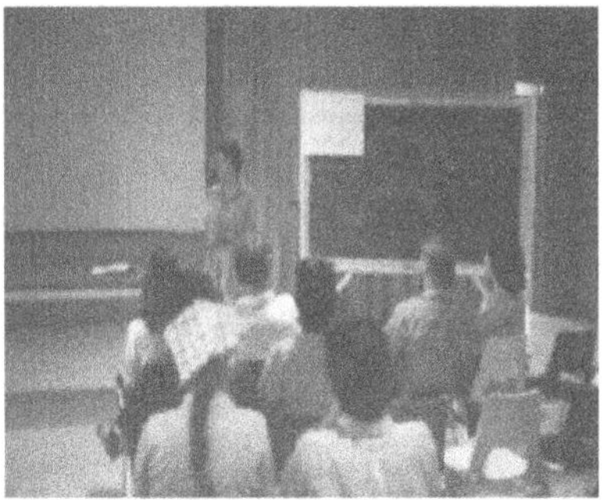

Fig. 3. U.S. childbirth preparation instruction, c. 1970s. Courtesy of The Schlesinger Library, Radcliffe Institute, Harvard University

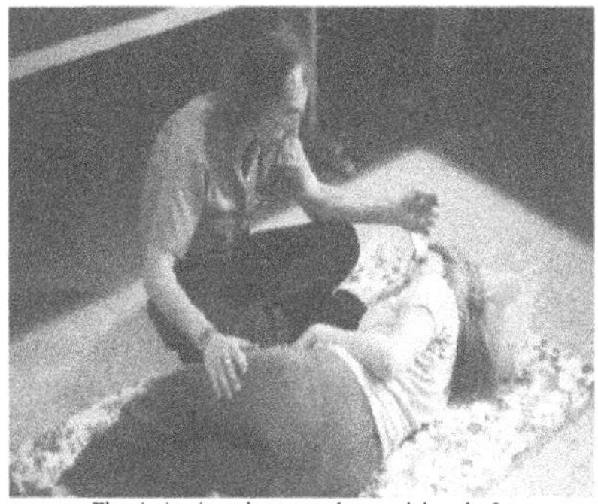

Fig. 4. An American couple practicing the Lamaze method, c. 1970s. Courtesy of The Schlesinger Library, Radcliffe Institute, Harvard University

Despite their diverse origins and different emphases, the shared, underlying assumption of Dick-Read, Vel'vovskii, Lamaze, and their allies was that labour pain was largely or wholly psychogenic in origin. Conveying a perspective very much like that of Dick-Read, one early Soviet promoter of psychoprophylaxis, obstetrician A. P. Nikolaev, quipped that 'if [there's a] head . . . in any way responsible for labour pain, it is not the head of the fetus but that of the mother.'[17] Lamaze shared these views, stating that 'the affective quality of a painful sensation lies in its subjective perception.'[18] Put simply, labour was experienced in the body, but interpreted in the mind. Soviet proponents of psychoprophylaxis were inclined to emphasise materialist, Pavlovian explanations of the relative strength or weakness of a woman's nervous system as the source of labour pain; for political and ideological reasons, their leftist French allies tended to rely on these same justifications. Like Dick-Read's supporters in Great Britain and the U.S., more conservative elements of the French medical profession favoured Freudian interpretations of the mind's role in obstetric pain. These obstetricians and psychologists came to see a woman's subconscious desires and early childhood experiences as the source of her physical suffering during childbirth.[19] Irrespective of the details, psychology, not anaesthesiology, was the answer.

For many women and their obstetric caregivers in France, the United States, and elsewhere, the assertion that the solution to labour pain lay in psychological training implied a corollary: women who experienced labour pain despite prenatal training demonstrated a psychological failing, a weak nervous system, or some other flaw that made them responsible for their own labour pain. Doctors' judgmental attitudes come through clearly in their evaluations of patient comportment during labour and birth. New York City obstetrician Benjamin Segal described the November 1961 birth of one Mrs. S.'s son as 'a complete failure':

> Judging by patient's attitude antenatally - one of inordinate sense of 'everything is all right' with no questions for the obstetrician, creating a cloak of safety in the method, safety from any harm - necessary for the patient's emotional insecurity (complete ten finger nail biting). One could expect poor results. This became manifest early in labour with tossing about, restlessness and moaning - long before any average patient trained or untrained would or might so respond even with obstetric abnormality. Also patient pushed in 2nd stage, it was done frantically and with groaning.[20]

For Segal and other devotees of psychoprophylaxis, failure meant that the parturient experienced pain and expressed that pain outwardly, through screaming, crying, grimacing, writhing or other behavioural signals. Overwhelmed and in despair, some women demanded the use of anaesthesia, the hallmark of failure.[21]

Advocates of psychoprophylaxis ascribed partial or total failure to two kinds of sources: those related to the method's application and those 'due to the woman herself.'[22] A noisy maternity ward, a hostile staff or poor preparatory instruction could all contribute to inadequate pain relief. More often than not, the obstetricians, psychologists, and childbirth educators who assessed patient performance attributed failure to 'the fragility [of a woman's] cortical equilibrium. The event that leads to failure can be in the distant past, recent, or at the time of labour itself,' asserted Pierre Vellay, an obstetrician at Les Bluets and Lamaze's closest collaborator.[23] Segal's remarks, above, make clear his scepticism that Mrs. S.'s pain had physiological, rather than psychogenic origin. He attributed its severity to her 'emotional insecurity.' That she expressed her pain through writhing and moaning early in her labour attested in his eyes to her need for drama. With this judgment came blame of the parturient for her own suffering and a refusal to entertain the possibility that the method itself may have been of limited efficacy.

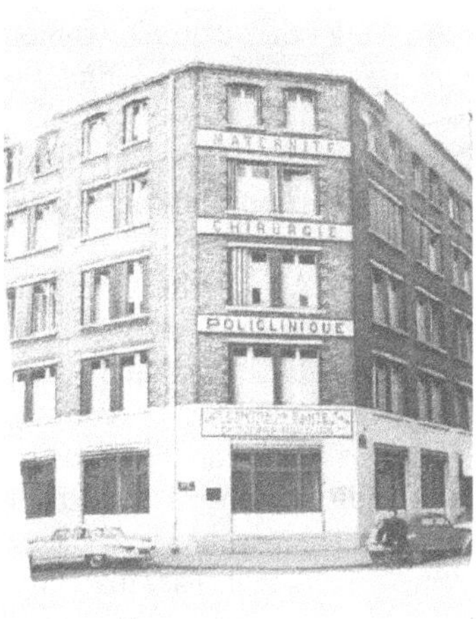

Fig. 5. Pierre Rouquès Metallurgists Polyclinic, c. 1950s. From Caroline Gutmann, *The Legacy of Doctor Lamaze: The Story of the Man who Changed Childbirth* (New York: St. Martin's Press, 2001). Reproduced with permission

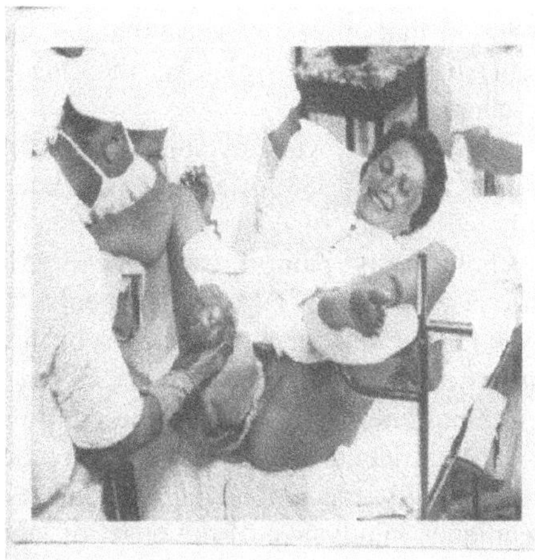

Fig. 6. French woman giving birth using psychoprophylaxis, attended by Pierre Vellay, c. 1960s. Courtesy of The Schlesinger Library, Radcliffe Institute, Harvard University

The ways in which medical personnel were quick to turn to psychological explanations for women's pain and suffering is well-illustrated by the post-partum experience of a Frenchwoman who gave birth at Les Bluets in the mid-1970s. She had an episiotomy that required a couple of stitches. Four months after her birth, however, she continued to have perineal pain and sought help. The gynaecologist at Les Bluets 'saw nothing there but told me that it was 'psychological.'' She returned several times complaining of pain and was repeatedly told that the problem was wholly in her mind. She began to fret about her mental state in light of what the doctors said, even telling herself 'I should see a psychiatrist if this continues.' After six months, she went to see a gynaecologist at another clinic. He found an infection where the thread from the stitches had neither been absorbed into the tissue nor been removed.[24] The quick resorting to a psychological explanation for this woman's pain is far from atypical. Recent studies demonstrate that women continue to receive less treatment for pain than men and are more frequently than men prescribed sedatives rather than pain relievers in response to complaints of pain.[25]

One is not surprised to find that women often internalized and mirrored the assessments of their performance by obstetric caregivers. Testimonials from French mothers in the 1950s speak about women's expectations for and experience of pain in childbirth. These birth stories are frequently marked by women's regret that they had let down their caregivers and themselves. They shoulder responsibility for their failures and express hope to do better the next time. What is conspicuously absent from birth stories of that era is any sense that anyone or anything other than the women themselves play a role in the inadequate pain relief they find in psychoprophylaxis.

Mrs. L., who gave birth to her first child at Lamaze's maternity ward in Paris in June 1953, offers a typical tale of a failed psychoprophylactic birth and the sense of regret that often accompanied this physically and psychologically painful experience. 'An hour after Anne's birth, I was furious with myself,' Mrs. L. laments. 'I had refused to push my baby out myself.' She describes her baby's birth as 'a painful test' that, rather than cause her to question the efficacy of psychoprophylaxis, led her to redouble her commitment 'to dominate and control [her] nerves' better on the occasion of her next labour and birth. Before recounting the birth itself, Mrs. L. takes responsibility for not having adequately practiced the psychoprophylactic techniques in advance of the onset of labour. She asserts that, paradoxically, though she appeared on the surface to have wanted to participate actively in childbirth, she 'had [unconsciously] decided from the first day of [her] pregnancy that [she] did not want to help in the birth of [her] baby.' Despite demonstrating calm and control throughout her labour, when it came time to birth the baby, Mrs. L. 'demanded to be put to sleep. The doctor told me to keep going and push, but I refused.' He obliged, but afterward, she writes, 'I . . . regret having asked for the mask' for anaesthesia.[26] What precisely led Mrs. L. to demand pharmacological pain relief we can never know, but from her testimony it is clear that she took upon herself sole responsibility for the course of her labour. She took pride in having done well initially, but also shouldered the blame for resorting to the use of drugs to aid her in her delivery.

American birth narratives from the 1960s break with the stories French women told about their experience of pain. They also diverge from the understanding of childbirth pain offered by Lamaze advocates in the American medical community. Even in the 1960s, when Dr. Segal and other ASPO leaders concurred with the French that labour pain was primarily psychogenic, American women showed an acceptance of pain as part of a normal, natural birth. The experience of pain, even severe pain, did not deter women from understanding their psychoprophylactic births as successful even if their obstetricians might have labelled them failures. For example, one Mrs. N. gave birth in New York City in 1964 and shortly afterward wrote a letter to her childbirth educator describing her birth experience. 'For me it was not childbirth without pain, . . . for I had the same sensations with my first [untrained] delivery and I remember them as painful. But this time I had something to do, I did it, and each contraction was a chance to do better.'[27] For Mrs. N. the presence of pain did not detract from the value of psychoprophylactic training, even if the method was being promoted as capable of rendering childbirth painless. Mrs. N. saw the value of psychoprophylaxis not in the elimination of pain, but in its impact on the attitude toward pain.

In Mrs. N.'s equanimity toward the presence of pain despite the use of psychoprophylaxis we may see evidence of Dick-Read's continuing influence. Unlike psychoprophylaxis's orthodox advocates, who stressed the mind's ability to eliminate pain through psychological conditioning, Dick-Read made it clear in his writings that birth is, at times, uncomfortable but that the pain need not cross into the realm of suffering. Natural childbirth preparation enabled many women to cope with rather than escape pain. In France, where Dick-Read's influence was minimal and where the psychoprophylactic method enjoyed far greater popularity, there seem to have been higher expectations for the absence of pain. In the United States, where nearly two decades of exposure to Dick-Read's theories about 'childbirth without fear' preceded the arrival of psychoprophylaxis, women appear to have sought not the elimination of pain, but tools for its management. While medical professionals like Dr. Segal may have subscribed to the same standards and expectations for the absence of pain as their French colleagues, expectant mothers seem to have remained under the continuing influence of Dick-Read's more modest aspirations for a joyous and fearless, not painless labour and birth.

Interestingly, American women's thinking at this juncture approached that of most medical professionals in the USSR after 1956, when destalinization led to more frank conversations about medical research methods and clinical practice. Soviet obstetricians became increasingly vocal about the limitations of psychoprophylaxis. No longer touting it as a virtual panacea for obstetric pain, they began to deemphasise the anaesthetic effect of psychoprophylaxis and to underscore the method's value as a means to promote calm, quiet, compliant behaviour in labouring women.[28] Hamstrung by the continuing underperformance of the pharmaceutical industry, Soviet obstetricians had few means at their disposal to alleviate women's suffering in childbirth once they became disenchanted with the anaesthetizing capabilities of psychoprophylaxis. Though archival records claim that psychoprophylactic training persisted through the late-Soviet era, anecdotal evidence suggests that not only did prenatal training all but disappear from the Soviet obstetric landscape but a cavalier and even cruel attitude toward women's pain and suffering persisted.[29] Prenatal lectures reportedly offered advice that was 'superficial, consisting mainly of homilies about the importance of walks and the dangers of sweets. Such crucial subjects as breathing and massaging the stomach during labour [were] rarely mentioned more than once.'[30] Dr. Ol'ga Valentinovna Grishchenko, a third-generation Kharkiv physician, observed that in the waning years of the USSR women were not compelled to attend childbirth preparation courses, and the double burden of working full time both inside and outside the home often kept them away.[31] In well-equipped urban hospitals, a woman screaming in pain might receive some medication if her fuss began to irritate the midwife or obstetrician, but otherwise women's suffering met with indifference, and horror stories abound about the squalor and inhumanity of Soviet maternity wards.[32]

Unlike their Soviet sisters, French women in the 1970s had the ability and opportunity to raise their voices in protest against conditions that they considered unacceptable. In the changed atmosphere of feminist empowerment, newly granted access to birth control (1967), and legalised abortion (1975), French women decried the idealization of psychoprophylactic births.[33] In contrast to an earlier generation that drove blame inward, they channelled their anger at the hospital staff, the physical layout of the maternity ward, the regimentation and organization of ward practices, and the limitations of the method itself. They denounced proponents of psychoprophylaxis for misleading women with fairy tales about the method's efficacy and benefits, touted as scientifically proven. A thirty-year-old mother of three, Veronique, described psychoprophylactic training as 'a disaster' that inadequately prepared women for the harsh reality of birth. In her estimation, filling women's heads with stories of easy, beautiful, and painless labour did little to ready women for birth. 'That is why I felt cheated during my birth. ... [T]here is a moment when suffering is unbearable, and I was enraged. Telling women such nonsense seems monstrous to me.'[34] It is unclear whether we see in Veronique's testimony a different attitude toward psychoprophylaxis among women who experienced pain, or we can merely hear her voice more clearly because it is not mediated by the doctors who cherry-picked women's testimony for publication in the 1950s. Veronique's birth story too was selected and edited, and must be understood in the context of the book in which it appeared: Maria-José Jaubert's scathing exposé of psychoprophylaxis as a 'myth.' However, a leap in the sheer quantity of negative comments regarding psychoprophylaxis suggests something more than mere editorial sleight-of-hand at work in the 1970s. Some of this increase in the volume of complaints may be attributable to the dramatic rise in the number of women using psychoprophylaxis. By the close of the 1970s, the Lamaze method was taught universally in French maternity hospitals.[35] Nonetheless, women's changing desires and expectations for themselves and their caregivers must also account for some of this increasingly voluble outcry against psychoprophylaxis.

The rise in patient dissatisfaction is evident in exit surveys completed within a week of giving birth at Les Bluets in the mid-1970s. Along with unsolicited letters, these unpublished documents offer a window into women's assessments made when they were fresh and when they thought they had the ears of those who could effect change. These sources attest to many satisfied new mothers at the clinic where psychoprophylactic practice in France originated, but complaints also surface about everything from poor food to rough toilet paper. Among their disappointments, many women underscored their lack of pain relief from psychoprophylaxis and their resentment that obstetric staff, at least on occasion, denied them pharmacological pain relief despite explicit requests. Rather than risk being refused access to anaesthesia if she needed it, a Madame E. left the care of Les Bluets before her baby's arrival: 'I would be terrified by the idea of giving birth in your clinic, thinking that no one would really help me, but instead test my training or judge if I had prepared well or poorly.'[36] The remarks of a Madame P. show just how much Madame E. was right to be fearful. In 1976, Madame P. wrote that 'after 6 centimetres dilation, the pain was intense. Despite the encouragement of the midwife about my 'good cooperation' and 'good preparation,' . . . I would have preferred an epidural, because I have not chosen to be a masochist.'[37] Not only does Madame P.'s testimony imply that the staff dismissed the severity of women's pain by denying access to pharmacological pain relief, but her reference to the midwife's compliment that she had shown 'good cooperation' reveals the way in which medical staff may have sought to ease their own burden by encouraging compliant behaviour with praise. Rather than yield to these expectations, French women in the 1970s fought against being straitjacketed into narrow definitions of the ideal patient, demanded pharmacological pain relief, sought obstetric care elsewhere when drugs appeared not to be forthcoming, and rejected personal culpability for their inability to find psychoprophylaxis an effective tool for pain management.

In France, demands for drugs translated into empowerment, but amid the U.S.'s highly medicalised way of birth it was the refusal of drugs that affirmed women's authority. In her seminal 1976 *Immaculate Deception*, Suzanne Arms sounded the clarion call to rebellion against what she characterised as the infantilisation and disempowerment of women in American birth practices. In a 2002 interview, Arms recalled the traumatic experience of her daughter Molly's birth in 1970 and how it inspired her to write her denunciation of conventional American obstetrics. The labour was

> a nightmare . . . and yet certainly all too typical. ... My labour was so manipulated; my body didn't know what to do. I was a very compliant patient. I let go of my entire college-educated, competent-woman persona and reverted, as many women do in labour, to my child self. In my case, my child self was a pleaser who tried to avoid blaming and shaming and abuse by reading the needs of the adults around me and doing what is needed in order to gain approval. I was a nice little girl from New Jersey, raised . . . to be docile.[38]

For those like Arms who experienced traumatic births, and for those inspired by their stories to seek a different kind of birth experience, childbirth without pharmacological pain relief offered a chance to find in the pain of labour a way to wrest control of birth from the almost exclusively male ranks of obstetricians and assert female power and authority. For American women with a budding feminist consciousness, unanaesthetised childbirth meant resistance to patriarchal obstetric authority. These beliefs dovetailed with the Zeitgeist among middle-class, educated, white women, 'arising out of the 'hippie,' 'back-to-the-land,' and 'natural living' movements of the late 1960s.'[39]

Arms reflected and nurtured a culture that lionised women who demonstrated an ability to endure the pain of birth. American women in the 1970s wrote and spoke about the hard work of labour and their triumph in the face of it as something profoundly empowering, not because they had managed to suppress or avoid pain but precisely because they had embraced the challenge of it and experienced it fully. Success in this context meant not the absence of pain but an ability to cope with and 'stay on top' of pain, at times extreme pain, which was taken to be a normal part of labour. American valorisation of pain elevated natural childbirth to a rite of passage for many educated, middle-class white American women and their partners. Writing in a 1970 newsletter for the Los Angeles chapter of ASPO, one new father captured the sense of natural childbirth as an attestation of a woman's strength and power. Describing his wife's giving birth, which he witnessed, he noted that

> within the borders of Lamaze control she was a she-wolf, fighting with all her soul and heart - and deeply enjoying it. ... [I]n delivery she tapped some mysterious source of power and unleashed a force unlike anything else I have ever seen. ... [S]he was Woman and by that I don't mean don't-muss-my-hair woman, or eek-a-mouse woman; I mean Woman of the earth and sky and origins, the creator, the living source of love and caring and strength. And in that wet-faced, vein-stretching baretoothed effort, she was truly beautiful.[40]

This young father's words, of course, suggest the link between the natural childbirth movement and the American counterculture, with its affinity for anti-materialist, anti-consumerist spirituality. This conceptualisation of the Lamaze method as something that could unleash mysterious and even mystical forces was a long way from what the Soviet developers of psychoprophylaxis or their French students ever intended. The Lamaze method as a spiritual, countercultural, or New Age phenomenon belongs very much and uniquely to the American context.

By the 1980s, U.S. medical professionals who advocated the Lamaze method had broken definitively with the orthodox view that psychoprophylaxis could eradicate pain. Unlike the earliest U.S. Lamaze activists, these obstetricians and childbirth educators publicly expressed a belief long held by many American mothers: psychoprophylaxis was a means to cope with, not eliminate pain. In a 1983 film produced by ASPO for classroom use, actress Patty Duke Astin narrated that the Lamaze method 'doesn't promise to get rid of pain, only to give you tools to manage it and the knowledge to understand the process. … As labour pro-gresses, contractions come closer together and may be hard, powerful and, yes, painful.'[41] This open admission that pain was a normal, near universal part of birth even with psychoprophylactic training was a far cry from the party line among Lamaze advocates in the 1960s and 1970s, when expectant mothers were promised that 'medication is not the only or ideal way to have a happy, painless birth.'[42]

The meaning and value of labour pain remained in flux, as a new generation of mothers put renewed value on pharmacological pain relief in childbirth. In 1981, only 22 percent of American women received epidural anaesthesia during labour. This figure climbed to nearly two-thirds by 1997. As of 2009, the number hovered around 75 percent, though some sources claim that rates are as low as fifty percent.[43] Accurate figures for France are difficult to identify, but at least one source puts the epidural rate there at approximately fifty percent as of 1996, indicating that French feminists' demands for anaesthesia in the late 1970s had ultimately met with satisfaction.[44] Though the rate for France may be lower than that for the U.S., it reflects similar changes in childbirth pain as cultural capital. The popularity of epidural anaesthesia in the U.S. and France attests to more than just pharmacological advances or the financial incentives for hospitals, anaesthesiologists, and drug companies alike to promote this particular, highly effective, but costly means of pain management. Cultural winds had shifted, and, regardless of the diverse reasons, no longer did a significant number of women seek to assert their power through the mastery of a psychological approach to obstetric pain management.

Surveying the history of mid-twentieth century psychological methods of obstetric anaesthesia, one is struck by the singularity of labour pain, long distinguished from other kinds of physical pain. In Genesis 3:16, God's punishment for Eve is 'in sorrow thou shall bring forth children,' a biblical passage that for centuries imbued the pain of childbirth with spiritual significance. The rise of obstetric anaesthesia in nineteenth-century Europe and North America opened up a debate over whether or not, for spiritual or other reasons, the pain of labour was an experience to be embraced or avoided. In the mid-twentieth century, supporters of the Read method and psychoprophylaxis answered that women need not suffer in childbirth. They saw the solution to that pain in women's minds, not in the latest pharmacological advances, and they rejected the idea of pain as a normal, natural part of childbirth. Stripped of any social value or biological function, labour pain became largely a litmus test of a woman's psychological health. As the view that pain was natural and normal began to reassert itself, the presence of labour pain came to attest in the U.S. to a woman's empowerment and even her spiritual depth, rather than psychological weakness. This romanticisation cannot be said to have characterized women's attitude toward childbirth pain in France, where many women were profoundly disappointed with the promises of 'painless childbirth' put forth by the proponents of psychoprophylaxis. In the context of a French obstetric culture reluctant to alleviate women's pain through pharmacological methods, feminist demands meant a cry for anaesthesia, an impulse in contrast to that of American women who sought to resist obstetric authority through a refusal to rely on drugs for pain relief. These divergent stances point toward the acute sensitivity of the meaning and value of childbirth pain to cultural and historical context.

Notes

[1] An International Travel Award from the University of Iowa's International Programs, funded in part by the Stanley-UI Foundation Support Organization, as well as travel funds from the University of Iowa's Department of History enabled me to participate in the 'Knowledge and Pain' International Conference, Scholion Center for Jewish Studies, The Hebrew University of Jerusalem, in May 2010. I appreciate the input and exceptionally stimulating environment provided by conference organizers and participants, as well as the suggestions for revision from Emily Burrill, Dan Coleman, Gigi Dillon, Anne Drapkin Lyerly, and Sarah Shields. A University of Iowa Faculty Scholar Award (2005-2008) supported much of the research for this chapter. Funds provided by the National Council for Eurasian and East European Research (NCEEER) and the International Research and Exchanges Board (IREX) in 2005-2006 under authority of a Title VIII grant from the U.S. Department of State sponsored part of the work leading to this study. Additional funding was provided by a Schlesinger Library Research Support Grant (2005-2006). None of these organizations or individuals bear responsibility for the views expressed within the text. Accountability for all errors lies with me alone. Unless otherwise noted, all translations are mine.

[2] See Elisabeth Bing with Libby Coleman, *My Life in Birth: The Memoirs of Elisabeth Bing* (Washington D.C.: Lamaze International, 2000).
[3] 'Interview with Elisabeth Bing,' *American Baby CBE Reporter: A Supplement to American Baby Magazine* (Spring 2001): 3.
[4] Elaine Zwelling, 'The History of Lamaze Continues: An Interview with Elisabeth Bing,' *Journal of Perinatal Education* 9 (2000): 20.
[5] Ibid., 19.
[6] 'Interview with Elisabeth Bing.'
[7] Zwelling, 'The History of Lamaze Continues,' 20.
[8] See Brigitte Jordan, *Birth in Four Cultures: A Crosscultural Investigation of Childbirth in Yucatan, Holland, Sweden and the United States* (Long Grove, IL: Waveland, 1992).
[9] In the first half of the twentieth century, childbirth education was often aimed not at the middle- and upper-class women who popularized it in the post-World War II era but at poor immigrant women. Founded in 1918, the Maternity Center Association (MCA; now known as Childbirth Connection), for example, operated in New York City's overcrowded, impoverished immigrant neighbourhoods in an effort to reduce maternal and infant mortality rates. In the 1940s, MCA became a proponent of Dick-Read's natural childbirth method and reached out to an entirely different demographic. *Maternity Center Association, 1918-1943* (New York: The Maternity Center Association, 1943).
[10] Grantly Dick-Read, *Childbirth without Fear: The Principles and Practices of Natural Childbirth*, 2nd rev. ed., (New York: Harper & Row, 1959), 143.
[11] For a hagiographic work on Dick-Read, see A. Noyes Thomas, *Doctor Courageous: The Story of Dr. Grantly Dick-Read* (New York: Harper, 1957). See also Mary Thomas, *Post-War Mothers: Childbirth Letters to Grantly Dick-Read, 1946-1956* (Rochester, N.Y.: University of Rochester Press, 1997); Margarete Sandelowski, *Pain, Pleasure, and American Childbirth: From the Twilight Sleep to the Read Method, 1914-1960* (Westport, Conn.: Greenwood Press, 1984), 85-138; Jacqueline H. Wolf, *Deliver Me from Pain: Anesthesia and Birth in America* (Baltimore: Johns Hopkins University Press, 2009), 151-55.
[12] I. Z. Vel'vovskii and A. P. Nikolaev, *Psikhoprofilaktika bolei v rodakh*, Moscow: Medgiz, 1954; Paula A. Michaels, 'Childbirth Pain Relief and the Soviet Origins of the Lamaze Method,' NCEEER Working Paper, (October 16, 2007): 1-31; John D. Bell, 'Giving Birth to the New Soviet Man: Politics and Obstetrics in the U.S.S.R.,' *Slavic Review* 40 (1981): 1-16.
[13] Marjorie Karmel, *Thank You, Dr. Lamaze: A Mother's Experiences in Painless Childbirth* (Philadelphia: Lippincott, 1959).

[14] On the history of psychoprophylaxis outside the USSR, see Paula A. Michaels, 'A Chapter from Lamaze History: Birth Stories and Authoritative Knowledge in France, 1951-1957,' *Journal of Perinatal Education* 19 (2010): 35-43; Paula A. Michaels, 'Comrades in the Labor Room: The Lamaze Method of Childbirth Preparation and France's Cold War Home Front, 1951-1957,' *American Historical Review* 115 (2010): 1031-60; Marianne Caron-Leulliez and Jocelyne George, *L'accouchement sans douleur: Histoire d'une révolution oubliée* (Paris: Ouvrières, 2004); Caroline Gutmann, *The Legacy of Dr. Lamaze: The Story of the Man Who Changed Childbirth* (New York: St. Martin's Press, 2001); Marilène Vuille, *Accouchement et douleur: Une étude sociologique* (Lausanne: Antipodes, 2000).
[15] Bing and Coleman, 88.
[16] Sunnye Strickland, Memo to the ASPO Board of Directors, September 20, 1972, Assession 2000-M58, carton 2, Lamaze International Records, Schlesinger Library, Radcliffe Institute, Harvard University, Cambridge, MA.
[17] Quoted in I. Velvovsky, V. Ploticher, K. Platonov, and E. Shugom, *Painless Childbirth through Psychoprophylaxis: Lectures for Obstetrician* (Honolulu: University of Hawaii Press, 2003), 130.
[18] Fernand Lamaze, *Qu'est-ce que l'accouchement sans douleur?* (Paris: La Farandole, 1956), 49.
[19] See Michaels, 'A Chapter from Lamaze History'; Michaels, 'Comrades in the Labor Room'; Vuille, *Accouchement et douleur*, 57-60.
[20] ASPO Outline Form Obstetrician's Report, November 11, 1961, Assession 2003-M153, Box 1, Lamaze International Records, Schlesinger Library, Radcliffe Institute, Harvard University, Cambridge, MA.
[21] In contrast to what obstetricians would have considered only a partial failure, 'complete failure' was characterized by agitation and cries throughout the entire period of dilation. As one French textbook for training childbirth educators and obstetric nurses described it, the labouring woman 'loses self-control from the beginning and she ceaselessly demands anaesthesia. She completely fails at expulsion and ends her birth by forceps under anesthesia' (Zila Rennert, Blanche Cohen, and Christiane Goirand, *L'enseignement de l'accouchement sans douleur: Comment le préparer et le diriger, gymastique pré et postnatale* [Paris: Vigot Frères, 1975], 197-98). In the 1950s and 1960s, demands for anaesthesia, especially in the United States, meant general anaesthesia, though sometimes local anaesthesia, such as pudendal or paracervical block, was used. In the 1970s and beyond, medical personnel in both France and the U.S. increasingly responded to labouring women's demands with epidural anaesthesia. In the USSR, however, women in labour

and birth rarely received pharmacological pain relief, even in the face of the total failure of psychoprophylaxis to alleviate their suffering.

[22] Pierre Vellay and Aline Vellay-Dalsace, *Témoignages sur l'accouchement sans douleur* (Paris: Seuil, 1956), 237.

[23] Ibid.

[24] Marie-José Jaubert, *Les bateleurs du mal-joli: Le mythe de l'accouchement sans douleur* (Paris: Balland, 1979), 71.

[25] See Diane E. Hoffman and Anita J. Tarzian, 'The Girl Who Cried Pain: A Bias against Women in the Treatment of Pain,' *Journal of Law, Medicine, and Ethics* 29 (2001): 13-27.

[26] Vellay and Vellay-Dalsace, *Témoignages*, 343-45.

[27] Mrs. N., Letter to Mrs. Ferris, 1964, Assession 2003-M153, Box 1, Lamaze International Records, Schlesinger Library, Radcliffe Institute, Harvard University, Cambridge, MA.

[28] See, for instance, Stenogramma vsesoiuznogo soveshchaniia po dal'neishemu razvitiiu psikhoprofilakticheskoi podgotovki beremennykh k rodam, Tsentral'nyii derzhavnii arkhiv vishchikh organiv vladi ta upravlinnia Ukraini, Kyiv, fond 342, Ministerstvo zdravookhraneniia Ukrainskoi SSR, opis 15, spravka 4267, February 10-14, 1956, arkush 46, 211, 239; Michaels, 'Comrades in the Labor Room,' 1053.

[29] Though there was wide regional variation, official rates of psychoprophylactic preparation in the 1960s in urban areas typically ranged from 50 to 75 percent. Rural areas often reported figures considerably lower, in some dwindling to as little as 20 percent (e.g., Kon'iunkturnye obzory sostoianiia akushersko-ginekologicheskoi pomoshchi naseleniiu Leningradskoi, Lipetskoi, Magadanskoi, Moskovskoi, Novgorodskoi i Novosibirskoi oblasti, 1963, Gosudarstvennyi arkhiv Rossiiskoi Federatsii, Moscow, fond A-482, Ministersvo zdravookhraneniia RSFSR, opis 50, delo 8546).

[30] Peter Osnos, 'Childbirth, Soviet Style: Labor in Keeping with the Party Line.' *Washington Post*, November 28, 1976, G13.

[31] Ol'ga Valentinovna Grishchenko, Interview by the author. Kharkiv, April 3, 2006.

[32] See Jean Ispa, 'Soviet and American Childbearing Experiences and Attitudes: A Comparison,' *Slavic Review* 42 (1983): 1-13; Ekaterina Belooussova, 'The 'Natural Childbirth' Movement in Russia: Self-Representation Strategies,' *Anthropology of East Europe Review* 20 (2002): 1-8; Grishchenko, 2006; Nataliia Vorontsova-Iurieva, 'Rody v SSSR,' in *Predmety sovetskoi zhizni*, June 19, 2007, viewed on August 20, 2010, http://community.livejournal.com/soviet_life/ 53730.html#cutid1.

[33] Marie-Françoise Lévy, 'Le mouvement français pour le planning familial et les jeunes,' *Vingtième siècle: Revue d'histoire* 75 (July-September 2002): 75-84; Claire Duchen, *Feminism in France: From May '68 to Mitterrand* (London: Routledge and Kegan Paul, 1986), 49-66.
[34] Jaubert, 132.
[35] P. A. Chadeyron, 'Comment accoucher dans le plaisir,' *La Généraliste*, November 21, 1979, 24.
[36] Madame E., Letter to Pierre Rouquès Metallurgists' Polyclinic administration, December 15, 1975, Box X-1, Collection l'Accouchement sans douleur [hereafter ASD Archives], Institut CGT d'Histoire Sociale de la Métallurgie, Paris.
[37] Madame P., Letter to Pierre Rouquès Metallurgists' Polyclinic administration, October 17, 1976, Box X-1, ASD Archives, Institut CGT d'Histoire Sociale de la Métallurgie, Paris.
[38] Elaine Zwelling, 'Activist for Change. An Interview with Suzanne Arms,' *Journal of Perinatal Education*, 11 (2002): 12.
[39] Ibid., 13.
[40] Theodore Sturgeon, 'Woman of Earth and Sky and Origins . . .,' *Los Angeles Chapter ASPO Newsletter* (April, 1970): 1.
[41] *The Lamaze Method: Techniques for Childbirth Preparation*, directed by Woody Robertson, produced by ASPO, 1983.
[42] BACE Training Exam for Instructors, 1972, Box 5, Folder 1, MC515, Boston Association for Childbirth Education Records, Schlesinger Library, Radcliffe Institute, Harvard University, Cambridge, MA.
[43] Advocates of natural childbirth put the figure of epidural anaesthesia rates at the high end, while those in the obstetrics and anaesthesiology communities tend to offer considerably lower figures; see Judith P. Rooks, 'Epidural Anesthesia as Used during Childbirth in the United States,' *Japanese Journal for Midwives* 54 (2000): 9-14; Wilhelm Ruppen, Sheena Derry, Henry McQuay, and R. Andrew Moore, 'Incidence of Epidural Hematoma, Infection, and Neurologic Injury in Obstetric Patients with Epidural Analgesia/Anesthesia.' *Anesthesiology*, 105 (2006): 394-99; Brenda Lane, 'Epidural Rates in the US and Around the World: How Many Mothers Choose to Use an Epidural to Provide Pain Relief?' *Suite101.com*, November 29, 2009, viewed on August 20, 2010, <http://childbirth-labour-delivery.suite101.com/article.cfm/epidural_for_labor>.
[44] Ruppen et al., 394.

Bibliography

Arms, Suzanne. *Immaculate Deception: A New Look at Women and Childbirth in America.* New York: Houghton Mifflin, 1975.

ASPO Outline Form Obstetrician's Report, November 11, 1961, Assession 2003-M153, Box 1, Lamaze International Records, Schlesinger Library, Radcliffe Institute, Harvard University, Cambridge, MA.

BACE Training Exam for Instructors, 1972, Box 5, Folder 1, MC515, Boston Association for Childbirth Education Records, Schlesinger Library. Radcliffe Institute. Harvard University, Cambridge, MA.

Beck, N. C. and D. Hall. 'Natural Childbirth: A Review and Analysis.' *Obstetrics and Gynecology* 52 (1978): 371-79.

Beck, N. C., E. A. Geden and G. T. Brouder. 'Preparation for Labor: A Historical Perspective.' *Psychosomatic Medicine* 41 (1979): 243-58.

Bell, John D. 'Giving Birth to the New Soviet Man: Politics and Obstetrics in the U.S.S.R.' *Slavic Review* 40 (1981): 1-16.

Belooussova, Ekaterina. 'The 'Natural Childbirth' Movement in Russia: Self-Representation Strategies.' *Anthropology of East Europe Review* 20 (2002): 1-8.

Bing, Elisabeth, with Libby Coleman. *My Life in Birth: The Memoirs of Elisabeth Bing*. Washington, D.C.: Lamaze International, 2000.

Caron-Leulliez, Marianne, and Jocelyne George. *L'accouchement sans douleur: Histoire d'une révolution oubliée.* Paris: Ouvrières, 2004.

Chadeyron, P. A. 'Comment accoucher dans le plaisir.' *La Généraliste*, November 21, 1979, 22-24.

Dick-Read, Grantly. *Childbirth without Fear: The Principles and Practice of Natural Childbirth.* 2nd revised edition. London: William Heinemann, 1943. New York: Harper & Row, 1959.

———. *Natural Childbirth.* London, Heinemann, 1933.

Duchen, Claire. *Feminism in France: From May '68 to Mitterrand.* London: Routledge and Kegan Paul, 1986.

Grishchenko, Ol'ga Valentinovna. Interview by the author. Kharkiv, April 3, 2006.

Gutmann, Caroline. *The Legacy of Dr. Lamaze: The Story of the Man Who Changed Childbirth.* New York: St. Martin's Press, 2001.

Hoffman, Diane E. and Anita J. Tarzian. 'The Girl Who Cried Pain: A Bias against Women in the Treatment of Pain.' *Journal of Law, Medicine, and Ethics* 29 (2001): 13-27.

'Interview with Elisabeth Bing.' *American Baby CBE Reporter: A Supplement to American Baby Magazine* (Spring 2001): 3.

Ispa, Jean. 'Soviet and American Childbearing Experiences and Attitudes: A Comparison.' *Slavic Review* 42 (1983): 1-13.

Jaubert, Marie-José. *Les bateleurs du mal-joli: Le mythe de l'accouchement sans douleur.* Paris: Balland, 1979.

Jordan, Brigitte. *Birth in Four Cultures: A Crosscultural Investigation of Childbirth in Yucatan, Holland, Sweden and the United States*, 4th rev. ed. Long Grove, IL: Waveland, 1992.

Karmel, Marjorie, *Thank You, Dr. Lamaze: A Mother's Experiences in Painless Childbirth.* Philadelphia: Lippincott, 1959.

Kon'iunkturnye obzory sostoianiia akushersko-ginekologicheskoi pomoshchi naseleniiu Leningradskoi, Lipetskoi, Magadanskoi, Moskovskoi, Novgorodskoi i Novosibirskoi oblasti, 1963, fond A-482, opis 50, delo 8564, Ministersvo zdravookhraneniia RSFSR, Gosudarstvennyi arkhiv Rossiiskoi Federatsii, Moscow.

Lamaze, Fernand. *Qu'est-ce que l'accouchement sans douleur?* Paris: La Farandole, 1956.

The Lamaze Method: Techniques for Childbirth Preparation. Directed by Woody Robertson. Produced by ASPO, 1983.

Lane, Brenda. 'Epidural Rates in the US and Around the World: How Many Mothers Choose to Use an Epidural to Provide Pain Relief?' *Suite101.com,* November 29, 2009. Viewed on August 20, 2010. <http://childbirth-labour-delivery.suite101.com/article.cfm/epidural_for_labor>.

Lévy, Marie-Françoise. 'Le mouvement français pour le planning familial et les jeunes.' *Vingtième Siècle. Revue d'histoire* 75 (July-September 2002): 75-84.

Madame E. Letter to Pierre Rouquès Metallurgists Polyclinic administration, December 15, 1975, Box X-1, Collection l'accouchement sans douleur, Institut CGT d'Histoire Sociale de la Métallurgie, Paris.

Madame P. Letter to Pierre Rouquès Metallurgists' Polyclinic administration, October 17, 1976, Box X-1, Collection l'accouchement sans douleur, Institut CGT d'Histoire Sociale de la Métallurgie, Paris.

Maternity Center Association, 1918-1943. New York: The Maternity Center Association, 1943.

Michaels, Paula A. 'A Chapter from Lamaze History: Birth Stories and Authoritative Knowledge in France, 1951-1957.' *Journal of Perinatal Education* 19 (2010): 35-43.

———. 'Childbirth Pain Relief and the Soviet Origins of the Lamaze Method.' NCEEER Working Paper, October 16, 2007, 1-31.

———. 'Comrades in the Labor Room: The Lamaze Method of Childbirth Preparation and France's Cold War Home Front, 1951-1957.' *American Historical Review* 115 (2010): 1031-60.

Mrs. N., Letter to Mrs. Ferris, 1964. Assession 2003-M153, Box 1, Lamaze International Records, Schlesinger Library, Radcliffe Institute, Harvard University, Cambridge, MA.

Osnos, Peter. 'Childbirth, Soviet Style: Labor in Keeping with the Party Line.' *Washington Post*, November 28, 1976, G13.

Rennert, Zila, Blanche Cohen and Christiane Goirand. *L'Enseignement de l'accouchement sans douleur: Comment le préparer et le diriger, gymastique pré et postnatale.* Paris: Vigot Frères, 1975.

Rooks, Judith P. 'Epidural Anesthesia as Used during Childbirth in the United States.' *Japanese Journal for Midwives* 54 (2000): 9-14.

Ruppen, Wilhelm, Sheena Derry, Henry McQuay and R. Andrew Moore. 'Incidence of Epidural Hematoma, Infection, and Neurologic Injury in Obstetric Patients with Epidural Analgesia/Anesthesia.' *Anesthesiology* 105 (2006): 394-99.

Sandelowski, Margarete. *Pain, Pleasure, and American Childbirth: From The Twilight Sleep to The Read Method, 1914-1960.* Westport, Conn.: Greenwood Press, 1984.

Stenogramma vsesoiuznogo soveshchaniia po dal'neishemu razvitiiu psikhoprofilakticheskoi podgotovki beremennykh k rodam February 10-14, 1956, fond 342, opis 15, spravka 4267, Ministerstvo zdravookhraneniia Ukrainskoi SSR, Tsentral'nyii derzhavnii arkhiv vishchikh organiv vladi ta upravlinnia Ukraini, Kyiv.

Strickland, Sunnye. Memo to the ASPO Board of Directors, September 20, 1972, Assession 2000-M58, carton 2, Lamaze International Records, Schlesinger Library, Radcliffe Institute, Harvard University, Cambridge, MA.

Sturgeon, Theodore. 'Woman of Earth and Sky and Origins . . .' *Los Angeles Chapter ASPO Newsletter*, April 1970, 1.

Thomas, A. Noyes. *Doctor Courageous: The Story of Dr. Grantly Dick-Read.* New York: Harper, 1957.

Thomas, Mary. *Post-War Mothers: Childbirth Letters to Grantly Dick-Read, 1946-1956.* Rochester, N.Y. : University of Rochester Press, 1997.

Vellay, Pierre and Aline Vellay-Dalsace. *Témoignages sur l'accouchement sans douleur.* Paris: Seuil, 1956.

Vel'vovskii, I. Z. and A. P. Nikolaev. *Psikhoprofilaktika bolei v rodakh.* Moscow: Medgiz, 1954.

Velvovsky, I., V. Ploticher, K. Platonov and E. Shugom. *Painless Childbirth through Psychoprophylaxis: Lectures for Obstetricians.* 1960; repr. Honolulu: University of Hawaii Press, 2003.

Vorontsova-Iurieva, Nataliia. 'Rody v SSSR.' *Predmety sovetskoi zhizni.* June 19, 2007. Viewed on August 20, 2010, <http://community.livejournal.com/soviet_life/ 53730.html#cutid1>.

Vuille, Marilène. *Accouchement et douleur: Une étude sociologique.* Lausanne: Antipodes, 1998.

——. 'La naissance de l'accouchement sans douleur.'' *Revue médicale de la Suisse romande* 120 (2000): 991-98.

Wolf, Jacqueline H. *Deliver Me from Pain: Anesthesia and Birth in America.* Baltimore: Johns Hopkins University Press, 2009.

Zwelling, Elaine. 'Activist for Change: An Interview with Suzanne Arms.' *Journal of Perinatal Education* 11 (2002): 11-24.

——. 'The History of Lamaze Continues: An Interview with Elisabeth Bing.' *Journal of Perinatal Education* 9 (2000): 15-21.

Part V

NARRATIVES

What Does Falling Ill Mean? Illness Narratives as Elucidation of Experience Expertise

Anna Leimumäki

Abstract
Falling seriously and chronically ill is a major emotional event that affects life and identity. I see narrative analysis as both a method for studying the processes of dealing with the experience of falling ill and as a way towards understanding the personal and shared meanings that such an experience provides. There is a strong demand in public discourse for future health care to be a client-oriented and efficient service system. Developing such a system requires knowledge of the clients' real needs - that is, knowledge from the patients' viewpoint. In this article I examine the process of narrativising illness experience mainly in relation to the medical script. In addition to the fluency of narrativisation, illness narratives include blanks, gaps, incoherence and obscurity. On all of these occasions, the speakers are struggling to define their relationship between experientiality and the accepted script, thus constructing the meanings of illness experience. I see narratives as a way of analysing experience expertise, and I hope that these diverse voices will in the future be heard more often in developing health care.

Key Words: Illness narrative, narrative devices, narrativisation, autobiographical narrative, medical script, experientiality, the narrative I, the experiencing I, experience expertise, client-orientation.

*****

Can narratives elucidate experience expertise? There is a strong demand in public discourse for future health care to be a client-oriented and efficient service system. Developing such a system requires knowledge of the clients' real needs - that is, knowledge from the patients' viewpoint. Even though narrative medicine has developed as a discipline in recent years,[1] we have been forced to realise that personal accounts of illness experiences have been excluded until quite recently from precisely those settings in which we might have expected them to be most relevant: for example in hospitals and clinics,[2] and in developing health care. Medical science has been the dominant frame there. According to Arthur Kleinman 'illness has a meaning and to understand *how it obtains meaning* is to understand something fundamental about illness, about care, and perhaps about life generally.'[3] My aim is to study the process of narrativising the experience of falling ill and the meanings given to this experience in narratives: a voice or voices of experience expertise. Even though these kinds of narratives deal with a personal experience, many common rules and conventions guide the process of handling and narrating an illness experience.[4] Narrating one's own personal experience brings together many influential cultural narratives from the medical to the psychological and religious.[5] Shlomith Rimmon-Kenan emphasises that illness narratives are essentially rhetorical and dialogical.[6] Both features relate to cultural and social interactions with the surrounding community.

Narrativising can be seen as a device for understanding and coming to terms with the illness experience by the patients themselves, and also for mediating it to others. Acting, thinking and narrating may be seen as standing in a circular relationship.[7] Narratives that surround us teach us about our world and how to narrate our place within it.[8] According to David Herman, narrative theory should be viewed as a subdomain of the cognitive sciences.[9] Thus, narrative devices should provide insight into the narrative process - into its fluency and into its difficulty. In cognitively-oriented literary research, narrativisation and narration resemble the process of understanding and analysing one's own experience. The similarity of these processes has been defined, for example, on the grounds of parallel prototypical elements[10] or prototypical narrative and narrativisation mechanisms.[11] Multi- and interdisciplinary narrative studies have often concentrated on the prototypical narrative frame or model by looking only for the conventional characteristics that support it.[12] Conventional here means a narrative that is coherent, linear and chronological. The speakers may aim at these conventions, often with limited success. More and more research has increasingly emphasised the structural and performative dimensions (not only the content) of meanings constructed in everyday narratives.[13] Still not much research has concentrated on literary narrative devices when studying oral narratives. Coordinating the processes of understanding, managing, mediating *and narrating* enables one to study this process with narratological tools. Studying specific narrative devices together with the contents of the narratives yields more potential for the analysis and interpretation of the meanings of the experience.

In this article my aim is to elucidate the process of narrativising illness experience mainly in relation to the medical script. My materials propose the medical script as a cultural story of treatment progression, functioning as a guiding frame to the speakers when they narrate - that is, understand, conceptualise, analyse, interpret - their subjective experiences. Medical discourse is often seen as displacing the everyday world in serious or life-threatening illness narratives.[14] The medical script involves the treatment progress but not the development of the ill person. Thus there are often contradictions in the narratives. From the medical point of view, there are objective knowledge and facts about health, illnesses and treatment;

they are there in the world of the ill person as well, but along with the experience and the meaning of these facts. Speakers have the possibility of strategically constructing their subjectivity in different ways in relation to the script in their narratives. This chapter points to occasions on which the speakers define the relationship between experientiality and the medical script and thus construct the meanings of illness experience. The focus is on the ways in which narratives open up the multidimensional narrativising process and elucidate the personal and cultural meanings of falling ill. Narratives are examined as a way of analysing experience expertise: the diverse voices of those who themselves have suffered from a disease.

According to Rita Charon, when we want to understand people in particular situations, we reach out for narratives or storytelling.[15] I have collected oral narratives of women and men suffering from a cardiovascular disease. I met each of them individually and asked them to tell me about their experience of falling ill and living with the disease. I hoped they would tell me about their experience in a way natural for them. After my request I tried to influence the course of the narrative as little as possible. Some narrators had learned of their cardiovascular disease only a few months previously, some had fallen ill many years ago. I recorded the narratives and transcribed them afterwards. My use of transcription and punctuation in these narrative texts follows the rhythm of the speech. I have also noted signs of emotions such as crying, laughter and sighs. I asked each interviewee to speak on the same topic - falling ill and being ill - but in the end I got very different kinds of narratives.

1. From Non-Narrative Experientiality to Narrative - Experience as Knowledge One Can Mediate

How can the experience of falling ill be captured in texts? How can we analyse and interpret verbally something that is largely non-verbal? What kind of phenomenon is experience? We can perhaps intuitively understand it, but can we define it theoretically? I shall here talk of a humanly important experientiality that is verbally constructed,[16] even though as a research object, 'experience' seems to be as slippery as a bar of wet soap.

Autobiographical narration goes together with the concept of 'the autobiographical pact': the narrator is committed to telling about her or his life truthfully to the audience.[17] The listeners or readers may expect the story to conform with the real life of the narrator. Ordinary narrators tend to think that they are telling about their lives as the events happened as as they were experienced - for them the narrative is a synonym for their past. To the researcher, however, a lived life is not identical to narrated experience. Verbal transition and conceptualisation occurs between these two poles; narratives are a way of studying this narrativisation process. The point of the process is to express something personal in a way that can be understood by others. According to Dorrit Cohn, narrative fiction can reveal aspects of other people's minds that we cannot reach in reality.[18] The reality effect is created by narrative techniques; narrative means construct an illusion of a direct presentation of experientiality.

At first the aim of narratology was to find general grammars of narration; components were also sought not only in literature but also in the oral narrative tradition (by Claude Lévi-Strauss and Vladimir Propp, among others). Subsequently, narratology focused on studying the specific devices available to literature. Nowadays all of these devices are seen as mobile parts of the cultural dialogue encountered by everyone. Thus the narrative tools for analysing fiction can also be applied to non-fictive texts like oral everyday narratives, even if the devices used by everyday narrators constitute, at least in part, a different kind of process and produce different kinds of meanings in the texts. Non-literary narratives, unlike literary ones, are not deliberately based on thematising problematic relationships between experiencing, interpreting and narrating the story and narration levels. Nonetheless, the narration is inevitably based on and works on these problems, and they cause the result of the narration to be less conventional than originally imagined. The speakers also test in their narratives the boundaries and relationships between experiencing, interpreting and narrating, for example when looking for phrases to express the content or the structure of their experience. Conventions are not necessarily the best way to express this from the speakers' viewpoints: one's own experientiality does not always fit into the conventional model; it often overflows it. Still, many speakers opt for conventional moulds. From a researcher's viewpoint, the interesting part of the study is based on this contradiction: conventionality on the one hand, and its challenge or deconstruction on the other.

It is not possible to narrate something from the past fully, as if everything that happened could be recounted in its full experientiality. Narration requires selecting and summarising, and there are always emphases involved.[19] As Anni Vilkko notes, selection is guided not only by personal reasons but also by cultural and narrative conventions.[20] According to David Herman, there are parallel prototypical elements in all narratives;[21] I first focus on them.

Most of the speakers, e.g., Hilkka who is quoted first, began their narratives by defining the outbreak of the illness as an unexpected event. According to Herman, a disruption and the resulting turn are essential prototypical elements in a narrative.[22] Illness narratives explicitly presuppose a turn from a healthy person to an ill one. So the turn is expected, but at the story level it is often constructed as an unexpected change, e.g.:

> The whole process was, a kind of surprise, for me, and for the whole, family and friends, they thought that I was, in good condition and, and really, I didn't have anything, I was even having a pause from the blood pressure medication, because the blood pressure had been all right and the pulse went quite down. And then it really came suddenly, well, I was quite tired at the beginning of the year. And, I was little surprised, that, what it is. But then, then it came like a bolt out of the blue. (Hilkka)

Hilkka characterises her sense of falling ill as a strong, unexpected experience. She expands her own point of view to include those outside her: she is focalising her own experience from the point of view of her family as well, trying to construct a collective, shared meaning for the event. Hilkka tells us that falling ill was a surprise for her family and friends: they had all regarded her as being in good condition. The story can be read against the medical script which includes opinions on the causes of cardiovascular disease, such as different kinds of risk factors related to life-style. Hilkka is commenting on the medical script and emphasizing her comments through the collective view-point: no one expected her to get sick or thought of her having an unhealthy life-style. She was 'in a good condition' and 'even having a pause from the blood pressure medication, because the blood pressure had been all right.'

She repeats the sense of unexpectedness a number of times, as if to reinforce the event's meaningfulness.[23] Sharing the experience of falling ill with her family may be very important to the narrator, but so is sharing it with the listener in a narrative situation. At the beginning of the story Hilkka opens the door into the storyworld and wants to show that her story is worth telling. An unexpected shift at the beginning makes the story worth hearing and makes the listener wish to learn more. At the beginning of the narration a point of view that guides the whole process of narrativisation is defined. In Hilkka's narrative, the meanings of falling ill are constructed on the basis of the question why - why did I fall ill?

Narratives are always constructed at a particular moment and in a specific situation. Herman defines situatedness as the second prototypical element of narrative;[24] according to Jens Brockmeier, the narrative present affects the whole narrative just as much as the past being dealt with.[25] Thus experientiality can be imported from the past to the present within the scope of a single narrative. A narrative can be analysed as a process that includes not only events, or their causes, but also their consequences.[26] In Hilkka's narrative, the theme of unexpectedness is repeated many times not only at the beginning but throughout: she can be seen as constructing the meaning of her illness as a process that required her to adjust again and again before reaching the present narrative moment. Illness narratives can provide essential knowledge about the illness process as a whole, as well as its effects on identity. At the end of her story Hilkka constructs the meaning of falling ill as a stage of life that was needed for her emotional maturity.

According to Herman, the third prototypical element is event sequencing: every narrative is structured by a time-course of particularised events.[27] At the beginning of the twentieth century, modernist writers such as Virginia Woolf and James Joyce sought credible represention of the mind and discovered new, fragmentary ways of describing consciousness in their novels. Later, so-called trauma fiction used similar techniques, for example fragmentedness and discontinuity, to express the way traumatic events are experienced in one's mind.[28] Narration has been seen as a way to create continuity between events, and events become linked together when speakers implicitly or explicitly use them to construct meanings.[29] For the listeners, or researchers of narratives, this convention provides a possibility of studying meaning-making from the specific viewpoint of the speaker. Usually everyday narrators at least try to create continuity and coherence in their narratives; most of the narrators in my materials did this by analysing their experience chronologically according to the medical script's treatment of events. We can see this in the narrative of Helena who first tells about her symptoms and visiting the doctor and then describes the tests and the debacle over medication:

> It began in this way, that, I got out of breath, and never ever have I got out of breath before . . . and then, suddenly, when I was having a walk, I got out of breath, well, I was horrified, what it is, but, I went to see the doctor, ok, there was my GP, who sent me to clinical tests and ecg and, ecg is just fine, yes, no concern, nothing, nothing, all those tests are just like they should be. ... Well, then, I am going on the second time, he did not give me but a statin, and, as things turned out, I started to listen to discussions about statins, for God's sake, that, yes, it will take off all your muscles, and I didn't like it at all, I was really terrified and stopped taking it, and, nevertheless, when I am going to see the doctor, it had came down, this cholesterol, I don't know why, but it had, and then, this doctor, he asked me, well, have you been taking the medicine, I said, well, I must confess that I haven't been taking it, I took twice and then I stopped, well, he nearly fainted and said to me that, well, what shall we do then, this is a serious matter that, he didn't tell me what kind if matter it was but he just said that

> it is a serious matter that you have not taken the medicine, when having a high cholesterol, do you have sudden deaths in your family and smiled strangely, I thought that aha, this concerns me this sudden death, it suits me bloody well, and I of course didn't take the medicine, after when my neighbour, he suddenly died, he was found with all clothes on in his flat on the floor, and he got out of breath, I thought that well, it is my destiny, that, bye, that's fine with me, I made my will quickly, left my whole corpse to the medicine and what's the matter, of course I didn't take those statins, bloody hell, why should I take them anymore when I'm going to die, well, I had a check-up then, yes, and again he said to me that you must take the medicine, well, I thought that you will see, I am not going to take them, I don't care a shit. (Helena)

Helena starts her story just like Hilkka; she describes her symptoms as unexpected. She is not looking for any kind of experiential sharing and common meanings with her family but rather with health care professionals. Deborah Tannen states that frequent use of adjectives indicates the narrator is evaluating and interpreting.[30] Helena is at least implicitly criticising the ongoing events all the time. The narrative is constructed as a debate between Helena and the medical script, especially the professionals in it. At the beginning there are many contradictions but at the end they find a shared meaning of the events.

Chronology is not the only way to organise an experience. Helena explains the course of events from her point of view and at the same time constructs its meanings. For instance, Helena narrates by using the negative expression that the doctor 'did not give anything but statin' for her symptoms, and the negative might indicate that she was expecting the doctor to do something else.[31] With this expression she can be seen as constructing a narrative connection and an explanation for the later events as well: she does not behave in a way that was expected - she neglects the medicines prescribed. Helena's narrative reveals that official narratives (such as medical ones) are not the strongest contenders in the everyday discursive field. Many kinds of narratives affect people and the decisions they make in their lives. Illness narratives provide a way of knowing what really matters to people.

Most of the narrators in my materials narrated their symptoms, tests, treatments or recoveries chronologically and at the end said something about the present. The events attached to the treatment process constituted the progressing plot, the frame for the illness narrative. Personal events, like Helena's disappointment with the doctor, or the stories she had heard about statins, constructed subjective meanings in the course of the plot. Of course these personal events were partly shared too. Hydén & Brockmeier note that researchers share a certain mode for interviewing people which is why research narratives resemble each other: they tend to constitute chronological and linear chains of events.[32] I tried to avoid affecting the course of the narratives by refraining from questions while my interlocutors were narrating. As a result, the narrators were able to choose the way and the means to express their experience of falling ill. Still, consciously or not, they chose a shared plot including common events. I call this plot the 'medical script': a cultural narrative of discovering illness, the progress of treatment and recovery. It affects not only the events the narrators chose to tell, but also the language they use for that purpose. Still, the script was not repeated in the same way every time; instead, the narrative was constructed around the script by way of describing, evaluating, criticising and commenting on it.

In his book *The Wounded Storyteller* Arthur Frank states that there are three plots in every illness narrative: *the restitution narrative, the chaos narrative and the quest narrative.* The restitution plot resembles the script normally included in my materials at least on the structural level. Frank describes this plot as 'I was in good condition yesterday, now I am ill, but tomorrow I will be fine again.' In my materials the narrators' common plot resembles the one that recurs in narratives told by health care professionals: the plot of the progress of treatment that appears in medical records. The restitution plot is constructed on the assumption of health and illness as opposites: health is a non-ill feeling and state of being.[33] I interpret the restitution plot as a cultural script of the progress of treatment that expresses the patients' assumption that the progress will continue. The script is repeated in many kinds of texts which deal with illnesses and the experience of falling ill in books, magazines, TV programs and movies. By repeating the script the narrator may be able to feel that she or he is entering a common story world. The speaker's experience is part of the socially and culturally shared world of suffering from a cardiovascular disease,[34] which enables one to discuss it with others. Although in the last quotation Helena showed a critical attitude towards health care professionals and towards commitment to the treatment, she was nevertheless analysing her experience through this script, too.

Recovery is described in the script mainly as a physical process: when the physical symptoms are removed, the person is cured. Frank defines the idea of being either healthy or ill as modernist.[35] This kind of script does not, however, correspond to the situation the narrators in my materials experienced: you could not be cured from a chronic disease, but you could still feel healthy. Helena's narrative has already given us a sense of the multiple meanings attached to the process of becoming ill. The experience of suffering from a serious chronic disease usually changes one's idea of the self and life. According to many studies, cardiovascular disease affects the patient not only physically but also in terms of reducing the experienced quality of their life.[36] Emotional pain, mental recovery, and adapting to a new situation often take far more time than physical recovery, as Hilja tells us in the next example:

> This was the biggest blow in my life. Well, I almost couldn't stand up to it, that, that now I am not capable of doing anything, so, that, that I am just creeping here inside and there in the yard, I took the waste out and some small bundle of papers or something, and there, that was my walk then. I can only take a very short walk at a time and then I must breath, and stop. So, I still have these kinds of things. And the heart, it is there, but never again, never the health will be like it used to be before. It's my past and it has gone. Of course, if like, if I could go on like this, like this here, could go on, could be here, [sighing], have some more time left, to be here. But the most significant thing was just this, I mean, giving up, giving up is the most shocking thing. It's like, like it would be only half of the health left because of that kind of mood, giving up hobbies, when nothing is left of them. (Hilja)

It is interesting that many of those who have a chronic disease continue telling the modernist restitution plot without questioning it explicitly.[37] So does Hilja in her narrative. First she tells about falling ill, then the progress of her treatment and physical recovery. But, as Hilja says herself in her story ('I always get back to the questions of giving up'), she returns over and over again to the meaning of falling ill as an enormous change in relation to her identity and life. Telling the script was surprisingly easy for most narrators in my materials, but they might have told about their falling ill many times already. In our culture it is more convenient or permissible to tell about falling ill as a set of concrete events than as subjective experiences.[38] However, in recent years there have been a lot of public discussions of sensitive themes such as depression in the media. Nowadays telling about one's life is part and parcel of our everyday culture owing to reality TV and social media.

Therefore I would claim that cultural conventions have changed, a fact my materials also attest to. Many of the narrators involved were quite open in telling about sensitive stages in their lives. Hilja does not explicitly mention 'death' in her narrative, but she is constructing a meaning to falling ill as giving up. She mentions her hope to be able to 'go on like this, like this here, could go on, could be here, [sighing], have some more time left, to be here.' This can be seen as an intimate discussion of the limits of life. Nevertheless, the cultural norms that have regulated the permissible way of telling about our experience of falling ill can still be detected. This is seen, for example, in the means which the interviewees used for describing their physical symptoms and the measures that were taken. Falling ill was proved by numbers and test results, and often it was told as something separate from the speaker's self - sometimes by using passive constructions and sometimes, as in the next example, an alienated clinical language:

> I was just thinking that maybe, I had had these kinds of problems already young. I had not considered that, that, it could lead to this kind of angina pectoris disease. When I was 44 years old, I had cardiac arrhythmia and low blood pressure and pulse. And then, when I was in the hospital, a cardiologist mentioned for the first time, that I would be a typical, well, a pace-maker-patient, they would like to set up a pace-maker for me. But I didn't want it, I just thought that if I had already lived 44 years without it, I could live on, too. I didn't pay much attention to my cardiac arrhythmia, it was the low blood pressure that made me feel uncomfortable, I had these fainting fits. They were very awkward, because I didn't know where and when I might faint. And I had, quite often, days, that I couldn't go to work, I felt dizzy all day long, in the morning I crawled to the bathroom, I couldn't stand up. But then I got medication for my low blood pressure. (Hilppa)

Ill people have learned to talk about the issues professionals usually ask about and in a way that the professionals want to hear about them. This can be a way of making sure one will be listened to, and that is how, I believe a common knowledge of illness practices has been formed. The devices used by the speakers can also be interpreted as expressing a wish to alienate the disease from one's self - a convention that takes many shapes.[39] Narrative can also provide an opportunity to try out new concepts for one's own story. The narrative can, in other words, offer new space for fitting alien words and new experiences into one's autobiographical identity. Cultural narratives will always be constructed and woven into autobiographical narratives. Through them it is possible to convert something new and alien into something familiar and shareable with someone else. A narrative resembling the cultural one is more likely to be recognised by members of the same culture.[40]

Herman defines *qualia*, experientiality, as the last prototypical element of a narrative.[41] According to Monika Fludernik, experientiality constitutes the base of narrativity - the basic theme underlying every narrative.[42] The question con-cerning the location of experientiality in narratives is a significant one. The concepts *experience* and *narrative* may lead to loose and overly general conclusions in the manner of 'life as narrative' and 'experience as narrative.' Life cannot be thought of as just a series of basic events placed together, but every time a life is related, a new narrative of it is created.[43] Narratives are social practises.[44] Experientiality cannot be interpreted through narrative texts without considering its contexts. For example, the narratives I gathered were largely shaped by the situation in which they were initially told - to the researcher and at the same time to the whole potential audience of the research.[45] Had they been told to, for instance, family members or only to professionals, they would have been different in some ways; people tell different versions of the same events on different occasions. Experience is a living and ongoing process, but as a research subject we can only have a freeze-frame of it in a narrative, or a text tied to its narrator in a specific narrative situation. However, as Lars-Christer Hydén has shown, autobiographical narration is a tool for performing and negotiating identity: instead of static spaces, both activities involve ongoing interactions with all that surrounds it.[46]

Listening to illness narratives enables us to understand what kind of experience it is to fall ill and to suffer from a disease. I see illness narratives as a way towards knowledge: towards understanding the processes of becoming ill from an experiential point of view. Experience can appear as a more chaotic event, and so narrating it demands reflection and presupposes distance from experientiality. Even though so far I have dealt with the prototypical elements of narrative and highlighted the role and the meaning of the script in my materials, I do not take narrative just as a prototypical form. Instead, I believe we should study narrative as a fluid form that consists of prototypical elements. For its speakers, narrative does not only provide a pattern for comprehending and telling about experientiality as a single coherent entity. Narrative may include the idea of the prototypical form the narrators are trying to attain in their narration, a form that makes mutual understanding between the speaker and the listener possible. However, oral narratives diverge from any coherent idea of form: they wander, break down from time to time, and lack definite closure. They express a process, and those are precisely the features we should be interested in: features that may be crucial when we study narrativising along with the process of understanding, interpreting and mediating experientiality. The idea of prototypical narrative as a coherent one often provides a structural background for narrating, but such results are achieved with varying success. Subjective experientiality is constantly narrated against the medical script, in different ways. Matti Hyvärinen notes that everyday narratives are usually told when the train of events has swerved away sufficiently from the speaker's expectations or from the canonical cultural narrative;[47] in this case, the common script of the progress of illness, treatment and recovery. Recounting a narrative is not a formula for taking control of experientiality but an attempt to understand and organise one's self, one's memories and one's life once again.

2. Different Versions of the Speaker - Falling Ill as a Process

In autobiographical texts there is usually an attempt to create continuity and/or a connection between the author, the narrator and the main character.[48] Undoubtedly all these concepts refer to the same speaking persona, but I claim that the speakers also question continuity. In oral narratives it is possible to define a) the speaking persona as the author, b) the textual version of the speaker (the narrating I) as the narrator, and the speaker in the past (the experiencing I) as the character. In my analysis the experiencing I mainly points at the character but also at the narrator as an experiencer: the speakers construct themselves not only as characters but also as narrators of a certain kind.

I mentioned above that experiencing appears as a more chaotic event when narrating involves at least some distance from the event. A theory of distance between the narrating I and the experiencing I is provided by Dorrit Cohn.[49] First-person narration, or memorizing narration, is usually presented in the past tense. One is narrating and, at the same time, interpreting and evaluating the past actions of the experiencing I, that is, of oneself in the past. The narrating I can also occasionally identify her- or himself with the position of the past experiencing I, in which case the narration switches to the present tense.

Narration devoted to the discourse of the experiencing I can be defined, for example, as *interior monologue.*[50] Experientiality is expressed as an ongoing process: it is continuous speech emanating from the mind. Several modernist writers, like Woolf and Joyce, tried to write narratives that would express subjective and individual experientiality. In her essay 'Modern Novels' Woolf characterised such a narrative technique as one that

> attempts to come closer to life and to preserve more sincerely and exactly what interests and moves them by discarding most of the conventions which are commonly observed by the novelists. Let us record the atoms as they fall upon the mind in the order in which they fall, let us trace the pattern, however disconnected and incoherent in appearance, which each sight or incident scores upon the consciousness. Let us not take for granted that life exists

> more in what is commonly thought big than in what is commonly thought small.[51]

Mental speech cannot be transferred as such from the experiencing mind to the text. There has to be something mediating the speech, and narrative theories have usually termed this mediator the third-person narrator. Classical narrative theories consider simultaneous first-person narration, where the narrating I would at the same time function as the experiencing I, as impossible: there has to be experiencing first and narration afterwards. However, this view has been called into question.[52] According to Päivi Kosonen, narratology is not helpful in analysing a narrator who is at the same time a living, experiencing subject and a narrative agent - in other words, an experiencing narrator.[53] In autobiographical narration experientiality cannot be restricted only to the object of the narration in the past, for narratives are also constructed in view of the experientiality of the narrative present.

Interior monologue expresses mental discourse in the form we assume it to have taken place. In fiction this kind of narration is not completely chaotic since the character often expresses thoughts progressing in time and constructed as a conceptual interpretation of simultaneous experientiality. In *The Distinction of Fiction* Cohn deals with, among other things, the interpretive problem evoked by first-person narration in the present tense: does the present tense really relate to the present moment or, indirectly, to the past?[54] Present-tense narration can also be a way of enlivening or dramatising the events. When the question raised by Cohn is reversed - does narration in the past tense only refer to the past or, indirectly, to the present too - we encounter the unsolvable problem characteristic of autobiographical narratives. Often the tenses employed do not refer to the moment of the action at all; the present tense may also be used when telling about events in the past. Even though the speaker may have employed the past tense, the present narrative moment inevitably affects the narration, and so the experientiality of the speaker has an effect on the narrative whole. Narratology does not give us precise tools for studying diverse kinds of experiential narration. Nevertheless, studying multidimensional narration may bring us closer to the experientiality expressed in narratives. In this respect, social sciences have often emphasised the coherence of narratives,[55] while in literary studies the focus has been on the difficulties of narrativisation in representing experientiality.

Narrativisation problems arise, for example, in Hilja's narrative below, when the narration moves from the past to the present tense as she switches into the narrative moment in the next quotation. The italicised sentence can be interpreted as living experientiality interrupting coherent narration much in the same way discourse belonging to the experiencing mind does in fiction: subjects or predicates may disappear, references will be blurred, pronouns become absent, tenses are confused. Narration is like mental discourse where the speaker searches for the right concepts. In oral narratives the speaker is not necessarily conscious of all the devices she or he is using in narration, but the experientiality of the narrative moment has an effect on the choices made. As Hilja tells about her hope that her life will continue, she does not say the word 'death,' but the thought about death is an absent other against which her narrativisation is constructed. The italicised sentence can be interpreted as Hilja's reflecting on her own experientiality, not as narrating about reflected experientiality:

> I can only take a very short walk at a time and then I must breathe, and stop. So, I still have these kinds of things. And the heart, it is there, but never again, never the health will be like it used to be before. It's my past and it has gone. *Of course, if like this, if I could go on like this, like this here, could go on, could be here, [sighing], have some more time left, to be here.* (Hilja)

To interpret present tense discourse as interior monologue, as an expression of the experiencing mind only, is inadequate in the case of oral narratives. It works for the italicised passage above but the rest of the quotation is clearly narrative. In the first sentence Hilja describes a situation that is typical in her life. By using these means - present-tense combined with description - as a speaker she invites her listener(s) to enter her situation: she constructs a freeze-frame of her life in front of the listener's eyes. Of course, narrative processes in autobiographical and fictional narratives differ from each other to an extent: in fiction the narrative devices are employed more deliberately whereas in everyday narration the narratives are also constructed in terms of the narrative situation, including emotional reactions. Still the narrative situation and the interaction with the listener or a reader affects the choice of narrative devices: the stories are always told to somebody, at least to an imagined person. We can perceive several structural consistencies between fictional texts and oral narratives. For example, the shift to present-tense narration can be seen as an exception from conventional retrospective narration and so as a sign of a turn, of something noteworthy. Fiction imitates everyday narration and the narration of the mind, while it also moulds and influences their options.

A character is the version of the speaker which is projected into the story, and the speaker's notion of this character may either conform with or differ from his or her own personality at the narrative moment. According to Jean Starobinski, it is possible to distinguish between several experiential-historical versions of the autobiographical I.[56] If the actors of the narrative whole (the experienced, the experiencing, and the narrative I) are separated from each other, a multidimensional analysis and interpretation of the speaker's self becomes possible. For example, Hilja represents herself in several versions. She was 'very keen on having many kinds of hobbies' but with the illness she becomes 'empty' and 'submissive.' Even if Hilja says that she is 'all the time getting back to these matters that [she has] been forced to forfeit,' she is constructing the possibility of a new turn, waiting for one more opportunity to represent a new version of herself in the future:

> I could have been thinking a year ago, that, well, it wouldn't have come to my mind that . . . but the illness, really, it makes a person humble. *They take from you even though you have nothing, when you are completely empty. You leave as an empty person, when I came here from the hospital I felt really empty*. And then indeed these, I am all the time getting back to these matters that I have been forced to forfeit, I have always been very keen on my hobbies, and then, suddenly, something like this. This was really a kind of thump, there had been nothing, that I could have known beforehand, no pain, until the sixth of April, in the evening, and I don't remember it myself but, but I didn't have, before that, any pain. I was not ill at all. (Hilja)

At the beginning of the quotation she distances herself from the past events and evaluates them from the standpoint of the narrative situation. The italicised sentence in the present tense can first be interpreted as Hilja's search for expressions that represent experientiality. After that she switches to the past tense when summing up the interpreted experience: 'I felt really empty.' The emptiness as an emotion is transferred from the present to the past tense. It then becomes a part of the past; in the present and especially in the future there will be room for other versions of the I as well.

Classical narrative norms regarding the impossibility of simultaneous experience and narration are also supported by the materials in my study. The language employed does not always reach the experientiality of the present or of the past. The less time has elapsed from the event of falling ill, the more the person has to rely on the script of treatment and recovery in arranging the experience; this makes the narrative resemble a medical illness narrative. Narratives like this tend to concentrate more on the illness than on the ill person.[57] Even though I had specifically asked the interviewees to tell me about their experiences of falling ill, instead of their emotions and thoughts they told me about the treatment and its effects on the disease.

If the experientiality of the events is still chaotic at the narrative moment, it may prevent the speaker from shaping the experience as a coherent narrative. Experientiality cannot then be formed into a progressive plot. Reflecting on one's own experientiality from a personal viewpoint demands distance from the events which some of the speakers in my materials did not yet command. The script may have appeared as a culturally suitable and mentally safe way of recounting the confusing or potentially embarrassing experientiality. In these kinds of narratives the character was not separated from the narrator, as the speaker did not see her or himself as distinct from the person who had fallen ill. One prototypical element of the narrative, the turn, was built into the narratives only as a change from being a healthy person to being ill. The narrated process did not include a change from falling ill to living with the illness.

The speaker's emotional state in the narrative situation may help in elucidating the experientiality, as we can see from Hannele's narrative below. Even though almost two decades have elapsed since her becoming ill, the speaker switches to the present tense when she discusses her still being shocked about it. Crying as an expression of emotion not only strengthens her interpretation of the event's meaning but also brings out the strong presence of experientiality at the narrative moment. The deconstruction of the structural coherence and contradictions in content may function precisely as expressions of an emotional state:

> I had a coronary on the ninth of June 1991, and I was, on a holiday, I got to go to the hospital, in a coronary, they were not able to do anything, to prevent it. Then I was on sick leave for almost five months. It was a catastrophe, I had to keep my firm closed all that time. *And, but I am, somehow, a kind of positive person, that I, well, because I am a religious person, so [crying], well, I always start to cry because I am so shocked.* So, well, I was putting my faith in God, because, this was a religious person in question, well, in any case, one knows that if leaving here is near, one will know where one is going. (Hannele)

Traumatic experience can be predominantly emotional; crying, among other things, may express emotional experientiality better than any words. According to Rita Charon, telling is performative, and she would like to expand the concept of narration to include, for example, gestures, physical changes and events in addition to verbal acts.[58] Language is able to express only verbal interpretations of experientiality. In Hannele's narrative, non-coherence can also be understood in relation to its content: Hannele's story of herself as a positive and trusting person due to her religiousness is not supported by the narration - it falls apart as the fear of death intervenes into the narrative. The re-lived shock and the crying, which deconstruct the narration at the structural level, tell us about Hannele's experiential chaos too. The gap between experientiality and language indicates not only the difficulty of narrativising experience but the occasional impossibility of comprehending and conceptualising existence on the whole.[59] The more intense and exceptional the experience is, the more awkward the attempts become to find verbal expressions for experientiality within the resources of familiar ordinary language. Hannele is accustomed to thinking of herself as a certain kind of person, but the emotional narrative situation repeatedly forces her to realign her sense of identity with the unexpected and disruptive event of falling ill. Hannele is still able to control the content, but experientiality affects the shape of her narrative.

3. Actual and Potential Narratives

Experiences do not exist in our memories as such: time, place and actors are brought into new formulas in the narrative situation.[60] It is possible to interpret the text as a process, or as strata of experientiality. The process can be explicated as the separation of the experiencing and narrating I - the character and the narrator, as well as in terms of the distinction between narration and narrative. On the level of narration the story events need not be represented in chronological order; they can be arranged in an order best suited to specific narrative aims.[61] Narratives are a way of organizing time and imposing order on a chaotic world, but they can also subvert that order.[62]

In my materials experientiality was often present when speakers started commenting on the script which was assumed as culturally proper and shared and their experientiality was narrativised against this script. The events included in the script were repeatedly evaluated and interpreted. According to Hydén, such evaluation tells us much about the speaker.[63] It is sometimes effected through comparisons and negations, e.g.:

> There was not anything strange there, nothing strange. It was quite painless and I was feeling ok, anything but strange . . . well, then, the night was great, I woke up in the morning, when my roommate started to talk to me, and then, nothing, everything was nice, and quite soon I was, at noon they moved me back here to the local hospital and follow-up treatment. Here, I think, everything was, there were just normal activities, were there, and then, I felt like being [laughing] a healthy man all the time, and I didn't

> have some, well, like I would had have any difficulties, I was, I went to the stairs too, maybe I wasn't allowed to go there but, but I didn't feel anything, nothing, unwell, nothing like that, any time at all. (Hannes)

As mentioned above, various narrative devices may help capture fragmented and even elided experience. The absence may be constructed into the narrative, for example, by negations, as in Hannes's narrative above. It seems that Hannes is telling the restitution narrative, but he does not construct the falling ill process by creating narrative connections between the events - he only tells about particular events. For example, there is no turn from a healthy to an ill person: Hannes is in a hospital, but not because of being ill - he 'felt like being a healthy man all the time'; there have been measures taken in the hospital, but they were 'just normal activities.' The narrator keeps telling us that everything was all right all the time, and nothing seemed strange to him. This partly contradicts the assumption that narratives must always be based on the turn towards something exceptional,[64] as here the narrator explicitly denies that anything exceptional had taken place. Actually, however, the narrator evaluates and interprets his experientiality of the events against the script plot which presupposes that something exceptional should occur - and that he should expect it to occur.[65] He even resists the script of his being seriously ill and subject to a high-risk treatment. In his narrative the conventional turn is effected in the evaluation process (the speaker actually denies too much too obviously): it is not realised at the level of story content.

There is no dearth of definitions for the concept of narrative in literary studies.[66] One authoritative way of proceeding is to see narrative as a strategy for coming to terms with time, process and change.[67] Narrativising offers a possi-bility of producing a certain kind of experience by using narrative means that are associated with temporal and sequential ordering. Successive events are often interpreted as standing in a causal relation to each other,[68] unnecessarily so. Events succeeding each other need not be causally connected from the speaker's point of view. Narration is a way to create continuity between events, and events become linked together when speakers implicitly or explicitly use them to construct meanings.[69] Earlier events make later ones possible even when they are not the only links in the chain.

In illness narratives the expected turn from health to illness need not always define identity shifts, as we saw with Hannes's narrative. Most speakers highlight this turn by linking together sudden symptoms and subsequent medical consultations. Many narrators say they were not able to interpret the symptoms correctly when they first appeared. Nevertheless, when they talk about the symptoms afterwards, they quite predictably link them to the illness and construct the expected turn on this basis. At the beginning of her narrative, Helena described her breathlessness as a symptom that made her consult the doctor, but breathlessness was only later interpreted as a fatal symptom because of the doctor's question, the expression on his face, and the memory of the dead friend who had had the same symptom.

Narrative connections can also provide a way to express implicit criticism.[70] Switching to the present tense though refering to past conversations, the speaker seems to be quoting, creating an illusion of *direct speech*.[71] The listener may be aware of having to rely on the speaker's memory but there is a strong cultural convention of regarding this kind of presentation as documentary. Hilkka's narrative below evaluates and resists the conventional medical script, providing a characterisation of the doctor by quoting, as it were, the doctor's speech. The doctor's and Hilkka's dialogue is arranged in a pattern of flawed turn-management: the doctor fails to acknowledge the narrator's turns to speak and instead proposes questions that neglect her state of mind, which was actually the reason for her wanting to see the doctor in the first place. The narrator asks for medication to improve her mental condition, but her request is ignored by the doctor who recommends taking various tests. Hilkka is suggesting that the doctor did not read her state of mind correctly despite her having just broken into tears in the waiting room. In this sense, Hilkka's narrative can be regarded in relation to Theory of Mind[72] according to which we could, and should, be cognitively capable of connecting mental states, emotions and behaviour when interpreting someone else's actions:

> It was, well, anyway, I was in such a mood that I said to him that, well, I just cried in the waiting room, I had to take heart medicine, and, but then, he didn't intervene but only asked me that, how have you slept, I said that I have slept about four or five hours with the help of sleeping pills. … I thought that any doctor would write this kind of prescription and then, when I went to see him but he said that he couldn't write it that he couldn't start this kind of antidepressant medicine that it should be done by your own GP. And then, but he took then, he said that we will take some blood tests which may be affecting it and he gave me the test, you know, and I answered it and, and then, after this I didn't get the medicine. (Hilkka)

As listeners or readers of this narrative we have no way of knowing the original conversation; nor is this essential since it is the narrative that creates the meanings: the narrative gives us Hilkka's experience of the event, the knowledge needed to understand her side of the matter. Speech belonging to an authority figure, such as the doctor, usually tends to be granted the status of convincing discourse regardless of its content;[73] Hilkka, however, reverses this regularity: by evoking the turn-takings and presenting the doctor's speech as quoted, she is actually questioning the authority of medical discourse. In their studies of illness narratives, Hydén and Brockmeier have claimed that the medical profession has long been suspicious of the patients' voice and instead trusts the so-called objective marks found in, for example, test results.[74] In Hilkka's narrative the medical voice and the patient's voice are linked together in a way that leads the listener to grasp the speaker's implicit criticism of this practice.

Everyday narrators may intentionally leave some parts of the story open, especially in ethically fraught passages where they may not have attained interpretations that they deem subjectively or culturally shareable. Conversely, the speakers may also fill in story-level blanks in their narration. In the case of illness narratives there are special kinds of blanks, moments in the course of the events that cannot be remembered because the speakers were unconscious or under the influence of drugs. In order to maintain continuity, the speakers sometimes fill in such blanks by using materials from someone else's narrative:

> I have heard that . . . after I'd fallen with a thump on my back and, my friend had started artificial respiration and apparently he didn't do it right, or hadn't known how to do it properly but, there was a nurse there, near and said to him that he was doing it the wrong way that, I have heard that my stomach had started to bulge out and. The nurse then, had given me artificial respiration and, I don't know how but somehow, we have talked about it many times, but, however the ambulance came 18 minutes later and, the heart had been at a standstill for 25 minutes, according to the medical record. And all the three veins were, like blocked up and. I remember nothing. (Henri)

According to Henri he is telling us something heard from others but his own telling is very vivid: it seems as if he witnessed the events too. He comments on and evaluates the events. We may question whether and in which ways narration serves to integrate one's identity, but it appears certain that construction of narrative continuity by such gap-filling may serve to overcome confusion. It may also be a way of dealing with a potential embarrassment, e.g.:

> I don't understand why I haven't, why they didn't tell me what I have been talking about then, I asked them, but I wasn't told. They didn't tell me what I have been waffling on there and then. Well, but it is, it is so strange, that I can't explain it, because it is like, I would like to know, awfully would like to know what has happened. (Hilja)

Cognitive narratology has often regarded narratives as integrative and therapeutic, especially in so far as narration offers ways of arranging separate events or chaotic experientiality both temporally and causally. The possibility to process - narrativise - the past, the present and future may have a restitutive function even when the plot is not coherent or connections not clear.

4. Narrativising as an Integration of Identity?

Narrating can be understood as identity work. To be a speaker is always an active role, involving strategies in which one constructs one's life story. Though Hilja's story begins with events concerning falling ill and then moves on to the progress of treatments, her narrative is more circular than linear. Giving up becomes a recurrent theme. Falling ill means to Hilja that she has to give up not just her old hobbies but her previous identity as well. Rimmon-Kenan has stated that falling ill is always a cause for a gap in the life story; the past, the present and the future will all be seen in a different light.[75] Chronic illness, such as cardiovascular disease, is the kind of experience where the structures of everyday life and the forms of knowledge are disrupted: it makes the person recognise the worlds of pain, suffering and even death, which are normally only seen as distant possibilities or the plight of others.[76] Hydén demonstrates how illness seems to produce a temporary chaos in the life of the ill person and how one's life story has to be subsequently reconstructed.[77] Since most people at least try to create coherence and continuity in their lives, they proceed to bridge the gap between their life story and their identity when narrating.

According to Rimmon-Kenan, identity is constructed of stories that we tell ourselves, those that other people tell about us, and cultural narratives.[78] I see the identity story in autobiographical narratives as consisting of a dialogue between different versions of the narrative I and the experiencing I. The identity story can be manifested in the illness narrative as a progressive negotiation of meanings, as in the next quotation:

> But the illness, really, it makes a person humble. They take from you even though you have nothing, when you are completely empty. You leave as an empty person, when I came here from the hospital I felt really empty. (Hilja)

Several narrators in my materials depict becoming ill as a humbling event. At the beginning of the previous quotation Hilja shares the common cultural meaning of falling ill as a humbling experience in the face of an unavoidable change. Then she tries to express her own personal notion of the event and the simultaneous change in her identity. She describes her feelings by using the present tense: 'You feel completely empty.' Presumably she is expressing her experientiality as it happened. By using the present tense and the second person mode she invites the listener to share her point of view, to identify with her experientiality. Then she proceeds to introduce her experientiality into past-tense narration and at the same time into her past: 'I felt empty.' The temporal dimension of narration enables the speaker to analyze and express experience and identity as processes in the narrative.[79] The speaker is first able to express her experientiality, then to conceptualise it and construct the meaning as part of her life story. The back-and-forth movement between the past and the present may be a device for constructing identity continuity, and identity and reality expand via experientiality to the narrative present.

Even though there is usually an attempt to maintain continuity between the speaker-narrator and the main character in autobiographical narratives, the speakers also distinguish between their past I and present I. Narrators may emphasise both the continuity and discontinuity when negotiating their identity in narration.[80] Narrativising can create fragmentation and coherence at the same time.[81] Some versions of the self may even be rejected. In any case, different versions are associated with changes.[82] The narrator can distance himself from the character and so evaluate the action and narrated events in his own voice:

> This depression and this kind of feeling unwell, it became worse and worse all the time. I do not understand, now I don't understand, then it was natural, that I had all the time a kind of feeling, that my life, I have lived it now, it is over. Nothing happens. (Henri)

Henri says that he does not understand his past feelings 'now,' at the present narrative situation, as opposed to the time when he became ill. Despite this he is able to conceptualise both his feelings of being unwell and his sense of an end of familiar life. His depiction of past experientiality - 'my life, I have lived it now, it is over. Nothing happens' - is quite similar to Hilja's description of falling ill as an experience of emptiness. In Hilja's narrative, verbal expressions of experientiality are used to construct continuity and coherence between the past and the present. Henri succeeds in verbalizing a parallel experience, but according to the narrator the past is differentiated from the present on the experiential level. The narrator himself does not identify and he does not expect the listener to identify with his past experientiality.

A cultural voice can also take part in the narrative negotiation. Experientiality is usually told in a way that is felt as culturally convenient.[83] While speakers explicitly give voice to attitudes and meanings that are culturally acceptable, they may implicitly tell things that are inconvenient and unacceptable as well. For example, distancing the illness from oneself has often been seen in a negative light - one has not adapted to the new situation - or it refers to the medical script in which the person is not even seen, only the disease is. But this convention can also give illness its own positive voice. Living with illness may involve negotiating the boundaries between the speaker and the disease as actors:

> But I have been forced to learn that the heart is the one who dictates the terms . . . if it says that listen to me, today I am not feeling well, then I have to be still and I can't try, can do almost nothing. It is not possible to go skiing or swimming, if the pump says that you have to be still and take it easy, listen to me and go to rest. (Hilppa)

There need not always be an essential change in the identity of the speaker in illness narratives. The gap caused by the illness may also be bridged by preserving identity, as it happens in Hilppa's and Hannes's narratives. In this case, there is no separate ill character constructed at the level of narration but the narrator deals with the changes undergone on the story level.

The narratological concept of *focalisation* indicates the point of view from which the story-world is perceived.[84] My materials also indicate that the narrower the temporal distance between the speakers' becoming ill and the narrative situation, the stronger the effect of the original illness on focalisation. The narrators were closer to the experiencing I than to a distinctive narrating I: the narratives were more like records of the events than their evaluations. On the other hand, due to the narrators' avoidance of strong emotional expressions, the narratives also resembled medical illness narratives dealing with treatment. The identity constructed in the narrative was dominantly that of an ill person, apparently because the illness affected both the focalisation and one's entire view of life. The speakers later implicitly or explicitly try to get rid of this emphasis - very few of them actually want to identify themselves only through the illness. They construct a character separate from the narrative I, and this character is the one who encounters illness in the beginning. Still the experiential expression of falling ill might paradoxically be more intense when more time has elapsed after the event. Narratives can capture the complexities of experience.[85]

When the latter is the case, the speakers are able to construct a personal point of view regarding the event. This is inter-woven with the speaker's identity change: apart from the life story, it is constructed into the identity story as well. The plot that Frank designates as that of the quest narrative can here be seen as gaining ground, crystallizing from restitution and chaos narratives.[86] Some personally meaningful theme now emerges to arrange the events, and the narrative I starts to focalise the experience. Religious feelings, for instance, might begin to construct the meanings of both falling ill and recovering, with the result of creating new continuity in the life and identity stories broken off by the illness, e.g.:

> Well, they were, there were many kinds of thoughts at that time but, I never thought why something like this would happen to me, why, but I thought that I needed, this is something that God is offering to me, this is, however, the way he loves me, he is teaching me something, humility, I have been very proud before, well, really, I have noticed this has changed me, as a person. (Hilkka)

Even though months have passed from the moment of falling ill, we can conclude from the use of the present tense that Hilkka is still processing her experientiality at the narrative situation. Probably she has narrated the experience many times, but each new telling provides another possibility of articulating the experience. As her narration shifts between the past and present tenses, she conveys in direct quotations what she thought in the past even though the thoughts must have been conceptualised only later: it was later that she interpreted herself as a person who had been proud before falling ill. Now, she tells us that she has become something else: she has learned to be humble. Even though the theme is the same as in Hilja's narrative, the attitude expressed is different: Hilja said that she had been forced to be humble whereas Hilkka felt that she had received the chance to learn to be humble. Falling ill, for Hilkka, was an interruption and a turn in her life, as well as a change of identity, but at the narrative situation it becomes a bridged gap. Bridging, or the learning process, reaches all the way to the narrative moment and the situation of the narrative I. Hilkka uses two different words when referring to the turn that the illness caused; 'that' indicates the part of the process further away than the part of process referred to by 'this.' The change has been woven into the identity story, and this provides the speaker with a more coherent idea of herself in the narrative situation. A quest for continuity is associated with the temporal dimension of narration and thus the narrative enables the speaker to reconstruct her identity in relation to the past, the present and the future.

5. Conclusion

Falling seriously and chronically ill is a strong emotional event that affects life and identity. I have tried to depict the many ways in which people attempt to narrativise such an experiential event against the medical script. I see narrative analysis as a method both for studying the processes of dealing with the experience of falling ill and for exploring the personal and shared meanings that such an experience provides.

Devices known from literary analysis may provide clues to the process of the narrativisation of actual experience, in this case illness experience. Awareness of these devices enables us to recognise the difficulties of narrativisation signalled by blanks, incoherence, gaps and obscurity. Guided by conventions, the speakers may try to tell coherent, logical and conclusive stories, but the narratives that emerge tend to be fragmented, contradictory and open - they tell us about the difficulties, sometimes insurmountable, in comprehending and conceptualizing existence in the world. The speakers may opt for patterns that they deem culturally convenient and shareable, but the points at which the conventional narrativisation vacillates, denies something or fails are crucial when studying the meanings of narrated phenomena.

Narrative and experience have met each other in different disciplines. Concepts and methods derived from the literary field have been applied to different kinds of non-literary research, often remaining abstract and metaphorical. The possibility of adopting them when analysing illness narratives, has allowed me to gain insight by taking advantage of their explanatory power.

Silent knowledge and experiential knowledge have become a subject of attention in recent years. Each ill person has experiential knowledge of what becoming ill means and how life will go on afterwards. Voices of experience expertise are not heard in places where health care service requirements are estimated and decisions are made. Health care professionals have amassed a wealth of physical and physiological information from patients into medical records but, at the same time, there has not been much data on patients as individuals and members of their communities. As a result, the regrettably narrow view of the meanings involved in becoming ill has maintained health care as a routine and bureaucratic service system; the restitution plot - or the medical illness narrative script - has directed the planning and carrying out of its operations. In my opinion, tools are needed to mediate the meanings of other kinds of plots, by studying the avenues that illness narratives could open up for experience expertise, in order to help in developing client-centred health care.

Notes

[1] See Rita Charon, *Narrative Medicine: Honoring the Stories of Illness* (Oxford: Oxford University Press, 2006).
[2] Elliot Mishler, 'Patient Stories, Narratives of Resistance and the Ethics of Human Care: A la recherche du temps perdu,' *Health* 9 (2005): 431-51.
[3] Arthur Kleinman, *The Illness Narratives: Suffering, Healing and the Human Condition* (New York: Basic Books, 1988), xiv (italics mine).
[4] See Lars-Christer Hydén, 'Identity, Self, Narrative,' in *Beyond Narrative Coherence*, ed. Matti Hyvärinen, Lars-Christer Hydén, Marja Saarenheimo and Maria Tamboukou (Amsterdam: John Benjamins, 2010), 33-48.
[5] Corinne Squire, 'Experience-Centered and Culturally-Oriented Approaches to Narrative,' in *Doing Narrative Research*, ed. Molly Andrews, Corinne Squire, and Maria Tamboukou (London: Sage, 2008), 50.
[6] Shlomith Rimmon-Kenan, 'In Two Voices, or: Whose Life/Death/Story Is It, Anyway?' in *A Companion to Narrative Theory*, edited by James Phelan and Peter J. Rabinowitz (Oxford: Blackwell, 2005), 408-409.
[7] See Matti Hyvärinen, 'Acting, Thinking, and Telling,' *Partial Answers* 4/2 (2006): 59-77.
[8] See Cate Watson, 'Tensions and Aporias in the Narrative Construction of Lives.' *Qualitative Research* 8 (2008): 333-37.
[9] David Herman, 'Narratology as a Cognitive Science,' *Image & Narrative*. 1. Cognitive Narratology, 2000. <http://www.imageandnarrative.be/in archive/narratology/davidherman.htm>, viewed on March 21, 2012.
[10] David Herman, *Basic Elements of Narrative* (West Sussex: Wiley-Blackwell, 2009).
[11] Monika Fludernik, *Towards a 'Natural' Narratology* (London: Routledge, 1996).
[12] See Matti Hyvärinen et al., editors, *Beyond Narrative Coherence* (Amsterdam: John Benjamins, 2010); Liz Stanley and Bogusia Temple, 'Narrative Methodologies: Subjects, Silences, Re-readings and Analyses,' *Qualitative Research* 8 (2008): 275-81.
[13] Hydén, 'Identity, Self, Narrative,' 33-48; Tarja Aaltonen, 'Mind-reading: A Method for Understanding the Broken Narrative of an Aphasic Man,' in *Beyond Narrative Coherence*, ed. Matti Hyvärinen et al., 49-66; Jarmila Mildorf, 'Sociolinguistic Implications of Narratology: Focalisation and 'Double Deixis' in Conversational Storytelling,' in *The Travelling Concept of Narrative*, ed. Matti Hyvärinen, Anu Korhonen, and Juri Mykkänen (Helsinki: Helsinki Collegium for Advanced Studies, 2006), 42-59; 'Thought

Presentation and Constructed Dialogue in Oral Stories: Limits and Possibilities of a Cross-Disciplinary Narratology,' *Partial Answers* 6 (2008): 279-300.

[14] See Alan Radley, 'The Aesthetics of Illness: Narrative, Horror and the Sublime,' *Sociology of Health and Illness* 21 (1999): 778-96.

[15] Charon, *Narrative Medicine*, 11.

[16] Cf. Squire, 'Experience-Centered and Culturally-Oriented Approaches to Narrative,' 42.

[17] Philippe Lejeune, *Signes de vie: Le pacte autobiographique 2* (Paris: Seuil, 2005), 31; Päivi Kosonen, 'Moderni omaelämäkerta kertomuksena,' in *Näkökulmia kertomuksen tutkimukseen*, ed. Samuli Hägg, Markku Lehtimäki, and Liisa Steinby (Helsinki: Suomalaisen Kirjallisuuden Seura, 2009), 288.

[18] Dorrit Cohn, *Transparent Minds: Narrative Modes for Presenting Conscious-ness in Fiction* (Princeton: Princeton University Press, 1978), 8.

[19] Rimmon-Kenan, 'In Two Voices, or: Whose Life/Death/Story Is It, Anyway?' 399-412.

[20] Anni Vilkko, *Omaelämäkerta kohtaamispaikkana: Naisen elämän kerronta ja luenta* (Helsinki: SKS, 1997), 93.

[21] Herman, *Basic Elements of Narrative*, 9.

[22] Ibid., 105.

[23] Arja Jokinen, 'Vakuuttelevan ja suostuttelevan retoriikan analysoiminen.' In *Diskurssianalyysi liikkeessä. Vuorovaikutus, toimijuus ja kulttuuri empiirisen tutkimuksen haasteina*, ed. Arja Jokinen, Kirsi Juhila, and Eero Suoninen (Tampere: Vastapaino, 1999), 154.

[24] Herman, *Basic Elements of Narrative*, 37.

[25] Jens Brockmeier, 'Language, Experience, and the 'Traumatic Gap': How to Talk About 9/11?' in *Health, Illness and Culture: Broken Narratives*, ed. Lars-Christer Hydén and Jens Brockmeier (New York: Routledge, 2008), 28.

[26] Ibid., 27.

[27] Herman, *Basic Elements of Narrative*, 75.

[28] See Anne Whitehead, *Trauma Fiction* (Edinburgh: Edinburgh University Press, 2004), 82-83.

[29] Noël Carroll, 'On the Narrative Connection,' in *New Perspectives on Narrative Perspective*, ed. Willie van Peer and Seymour Chatman (New York: State University of New York Press, 2001), 21-41.

[30] Deborah Tannen, 'What's in a Frame? Surface Evidence for Underlying Expec-tations,' in *Framing in Discourse*, ed. Deborah Tannen (Oxford: Oxford University Press, 1993), 36.

[31] Ibid., 35.

[32] Lars-Christer Hydén and Jens Brockmeier, 'Introduction: From the Retold to the Performed Story,' in *Health, Illness and Culture: Broken Narratives*,

ed. Lars-Christer Hydén and Jens Brockmeier (New York: Routledge, 2008), 1-15.
[33] Arthur Frank, *The Wounded Storyteller: Body, Illness, and Ethics* (Chicago: University of Chicago Press, 1995), 9.
[34] See Tarja Aaltonen, *Sanatonko tarinaton? Afaatikon intersubjektiivinen maailma ja kertoen rakentuva identiteetti.* Akateeminen väitöskirja. Miina Sillanpään Säätiön Julkaisuja A: 5 (Helsinki: MSS, 2002), 11.
[35] Frank, *The Wounded Storyteller*, 9.
[36] Peter Währborg, 'Quality of Life after Coronary Angioplasty or Bypass Surgery. 1-Year-Follow-Up in the Coronary Angioplasty versus Bypass Revascularisation Investigation (CAPRI) Trial,' *European Heart Journal* 20 (1999): 653-58.
[37] Frank, *The Wounded Storyteller*, 10-12.
[38] Jukka Valkonen, *Tarinametafora sydäninfarktista kuntoutumisessa.* Kuntoutussäätiön tutkimuksia 45 (Helsinki: Kuntoutussäätiö, 1994), 61.
[39] See Michael Bury, 'Chronic Illness as Biographical Disruption,' *Sociology of Health and Illness* 4 (1982): 167-82.
[40] Aaltonen, *Sanatonko tarinaton?* 13.
[41] Herman, *Basic Elements of Narrative*, 137.
[42] Fludernik, *Towards a 'Natural' Narratology*, 13.
[43] Watson, 'Tensions and Aporias,' 333-37.
[44] Anna De Fina and Alexandra Georgakopoulou, 'Analysing Narratives as Practices,' *Qualitative Research* 8 (2008): 379-87.
[45] Squire, 'Experience-Centered and Culturally-Oriented Approaches to Narrative,' 44.
[46] See Hydén, 'Identity, Self, Narrative,' 33-48.
[47] Matti Hyvärinen, ''Life as Narrative' Revisited,' *Partial Answers* 6 (2008): 261-77.
[48] See Kosonen, 'Moderni omaelämäkerta kertomuksena,' 284-85.
[49] Cohn, *Transparent Minds*, 143.
[50] Gerard Génette, *Narrative Discourse: An Essay in Method*, trans. Jane E. Lewin (Ithaca: Cornell University Press, 1980), 192-93; Franz K. Stanzel, *A Theory of Narrative*, trans. Charlotte Goedsche (Cambridge: Cambridge University Press, 1984), 225-26.
[51] Virginia Woolf, 'Modern Novels,' in *The Essays of Virginia Woolf.* Vol 3: *1919-1924*, ed. Andrew McNeillie (London: Hogarth Press, 1988 [1919]), 33-34.
[52] Cohn, *Distinction of Fiction*, 96-97.
[53] Kosonen, 'Moderni omaelämäkerta kertomuksena,' 291.
[54] Cohn, *Distinction of Fiction*, 102-104.
[55] Hyvärinen, et al., *Beyond Narrative Coherence*, 1-2.

[56] See Kosonen, 'Moderni omaelämäkerta kertomuksena,' 286.
[57] See Shlomith Rimmon-Kenan, 'The Story of 'I': Illness and Narrative Identity,' *Narrative* 10 (2002).
[58] Rita Charon, 'Narrative Medicine: Attention, Representation, Affiliation,' *Narrative* 13/3 (2005): 261-70; see also Hydén and Brockmeier, 'Introduction: From the Retold to the Performed Story,' 1-15; Lars-Christer Hydén, 'Narratives in Illness: A Methodological Note,' *Qualitative Sociology Review* 4 (2008): 49-58.
[59] Brockmeier, 'Language, Experience, and the Traumatic Gap,' 16-35.
[60] See Lisa Zunshine, *Why We Read Fiction: Theory of Mind and the Novel* (Columbus: Ohio State University Press, 2006); Carroll, 'On the Narrative Connection,' 21-41.
[61] See Rimmon-Kenan, 'In Two Voices, or: Whose Life/Death/Story Is It, Anyway?' 399-412.
[62] See Watson, 'Tensions and Aporias,' 333.
[63] Hydén, 'Identity, Self, Narrative,' 33-48.
[64] See Hyvärinen, ''Life as Narrative' Revisited,' 261-77; Herman, *Basic Elements of Narrative*, 105.
[65] See Tannen, 'What's in a Frame?' 35-36.
[66] See Pekka Tammi, 'Against Narrative ('A Boring Story'),' *Partial Answers* 4 (2006): 19-40.
[67] David Herman, Manfred Jahn, and Marie-Laure Ryan, editors, *Routledge Encyclopedia of Narrative Theory* (London: Routledge, 2005), ix.
[68] Marie-Laure Ryan, 'Narrative,' in *Routledge Encyclopedia of Narrative Theory*, ed. David Herman, Manfred Jahn and Marie-Laure Ryan (London: Routledge, 2005), 344-48.
[69] Carroll, 'On the Narrative Connection,' 21-41.
[70] See Mishler, 'Patient Stories,' 440.
[71] See Meir Sternberg, 'Proteus in Quotation-Land: Mimesis and the Forms of Reported Discourse,' *Poetics Today* 3 (1982): 107-56; Mildorf, 'Thought Presentation,' 289.
[72] Zunshine, *Why We Read Fiction*, 6-8.
[73] See Jokinen, 'Vakuuttelevan ja suostuttelevan retoriikan analysoiminen,' 135.
[74] Hydén and Brockmeier, 'Introduction: From the Retold to the Performed Story,'1-15.
[75] Rimmon-Kenan, 'The story of 'I.''
[76] See Bury, 'Chronic Illness as Biographical Disruption,' 169.
[77] Hydén, 'Identity, Self, Narrative,' 33-48.
[78] See Rimmon-Kenan, 'The story of 'I.''

[79] Cf. Paul John Eakin, 'What Are We Reading When We Read Autobiography?' *Narrative* 12/2 (2004): 121-32.
[80] Hydén, 'Identity, Self, Narrative,' 33-48.
[81] See Rimmon-Kenan, 'The story of 'I.''
[82] Hydén, 'Identity, Self, Narrative,' 33-48.
[83] See Vilkko, *Omaelämäkerta kohtaamispaikkana*, 92.
[84] Génette, *Narrative Discourse*, 189-90.
[85] See Joanne Hall, 'Narrative Methods in a Study of Trauma Recovery,' *Qualitative Health Research* 21 (2011): 3-13.
[86] Frank, *The Wounded Storyteller*, 115.

Bibliography

Aaltonen, Tarja. 'Mind-reading: A Method for Understanding the Broken Narrative of an Aphasic Man.' In *Beyond Narrative Coherence.* Edited by Matti Hyvärinen, Lars Christer Hydén, Marja Saarenheimo and Maria Tamboukou, 49-66. Amsterdam: John Benjamins, 2010.

———. *Sanatonko tarinaton? Afaatikon intersubjektiivinen maailma ja kertoen rakentuva identiteetti.* Akateeminen väitöskirja. Miina Sillanpään Säätiön Julkaisuja A: 5. Helsinki: MSS, 2002.

Brockmeier, Jens. 'Language, Experience, and the 'Traumatic Gap': How to Talk About 9/11?' In *Health, Illness and Culture: Broken Narratives.* Edited by Lars-Christer Hydén and Jens Brockmeier, 16-35. New York: Routledge, 2008.

Bury, Michael. 'Chronic Illness as Biographical Disruption.' *Sociology of Health and Illness* 4/2 (1982): 167-82.

Carroll, Noël. 'On the Narrative Connection.' In *New Perspectives on Narrative Perspective.* Edited by Willie van Peer, and Seymour Chatman, 21-41. New York: State University of New York Press, 2001.

Charon, Rita. 'Narrative Medicine: Attention, Representation, Affiliation.' *Narrative* 13 (2005): 261-70.

———. *Narrative Medicine: Honoring the Stories of Illness.* Oxford: Oxford University Press, 2006.

Cohn, Dorrit. *The Distinction of Fiction*. Baltimore: The Johns Hopkins University Press, 1999.

———. *Transparent Minds: Narrative Modes for Presenting Consciousness in Fiction*. Princeton: Princeton University Press, 1978.

De Fina, Anna and Alexandra Georgakopoulou. 'Analysing Narratives as Practices.' *Qualitative Research* 8 (2008): 379-87.

Eakin, Paul John. 'What Are We Reading When We Read Autobiography?' *Narrative* 12/2 (2004): 121-32.

Frank, Arthur. *The Wounded Storyteller: Body, Illness, and Ethics*. Chicago: University of Chicago Press, 1995.

Fludernik, Monika. *Towards a 'Natural' Narratology*. London: Routledge, 1996.

Génette, Gerard. *Narrative Discourse: An Essay in Method*. Translated by Jane E. Lewin. Ithaca: Cornell University Press, 1980.

Hall, Joanne. 'Narrative Methods in a Study of Trauma Recovery.' *Qualitative Health Research* 21 (2011): 3-13.

Herman, David. *Basic Elements of Narrative*. West Sussex: Wiley-Blackwell, 2009.

———. 'Narratology as a Cognitive Science.' *Image & Narrative*. 1. Cognitive Narratology, 2000. <http://www.imageandnarrative.be/inarchive/narratology/davidherman.htm>, Viewed on March 21, 2012.

Herman, David, Manfred Jahn and Marie-Laure Ryan, editors. *Routledge Encyclopedia of Narrative Theory*. London: Routledge, 2005.

Hydén, Lars-Christer. 'Identity, Self, Narrative.' In *Beyond Narrative Coherence*, edited by Matti Hyvärinen, Lars Christer Hydén, Marja Saarenheimo and Maria Tamboukou, 33-48. Amsterdam: John Benjamins, 2010.

———. 'Narratives in Illness: A Methodological Note.' *Qualitative Sociology Review* 4 (2008): 49-58.

Hydén, Lars-Christer, and Jens Brockmeier. 'Introduction: From the Retold to the Performed Story.' In *Health, Illness and Culture: Broken Narratives*, edited by Lars-Christer Hydén and Jens Brockmeier, 1-15. New York: Routledge, 2008.

Hyvärinen, Matti. 'Acting, Thinking, and Telling.' *Partial Answers* 4/2 (2006): 59-77.

———. 'Life as Narrative Revisited.' *Partial Answers* 6/2 (2008): 261-77.

Hyvärinen, Matti, Lars-Christer Hydén, Marja Saarenheimo, and Maria Tamboukou, editors. *Beyond Narrative Coherence*. Amsterdam: John Benjamins, 2010.

Jokinen, Arja. 'Vakuuttelevan ja suostuttelevan retoriikan analysoiminen.'In *Diskurssianalyysi liikkeessä. Vuorovaikutus, toimijuus ja kulttuuri empiirisen tutkimuksen haasteina*, edited by Arja Jokinen, Kirsi Juhila and Eero Suoninen, 126-59. Tampere: Vastapaino, 1999.

Kleinman, Arthur. *The Illness Narratives: Suffering, Healing and the Human Condition*. New York: Basic Books, 1988.

Kosonen, Päivi. 'Moderni omaelämäkerta kertomuksena.' In *Näkökulmia kertomuksen tutkimukseen*, edited by Samuli Hägg, Markku Lehtimäki and Liisa Steinby, 282-293. Helsinki: Suomalaisen Kirjallisuuden Seura, 2009.

Lejeune, Philippe. *Signes de vie. Le pacte autobiographique 2*. Paris: Seuil, 2005.

Mildorf, Jarmila. 'Sociolinguistic Implications of Narratology: Focalisation and 'Double Deixis' in Conversational Storytelling.' In *The Travelling Concept of Narrative*, edited by Matti Hyvärinen, Anu Korhonen and Juri Mykkänen, 42-59. Helsinki: Helsinki Collegium for Advanced Studies, 2006.

———. 'Thought Presentation and Constructed Dialogue in Oral Stories: Limits and Possibilities of a Cross-Disciplinary Narratology.' *Partial Answers* 6 (2008): 279-300.

Mishler, Elliot. 'Patient Stories, Narratives of Resistance and the Ethics of Human Care: A la recherche du temps perdu.' *Health* 9 (2005): 431-51.

Radley, Alan. 'The Aesthetics of Illness: Narrative, Horror and the Sublime.' *Sociology of Health and Illness* 21/6 (1999): 778-96.

Rimmon-Kenan, Shlomith. 'In Two Voices, or: Whose Life/Death/Story Is It, Anyway?' In *A Companion to Narrative Theory*, edited by James Phelan and Peter J. Rabinowitz, 399-412. Oxford: Blackwell, 2005.

———. 'The story of 'I': Illness and Narrative Identity.' *Narrative* 10 (2002), 9-27.

Ryan, Marie-Laure. 'Narrative.' In *Routledge Encyclopedia of Narrative Theory*, edited by David Herman, Manfred Jahn and Marie-Laure Ryan, 344-48. London: Routledge, 2005.

Squire, Corinne. 'Experience-Centered and Culturally-Oriented Approaches to Narrative.' In *Doing Narrative Research*, edited by Molly Andrews, Corinne Squire and Maria Tamboukou, 41-63. London: Sage, 2008.

Stanley, Liz, and Bogusia Temple. 'Narrative Methodologies: Subjects, Silences, Re-readings and Analyses.' *Qualitative Research* 8 (2008): 275-81.

Stanzel, Franz K. *A Theory of Narrative*. Translated by Charlotte Goedsche. Cambridge: Cambridge University Press, 1984.

Sternberg, Meir. 'Proteus in Quotation-Land: Mimesis and the Forms of Reported Discourse.' *Poetics Today* 3 (1982): 107-56.

Tammi, Pekka. 'Against Narrative ('A Boring Story').' *Partial Answers* 4 (2006): 19-40.

Tannen, Deborah. 'What's in a Frame? Surface Evidence for Underlying Expectations.' In *Framing in Discourse*, edited by Deborah Tannen, 20-56. Oxford: Oxford University Press, 1993.

Valkonen, Jukka. *Tarinametafora sydäninfarktista kuntoutumisessa*. Kuntoutussäätiön tutkimuksia 45. Helsinki: Kuntoutussäätiö, 1994.

Vilkko, Anni. *Omaelämäkerta kohtaamispaikkana: Naisen elämän kerronta ja luenta*. Helsinki: SKS, 1997.

Watson, Cate. 'Tensions and Aporias in the Narrative Construction of Lives.' *Qualitative Research* 8 (2008): 333-37.

Whitehead, Anne. *Trauma Fiction.* Edinburg: Edinburgh University Press, 2004.

Woolf, Virginia. 'Modern Novels.' In *The Essays of Virginia Woolf.* 6 vols. Vol. 3: *1919-1924*, edited by Andrew McNeillie, 30-37. London: Hogarth Press, 1988 [1919].

Währborg, Peter. 'Quality of Life after Coronary Angioplasty or Bypass Surgery. 1-Year-Follow-Up in the Coronary Angioplasty versus Bypass Revascularisation Investigation (CAPRI) Trial.' *European Heart Journal* 20 (1999): 653-58.

Zunshine, Lisa. *Why We Read Fiction: Theory of Mind and the Novel.* Columbus: Ohio State University Press, 2006.

Place and Space in Christine Brooke-Rose's *Life, End of*

Shlomith Rimmon-Kenan

Abstract
Christine Brooke-Rose's *Life, End of* is a literary narrative, based on the author's autobiographical experience, of the suffering caused by a combination of a cardio-vascular condition with a neurological illness - polyneuritis. This chapter[1] focuses on one aspect of her trajectory: the superposition of a constriction of what Michel de Certeau calls 'place' and an expansion of what he calls 'space.' For de Certeau, 'place' is an institutionalized location, planned 'from above,' governed by the law of the 'proper,' and static. By contrast, 'space' is a location experienced 'from within,' subjectively created by the movements operating in it, and dynamic. *Life, End of* traces the shrinking of place available to the ill protagonist who can no longer drive a car, can no longer use the upper floor of her house, has difficulties in negotiating even areas needed for the most elementary activities, like the bathroom. The confinement of place, however, is countered by an expansion of space in three main ways: 1) books and television provide intertextual spaces that open up onto the world; 2) imagination (e.g. of the 'figures' she sees on the wall opposite her) expands the horizon beyond the boundaries of physical place; 3) the writing of the text we read, with its proliferation of language and abundance of puns, many of them multilingual. I situate the analysis within the debate between Elaine Scarry and David Morris concerning the relation between pain and language. While Scarry maintains that physical pain does not only resist language but actively destroys it, Morris emphasizes the meaning-generating quality of pain. Brooke-Rose's text is more in tune with Morris's position, opening up a linguistic space of meaning and play within the constriction imposed by suffering. Therein lies its phoenix-like quality.

Key Words: Illness narratives, narratology, space (constriction of), space (expansion of), language (proliferation of), Phoenix-like quality, Michel De Certeau, Elaine Scarry, David Morris, Arthur Frank.

*****

'House to flat to room to bed to coffin to urn'[2] is the way Christine Brooke-Rose's *Life, End of*, a self-reflexive, self-conscious text oscillating between the fictional and the autobiographical, describes the process of a life-time - not in terms of 'a succession of events,'[3] but in those of a movement from one space to another. The above master-narrative (if it can be labelled thus) competes with another generalizing statement earlier in the book, representing a doubly-directed movement: 'The immediate environment always shrinks, from house to flat to room to bed to coffin to earthworm-tums then grows again to compost to earth to planet to universe' (12). This twofold movement of shrinking and expansion is again couched in predominantly spatial terms.

These concise summaries of the human trajectory could serve as a springboard for an interrogation of the narratological privileging of time over space. These days, however, there is no need to defend the generative role of space in narrative and its inseparability from time: this insight has recently been given persuasive reformulations by David Herman,[4] Susan Stanford Friedman,[5] and Ruth Ginsburg.[6] I say 're-formulations,' because the position itself has already been argued for in earlier studies such as Bakhtin's[7] and the Tartu school's, including Jurij Lotman's *The Structure of the Artistic Text.*[8] However, classical narratology has continued, by and large, to privilege time over space. Today, in what Herman calls postclassical narratology,[9] this is no longer the case. Hard as it is for my past self, my present work takes the generative force of space in narrative as a given. On this basis, I make three propositions about illness narratives: a) because such narratives represent situations of extreme physical limitations, they often foreground spatial and spatiotemporal configurations; b) a chronotopic perspective detects in many illness narratives a tendency to relate a shrinking of space with an expansion of narrative time - Tolstoy's 'The Death of Ivan Ilyich' is the classical example of this phenomenon in literature; c) a superposition of a constriction of what Michel de Certeau calls 'place' and an expansion of what he calls 'space' often characterizes illness narratives. My chapter will focus on the third of the above issues, in conjunction with Brooke-Rose's *Life, End of.*

De Certeau's distinction between 'place' and 'space' differs from common usage, which either sees the two as synonymous or considers place as a particular portion of space. According to De Certeau, 'place' is an institutionalized location, planned 'from above,' governed by the law of the 'proper,' static. By contrast, 'space' is a location experienced 'from within,' subjectively created by the movements operating within it, dynamic:

> A place (*lieu*) is the order (of whatever kind) in accord with which elements are distributed in relationships of coexistence. It thus excludes the possibility of two things being in the same location (*place*). The law of the 'proper' rules in the place; the elements taken into consideration are beside one another, each situated in its own 'proper' and distinct location, a location it defines. A place is thus an instantaneous configuration of positions. It implies an indication of stability.

> A *space* exists when one takes into consideration vectors of direction, velocities, and time variables. Thus space is composed of intersections of mobile elements. It is in a sense actuated by the ensemble of movements deployed within it. Space occurs as the effect produced by the operations that orient it, situate it, temporalize it, and make it function in a polyvalent unity of conflictual programs or contractual proximities. On this view, in relation to place, space is like the word when it is spoken, that is, when it is caught in the ambiguity of an actualization, transformed into a term dependent upon many different conventions, situated as the act of a present (or of a time), and modified by the transformations caused by successive contexts. In contradistinction to the place, it has thus none of the univocity or stability of a 'proper.'[10]

In what follows, the term 'space' will be used according to this definition and not - as heretofore - as a synonym of place, location, site, etc. De Certeau's distinction is not always as watertight as some may wish it to be: 'space' and 'place' may, for instance, be more profitably conceived of as two aspects of the same phenomenon rather than as a pair of binary opposites. Nevertheless, I find it illuminating in the analysis of illness narratives: in particular, it may provide insights into Brooke-Rose's attempts to deal with her own pain.

1. The Past: Space as Practiced Place

As the title of Brooke-Rose's text clearly suggests, the narrative present revolves around the end of life - a temporal characterization whose spatial dimensions I explore in this chapter. The narration of the deteriorating course of a cardio-vascular condition combined with a neurological illness (polyneuritis) is frequently interrupted by non-chronological analepses that, taken together, conjure up a life-story. The protagonist is a woman of about eighty, a teacher of languages, who was often subjected to geographical displacements in her childhood, later experienced World War II from the point of view of the Germans while situated in the British Intelligence Service, and then spent her adult life writing, teaching and travelling freely in the world. These and other details are very close to the biography of the author, Christine Brooke-Rose, novelist, narratologist and retired university professor - and the text explicitly points to the near-identity of the two.

The protagonist-narrator's life-story emerging from the fragmented analepses is often rendered in terms of place or space. For example, during a poignant half-hallucinatory scene in the narrative present, in which she superimposes an earlier, larger house upon the one where she is imprisoned in her illness, the protagonist reviews her life as a sequence of locations in which she has lived:

> But why this haunting by a late and previous house? Why not the Paris flat, with its inebriating second life, slight loves and warm friendships? Why not the Hampstead flat with its views over all London and its seven remaining years of marriage and late collapse? Why not the earlier fifteen years of that marriage, idyllic in a rent-controlled Chelsea lodging, one and a half rooms with toilet and bathroom on the landing shared by all? And so on. (95)

These different places, stable and static in themselves, planned and built by others, become both dynamic and subjectively meaningful as a result of the experiences with which the character associates them. Significantly, these are also experiences in which the spatial dimension corresponds to the temporality of periods in the character's life.

The analepsis that most palpably dramatizes the transformation of a given place into a subjectively meaningful and creative space recalls the different ways the protagonist and her neighbour furnish two identically structured flats. The description is long, its very length emphasising the centrality of space in *Life, End of*:

> Their two flats are both shaped like prows, getting narrower and narrower after a fairly wide entrance made of small hall, small bathroom and kitchen on the left overlooking the courtyard with its two other entrance stairs, and a largish bedroom to the right, overlooking a narrow sidestreet. The hall then opens out into the living-room, which slowly shrinks into no-space, but prolongs the tall windows of the bedroom into four more, the end of the room a tiny space two arms wide, almost unfurnishable... And these identically odd flats are adapted, decorated and furnished into extremes of difference, expressing their owners' deep similarities in the initial choice mingled with astonishing particularities in the transformation. The only element the two flats have in common apart from the shape is the original Chinese-looking beige wallpaper. The top one is carpeted in dark brown, with tall matching velvet curtains in the bedroom against blood-red padded walls; the tall velvet curtains are continued in the living-room in warm colours grading off from violet to crimson to orange to yellow-gold. At the far end there's now a deep radiator

> across the short end-wall, below a Second Empire mirror framed in gold-painted wood, much damaged, with a large top crest. The mirror, too, is deficient, the tin-foil worn out here and there, but nevertheless prolonging the effect, not only of the curtain colours but of the tiny desk in the narrow part, facing the room, with an ex-door recess in the thick inner wall for books; then, the baby grand, beyond which are high book-shelves behind a sofa at the wide end and a bergère and huge floor cushions in the same velvets as the curtains, and books and files all along the inner wall. But the mirror can't see, in the tiny entrance-hall, a folding black dinner-table between two velvet crimson chairs, the other two nestling somewhere according to need. Nor can it see, on this side of the baby grand, the two guitars, brought over from Spain and London and now leaning against its inner curve like a pair of open legs with huge feet shod in rackets. The mirror cannot reflect all this, but tries.
>
> Her flat on the contrary shortens the narrowing room with a wall and door into a linen store-room. So the long room is no longer long, though still a trapeze. The carpeting is mustard, the curtains white lace with goldenish and white surrounds, the furniture all an elegant but unsinkable-in Louis XV style, a dining-table permanently there, instead of the piano, welcoming, surrounded by four chairs, not a makeshift hall affair. The books and desk are tucked away in the bedroom with a put-up bed. So that the effect is light. Light and airy versus dark and cosy. White and gold versus glowing warm colours, elegance and outsideness versus comfort and innerness, books absent from the salon below but furnishing the living-room above. Each of their six windows, making twelve, are planted with hanging geraniums, adding gaiety to this façade of the white old house along one of the two streets that join at the corner. (80-81)

This is merely a descriptive pause, many classical narratologists would argue. But de Certeau would maintain that the passage is a rendering of a space: 'Space occurs as the effect produced by the operations that orient it, situate it, temporalize it, and make it function in a polyvalent unity of conflictual programs or contractual proximities.'[11]

'A space,' de Certeau also says, 'exists when one takes into consideration vectors of direction, velocities, and time variables.'[12] Clearly, the protagonist's spatial mobility as well as temporal facility in the past was enhanced by the possession of a car, 'symbol and instrument of independence' (90), which she had to give up as a result of the loss of sensitivity in her legs. On the other hand, the dreaded symbol of dependence, passivity, submission to impersonal systems is the place bluntly called in French slang the *mouroir* (euphemistically labelled 'a retirement community' in the U.S.).

2. The Present: 'Imprisoned in Two Rooms'

The two illnesses with which the text opens, complicated by additional incapacities that develop later, turn the narrative present into a battlefield between repeated attempts to negotiate place creatively and make it into an inhabitable space and the shrinking of territory, coupled with limitations of movement. Without the use of the first person, which would conjure up subjectivity, the opening page dwells on the physical details involved in leaning against various objects in the bathroom in order to accomplish the seemingly simple act of washing. What is foregrounded is the body as site:

> The head top leans against the bathroom mirror so that the looking glass becomes a feeling glass. But what does it feel? This position is for body-balance during the brushing of teeth and the washing of face neck arms and torso. Below is for the biddy, and the feet, if sitting on a stool. But especially the torso. For in fact the teeth can also be brushed if the loins touch the washbasin however cold, or the hand grips the edge, on condition neither is wet.
>
> And then the drying of the body-parts, one hand on the tall towel-radiator, the other on the lower part of the towel to dry the lower body. Dressing means sitting on the bed, entering pants, rising, legs in calf-love with the bedside, to slide the pants then trousers past the bottom before swiftly sitting again. The feet feel where the entrances are, whether of pants or slippers.
>
> Standing, on its own, without support somewhere, causes a tidal wave of nothingness in the head and a limping rush to the nearest armchair or bed. That means that nothing, nothing at all, no action or gesture, can now be done with two hands, if standing. That's a lot of gestures to unlearn. (7)

The text describes in great detail the creative transfer of the protagonist's office downstairs, because climbing to the study, a room which offers an opening to the outside world with a superb view toward the distant mountains, has become impossible. Her library, however, remains largely upstairs, so that 'Writing, the old use of the office, is over. At an end. Like life' (16). Also described in detail is the purchase of a trolley table to help her negotiate inaccessible areas within the now small flat (44 and passim). This solution, however, requires acrobatics every time a tray needs to be transferred from the kitchen to the wheeled table (55). An analogy between this sequence and the master narrative, 'House to flat to room to bed to coffin to urn' (95), is explicitly formulated: 'From table to tray to trolley to templates. Recalling the coffin sequence' (59; see also 102). The acrobatics, in turn, causes two falls, one leading to a double sprain, the other to a fracture that necessitates a hip replacement. Movement is now further restricted, and, with it, the scope of desire shrinks: 'But if zimmimg alone to the bathroom is now the highest ambition and deepest desire, this confirms that there are moments in life when only the immediately preceding achievement and the immediately subsequent wish are relevant' (90). The ultimate aim of all the dangerous and tedious acrobatics is to reach the armchair or the bed.

3. Nevertheless: 'The Armchair, the World'

Like the twofold master narrative, the day-to-day present is also characterized not only by a shrinking but also by an expansion, an opening into alternative spaces. This doubleness is conveyed in a nutshell by the sentence 'And at last, the armchair, the world' (25). At first sight, 'the world' seems to be a synonym of 'the armchair,' suggesting that the protagonist's world at present is limited to this resting place, but possibly also alluding to the notion of the 'armchair traveller.' As the paragraph progresses, the relationship between the armchair and confinement is perceived as one of contrast, pinpointing the armchair as the site from which 'the world takes over' (25), thus becoming a space rather than a place.

'The world takes over' in at least two forms, one mediated by technology, the other by the imagination. In the past, technological mediation included airplanes, a car, e-mail communication with friends. At present, it is almost exclusively limited to television and books. Many discussions of the world in *Life, End of*, concerning issues such as wars, natural disasters, the unemployed, the homeless, AIDS, globalization, the death of languages, the decline of education, start off from a television programme. They are filtered not only through the protagonist's consciousness but also through her commentary on both the content and the (ab)uses of the medium. One television programme can be seen as a *mise en abyme* of the double movement of constriction and expansion: 'Black holes, says a tele-scientist, can, in this case, now forgotten, become creative' (62; see also 90). Applied to the protagonist's situation, this would suggest that a shrinking or effacement may provoke an emergence into space - a phenomenon impressively dramatized by the very springing of the text we read out of the suffering and limitations of illness.

Books are older friends than television, and they are particularly enjoyed when read for pleasure rather than for purposes of teaching, writing a paper, or preparing a conference lecture. A whole network of literary allusions, an intertextual space,[13] develops in *Life, End of,* and plays an important role for 'the invalid':

> For of course, since the world can't be visited any I more in what is called reality, there is no withdrawal but a lapping up of familiar illusion to forget the real. Or maybe to compare it, distantly, with memory. Is that what death is like? (26).

If older and newer technological mediations open up spaces beyond the armchair and the bed, imagination also expands the horizon beyond the boundaries of physical place. From her position in bed the protagonist imagines 'ghosts,' created by an interweaving of stones and plants, as well as a play of light and shade on the wall opposite her. The figures she sees span the broad cultural history of which her mental world is made, e. g.:

> To the left of Christ is a duchess in a wonderland headdress, and to the right Beethoven, broadfaced and aureoled in hair, scowling down furiously deaf at the score of Leonora being turned into Fidelio. But a slant of sun under the nose changes Beethoven into one of the zwei Grenadiere after being in Russland gefangen. Words by Heine, set by Schuman, learnt as a child. Or maybe Flambeau uttering Et nous les petits les obscurs les sans grades (24; see also 47, 55, 73, 95, 100-101).

That such scenes enact the coupling of restriction and expansion, one of the governing principles of *Life, End of,* is explicitly stated: 'This after all is the world, the universe, seen from the bed' (73).

For the protagonist, spatial expansion, whether with the help of technology or that of the imagination, is a means of saving her sanity and struggling against the destructive impact of illness, with its constriction of place. In the text's recurrent formulation: 'It is the brain, it is the brain endures' (e.g., 12).

4. The Space of Language

Within the broader context of illness narratives, I associate this affirmation with the prevalent emphasis on some kind of triumph or epiphany within the experience of illness. I have argued elsewhere that while the possibility of a 'phoenix-like' quality is a comfort to many patients, to people surrounding them, to readers and publishers, it also threatens to deprecate 'those who fail to rise out of their own ashes.'[14] However, *Life, End of* does offer a kind of phoenix quality through its play with language. As a result of her polyneuritis, the character's legs 'flinch wince jerk lapse collapse give way stagger *like language when it can't present the exact word needed*' (9; my italics). The very name of the illness is subject to repetitive puns in the text: 'Pollyana' (e.g., 88), 'Polly New Writis' (e.g., 88). The character's cardiovascular condition, causing her lacerations in the chest, is also subject to puns: 'The Cardiovasco de gamma network still functions' (10), 'vasco de Charmer' (36), 'the cardio-vasco de Harmer' (59) 'Vasco de Drama' (88), 'Vasco de Lamma, what are you waiting for?' (111). *Life, End of* is full of puns, some bi-lingual, on almost every subject, a proliferation of language that may be one way of dealing with pain. 'The happiness of wordplay' (51) is here not only an attempt to counter pain but also a way of expressing it.

In discussions of pain, there are two polar schools of thought concerning the relation between pain and language. Perhaps the best known advocate of the first view is Elaine Scarry, according to whom '[p]hysical pain does not simply resist language but actively destroys it, bringing about an immediate reversion to a state anterior to language, to sounds and cries a human being makes before language is learned.'[15] An eminent representative of the second view is David Morris, who engages directly with Scarry's thesis but stresses the meaning-generating quality of pain. 'It is the neglected encounter between pain and meaning,' he says at the beginning of *The Culture of Pain*, 'that lies at the center of this book and that the voices captured and created in writing from Homer to Beckett so powerfully help us to recover.'[16] He agrees with Scarry that pain, especially chronic pain, 'passes much of its time in utter inhuman silence,'[17] but nevertheless argues that 'individuals and cultures tend to construct - rather than simply feel - their pain.'[18] Similarly, he states that '[i]t seems we cannot simply suffer pain but are compelled to make sense of it.'[19] From this perspective, while Scarry implicitly considers pain a sensation, Morris views it as a perception in which meaning plays a constitutive role: 'Here is perhaps the most difficult thought to accept about pain. We experience pain only and entirely as we interpret it';[20] interpretation is historically and culturally bound, so that 'the same' pain means something different in different contexts. One such context is the religious. Interestingly, in the course of describing the protagonist's pain, the narrator of *Life, End of* adds: 'Pain is from Old French *pener*, to punish. For what? *Nulla poena sine lege*' (10). The text's many allusions to works of literature, music, the visual arts also situates it within various cultural contexts, endowing suffering with changing meanings. From all points of view, Brooke-Rose's text seems to be more in tune with Morris's position than with Scarry's, opening up a linguistic space of meaning and play within the constriction imposed by suffering. The text's title is thus an appropriate conclusion for my discussion: formatted like an item in an index, *Life, End of* is a triumph of language and wit over the painful process of the end of life.

Notes

[1] An earlier version of a part of this chapter was presented at a conference of the Narrative Society in Washington, D. C.
[2] Christine Brooke-Rose, *Life, End of* (Manchester: Carcanet, 2006), 95. All parenthetic references in the chapter are to this edition.
[3] Shlomith Rimmon-Kenan, *Narrative Fiction: Contemporary Poetics* (London: Methuen, 1983), 2.
[4] David Herman, *Story Logic: Problems and Possibilities of Narrative* (Lincoln: University of Nebraska Press, 2002).
[5] Susan Stanford Friedman, 'Spatialization: A Strategy for Reading Narrative,' *Narrative* 1 (1993): 12-23; 'Spatial Poetics and Arundhati Roy's *The God of Small Things*,' in *A Companion to Narrative Theory*, ed. James Phelan and Peter Rabinowitz (Oxford: Blackwell, 2005), 192-203.
[6] Ruth Ginsburg, 'Ida Fink's Scraps and Traces: Forms of Space and the Chronotope of Trauma Narratives,' *Partial Answers* 4 (2006): 205-218.
[7] M. M. Bakhtin, 'Forms of Time and of the Chronotope in the Novel,' in *The Dialogic Imagination*, trans. Caryl Emerson and Michael Holquist (Austin: University of Texas Press, 1981 [1937-1938]), 84-258.
[8] Jurij Lotman, *The Structure of the Artistic Text*, trans. R. Vroon (Ann Arbor: University of Michigan Press, 1977 [1970]).
[9] David Herman, 'Introduction,' in *Narratologies: New Perspectives on Narrative Analysis*, ed. David Herman (Columbus: Ohio State University Press, 1999), 1-30.
[10] Michel de Certeau, *The Practice of Everyday Life* (Berkeley: University of California Press, 1984), 117. For an interesting use of de Certeau's theory in the analysis of poetry, see Eynel Wardi, 'On Place and Space in Shirley Kaufman's Sanctum,' *Partial Answers* 2 (2004): 175-201.
[11] De Certeau, *Practice of Everyday Life*, 117.
[12] Ibid.
[13] For this concept, see Stanford Friedman, 'Spatialization,' 1993.
[14] Arthur Frank. *The Wounded Storyteller: Body, Illness, and Ethics* (Chicago: University of Chicago Press, 1995), 135.

[15] Elaine Scarry, *The Body in Pain: The Making and Unmaking of the World* (Oxford: Oxford University Press, 1985), 215.
[16] David B. Morris, *The Culture of Pain* (Berkeley: University of California Press, 1991), 3.
[17] Ibid.
[18] Ibid., 52.
[19] Ibid., 18.
[20] Ibid., 29.

Bibliography

Bakhtin, M. M. 'Forms of Time and of the Chronotope in the Novel.' In *The Dialogic Imagination.* Translated by Caryl Emerson and Michael Holquist, 84-258. Austin: The University of Texas Press, 1981 [1937-1938].

Brooke-Rose, Christine. *Life, End of.* Manchester: Carcanet, 2006.

De Certeau, Michel. *The Practice of Everyday Life.* Berkeley: University of California Press, 1984.

Frank, Arthur W. *The Wounded Storyteller: Body, Illness, and Ethics.* Chicago: University of Chicago Press, 1995.

Friedman, Susan Stanford. 'Spatialization: A Strategy for Reading Narrative.' *Narrative* 1 (1993): 12-23.

———. 'Spatial Poetics and Arundhati Roy's *The God of Small Things.'* In *A Com-panion to Narrative Theory*, edited by James Phelan and Peter Rabinowitz, 192-203. Oxford: Blackwell, 2005.

Ginsburg, Ruth. 'Ida Fink's Scraps and Traces: Forms of Space and the Chronotope of Trauma Narratives.' *Partial Answers* 4 (2006): 205-218.

Herman, David. 'Introduction.' In *Narratologies: New Perspectives on Narrative Analysis*, edited by David Herman, 1-30. Columbus: Ohio State University Press, 1999.

———. *Story Logic: Problems and Possibilities of Narrative.* Lincoln: University of Nebraska Press, 2002.

Lotman, Jurij. *The Structure of the Artistic Text.* Translated by R. Vroon. Ann Arbor: University of Michigan Press, 1977 [1970].

Morris, David B. *The Culture of Pain.* Berkeley: University of California Press, 1991.

Rimmon-Kenan, Shlomith. *Narrative Fiction: Contemporary Poetics.* London: Methuen, 1983.

Scarry, Elaine. *The Body in Pain: The Making and Unmaking of the World.* Oxford: Oxford University Press, 1985.

Wardi, Eynel. 'On Place and Space in Shirley Kaufman's 'Sanctum.'' *Partial Answers* 2 (2004): 175-201.

Representations of Dementia in Narrative Fiction

Rebecca Anna Bitenc

Abstract
This chapter explores the way literary representations of dementia enhance our understanding of what it is like to experience this disease, the light that dementia narratives throw on the particular plight of the sufferer. How does knowledge, in the sense of awareness of one's cognitive decline, interact with emotional pain? How does narrative technique contribute to an empathic engagement with the character afflicted by dementia? What are the ethical implications of both writing and reading about this condition? The main part of the chapter is devoted to a close analysis of two fictional narratives, *Out of Mind* by J. Bernlef (1988) and the more recent debut novel *Still Alice* by Lisa Genova (2007). Aware of the discrepancy between fictional worlds and the 'actual' world, this chapter nevertheless outlines the potential value of narrative fiction as a means of improving one's understanding of another person's mind and another person's pain.

Key Words: Dementia, early-onset Alzheimer's, novels, personhood, self-awareness, stigmatisation, empathy.

*****

1. Introduction

Dementia has become a major concern of our times. Not only is it ubiquitous across virtually all media - magazines, newspapers, blogs, cinema, radio, TV and even opera - but most people will at some point in their life come into contact with this disease. Its increasing incident rate has earned dementia the title of 'disease of the century.'[1] Often it is depicted as 'worse than death' because of its progressive neurodegenerative nature. People with dementia are forced to witness the decline of their own mental faculties, the loss of language and of memory - all that is intimately bound up with their personal identity and that supposedly defines what it is to be human. At the same time, spouses and children witness their partner's or parent's decline, must deal with abrupt changes in their personality, and have to face the painful experience of no longer being recognized by the person they love.

Dementia, as a disease characterized by cognitive deterioration, begs the question of how knowledge and pain interact. First, is it, indeed, true that knowledge 'increaseth sorrow'?[2] One will often hear that a person with dementia is at least spared the knowledge of his or her deterioration - a statement that sees the particular pain located more with the care-givers than the sufferer, and one that also (perhaps falsely) implies that a person with dementia completely loses self-awareness. However, sufferers' testimonies suggest that self-awareness of one's decline is precisely what makes the progress of dementia such a painful experience. How are self-awareness and emotional pain linked in this disease? Is there a point where the loss of knowledge takes on a redeeming or perhaps 'palliative' quality? Second, as dementia, like other mental diseases, is stigmatized in present-day society,[3] sufferers often attempt to hide the first signs of their deterioration rather than share their experience with others. This withdrawal from the society of others and the avoidance of cognitively taxing situations can exacerbate the distress of the sufferer, leading to loneliness and depression and a reduced sense of self-worth.[4] Furthermore, this can lead to the disease remaining undiagnosed for a long time. When family and friends finally recognize the true situation, the disease might already have progressed too far to make verbal communication about what it is like to suffer from dementia possible. What, then, can we, as outsiders, know about the pain of another, especially a person with dementia? If the answer is little at best, then how far can literature offer an imaginative insight into another person's mind and, with it, into another person's pain?

While I do not wish to minimize the disruptive force of this disease, to view dementia as outlined above comes dangerously close to subscribing to common tropes that dehumanize people with dementia - 'the living dead,' 'zombies,' 'lower primates' or 'vegetables.'[5] Such tropes strip people with dementia of their status as persons. They underline the importance our society accords to cognitive functioning as well as the dominance of reductionist philosophical models of personhood. They suggest that a meaningful life ends when a person has lost the capacity to remember and communicate his or her experience. While narrative fiction clearly cannot answer the question whether people with dementia lose their 'self,' it is singularly placed in that it simulates inside views, staging surmises about 'how another mind thinks, another body feels'[6] - in this case, what it might feel like to have dementia. This article seeks to explore the extent to which literary representations of dementia can enhance our understanding of what it is like to experience dementia. Furthermore, an inside view of an afflicted literary character potentially leads to an ethical engagement with the demented Other, causing us to acknowledge our basic similarity when recognizing the continuing inner life of the sufferer.

As might be expected, the form as well as the function of literary representations of dementia vary across different genres. Before concentrating on a close analysis of two particular dementia narratives, *Out of Mind* by J. Bernlef (1988)[7] and *Still Alice* by Lisa Genova (2007), I shall give a brief overview of the functions of dementia in contemporary narrative literature. This excursion will highlight the fact that the repertoire of ideas about dementia in narrative discourse does not *per se* produce a better understanding of what it is like to experience dementia: I argue that the latter effect may be achieved owing to artistic interactions of narrative technique and narrative content.

2. From Illness Narratives to Crime Stories

Over the last few decades, care-givers' (auto)biographies, by far the largest bulk of literature on dementia, have demonstrated that illness narratives can play an important role in dealing with the disease.[8] This is also true of a small number of autobiographies by people with dementia, which may, in addition, serve a political function. Illness narratives in general have been described as 'postcolonial acts'[9] in that they represent 'the demand to speak rather than be spoken for and to represent oneself rather than be represented, or in the worst cases, rather than being effaced entirely.'[10] This is particularly relevant to autobiographies by people with dementia[11] which 'speak from a subject position that is usually perceived to preclude first person narration. Indeed, they speak from a place which is popularly perceived to represent the ends of meaningful personhood per se.'[12] However, they necessarily end once the decline of the author's linguistic abilities makes written or coherent verbal expression impossible. Thus, they leave a crucial gap in our knowledge of what it is like to experience advanced dementia. Imaginative literature attempts to close this gap.

However, rather than exploring the possibility that narrative fiction offers to inhabit another person's consciousness imaginatively,[13] in a large number of novels dementia functions merely as a structuring device or as a theme. For instance, in the crime novel *Small World* by Martin Suter (1997) the protagonist's dementia creates suspense and constitutes the primary plot drive. In this novel Alzheimer's disease plays the role of detective: as the protagonist Konrad Lang progressively loses his recent memories, long-lost childhood memories resurface, leading him to remember a crime committed in his early infancy. Alzheimer's also serves as a structural device in Nicholas Sparks's *The Notebook* (2008), where the dementia narrative serves as a frame for a love story. In fact, the onset of dementia often triggers the narration of past love stories or family secrets, frequently in the form of the afflicted person's flashbacks. Thus, dementia is also frequently linked to the themes of love, memory, family heritage and family relationships.[14]

Finally, dementia is also depicted, less for its own sake than as a lens to criticise dominant social practices or beliefs. For example, in Jonathan Franzen's *The Corrections* (2001) we are presented with an inside view of what it is like to experience Parkinson's and the accompanying symptoms of dementia. The disease not only has personal meaning for the head of the Lambert family - formerly an authoritarian patriarch he is now no longer even capable of controlling his hands or his bladder - but can be read as a criticism of the American dream according to which the individual is responsible for his or her success and is supposed to be always able to *improve* his or her situation. Neurodegenerative diseases such as Parkinson's or Alzheimer's expose this world view as an illusion.[15]

By contrast, the two novels which I discuss here focus primarily on representing dementia through the mind of the sufferer. In both, dementia is at the centre of the narrative, rather than performing some type of secondary function. The novels show how dementia, which entails the loss of memory, language and arguably one's identity, affects the sufferer's sense of self and his or her relationship to others; they do so through narrative techniques that have the potential, albeit an inescapably limited one, to further our understanding of such an experience.

3. *Out of Mind* - the Implications of a Demented Narrator

J. Bernlef's *Out of Mind* (1988) is a rare instance of the use of a narrator with dementia.[16] The narrative represents Maarten's struggle to comprehend his condition, which remains undiagnosed throughout the novel. The title of the novel guides the reader to expect some form of insanity. We are presented with a first-person narrator who is unsure about setting and events, who says 'Maybe,' 'I don't understand,' 'I don't know' (1). As the whole text resembles a kind of immediate diary-entry of Maarten's experience, the symptoms form part of the narrative. Maarten minutely describes his experiences and thoughts, concealing nothing. If he experiences a distorted reality his detailed descriptions (of other characters' clothing, or of the setting) allow the reader to understand what is happening and to recognize characters even when Maarten can no longer recognize them. Due to his declining cognitive faculties, however, his narrative becomes more and more enigmatic and idiosyncratic and thus more difficult for the reader to decode. One could argue that the effort the reader has to put into making sense of Maarten's narrative is mimetic of the effort Maarten has to make to understand his reality. Leona Toker uses the term 'parallel experience'[17] to describe the effect of such narrative technique on the reader. Thus, the reader is placed in an 'intellectual predicament analogous to that of the characters':[18] here, both experience a sense of disorientation, the narrator-character with regard to his (fictional) reality and the reader in decoding the narrator's words.

The use of the present tense contributes to the sensation of being plunged into Maarten's immediate thought processes. In contrast to retrospective first-person narratives, here there is no distance between the narrating I (who has a fuller understanding of events retrospectively) and the experiencing-I. The reader is presented directly with Maarten's confusion, fear and delusions. The use of 'concurrent narration'[19] facilitates the representation of Maarten's *perception* and his *experience* of the symptoms of dementia. This is true of one of Maarten's first serious delusions about reality. He is simultaneously aware and unaware of the strangeness of the situation: 'I am the first to arrive, I can tell from the virgin snow all around. It is *perhaps a rather strange* and yet quite suitable place for an IMCO meeting, so close to the sea' (33; my emphasis); 'from time to time I glance briefly over my shoulder, because for the secretary to a meeting to be forcing a door open is not an everyday event, *I realize that*' (34; my emphasis). When he suddenly recovers full insight into his situation - that he is retired and in fact breaking into a holiday residence - he is overcome by nausea: 'What am I doing here?' (35-36). The present tense heightens the immediacy of the experience and also builds up the dramatic tension. That Maarten narrates this in the present tense, rather than retrospectively in the past tense, after having realized his mistake, allows the reader to follow the workings of his mind, and emphasises the acute pang he experiences when he becomes aware of his delusion.

As Maarten's decline affects his narrative, its logical coherence threatens to disintegrate. However, a number of techniques ensure that despite the narrator's decline the narrative transmission does not break down. For instance, the use of brackets is one important formal element that establishes a channel of communication between the more lucid version of Maarten and the reader. In a sense, the brackets represent Maarten's remaining metacognitive functions, his knowledge about his thinking processes and his general awareness of what is happening. As such, they present a textual space for Maarten to express his anguish and pain at his disintegrating faculties. At times, however, the conflict between Maarten's function as *the narrator* and as *a character experiencing dementia* leads to a certain dissonance. The reader is inclined to wonder whether this is indeed a realistic representation of how a person with advanced dementia thinks. Sometimes the brackets read more as an explanatory note by what Wayne C. Booth has called the 'implied author.'[20] As the (implied) author becomes more visible, the illusion of penetrating the narrator's mind is dispelled, which can lead to a lapse in the reader's suspension of disbelief. Potentially, this has a distancing effect, as it calls the reader's attention to the fact that the narrator is a fictional construct. It thus invites us to consider the limits to representing dementia from an inside perspective in narrative form; such intellectual activity competes with emotional involvement.[21]

From the outset, Maarten is clearly both aware of and preoccupied with his mental decline. After his first experience of a time-lapse, in which he believes himself back in his kindergarten days, he finds himself utterly unable to explain his present situation (6). He describes his confusion using a number of metaphors and images. For instance, he compares himself to 'a ship, a sailing vessel that is becalmed. And then suddenly there is a breeze, I am sailing again' (54). Furthermore, he uses a car simile to describe his impaired thinking process: 'Something inside me thinks and then stops halfway. Starts on a totally different track and then halts again. Like a car engine that keeps stalling' (82). Later, he experiences his disease not only as something that disrupts his thoughts or actions but as essentially a disintegration of his personality: he experiences his deterioration as 'sinking' (cf. 55) or 'leak[ing]' respectively: 'Every day something disappears, every day there's something gone. It leaks everywhere' (84). The use of metaphors suggests aspects of Maarten's experience that are otherwise inexpressible. By decoding the metaphor, visualizing its images and thinking of the connotations that it evokes, the reader can achieve a new way of seeing or conceptualizing this experience of deterioration.

Out of Mind also draws attention to what it feels like to be suffering from agnosia.[22] As his memory functions become more and more impaired, Maarten has trouble recognizing people's facial expressions and with time even their faces. His observation that '[t]o see something you must first be able to recognize it. Without memory you can merely look, and the world glides through you without leaving a trace' (41) is ironically a pertinent description of the problem faced by those with dementia. Maarten finds it increasingly difficult to attach meaning to facial expressions. He has lost the necessary memories, and his theory of mind[23] is seriously impaired. For example, he has forgotten about the death of a friend's husband and cannot understand her reaction when he inquires about him (28; cf. also 52, 67). He senses his *faux-pas* but cannot understand it and thus increasingly feels excluded from interactions with others. Furthermore, the narrative highlights how unsettling it can be to encounter people who to the protagonist-narrator appear to be complete strangers in his own home.

As Maarten's dementia progresses, he begins to live more and more in the past, especially the time-frame of World War II. These memories are so deeply engrained in his personality that they become his primary way of making sense of his life. At the same time, the war metaphorically represents his experience of dementia:

> there's even a war on now ... will it never end? ... occupied from within ... my liberators have occupied me, that's what it is ... more and more censorship ... hardly anything still gets through. (124)

On the story level, Maarten might be trying to make sense of the fact that everybody around him is speaking English ('my liberators'). This passage can be read as representing Maarten's feelings towards his doctors and nurses who exercise a large amount of constraint over him ('have occupied me'). But we are also invited to read this passage as depicting the war that is going on in his head. 'Dementia as war' is, in fact, a common metaphor to conceptualize this neurodegenerative disease. Maarten experiences his declining cognitive faculties as censorship that allows less and less to get through to the functioning parts of his brain.

Residues of his past experience and memories continue to transpire throughout his advanced dementia. Although for the most part he feels strongly dissociated from his body and speaks of himself as 'he' or 'it,' he can still remember playing the piano, especially the feeling associated with playing by heart: 'that blissful feeling that your body is playing you' (128); a memory, significantly, of feeling *one* with his body. One might want to draw a parallel to Kontos's idea of embodied self-hood in dementia,[24] highlighting how memories and selfhood are engrained in the bodies of people and do not depend solely on higher-order cognitive functioning.

Together with memory loss, language decline and aphasia are among the most important diagnostic criteria in dementia. Maarten's deteriorating language faculties are mimetically represented in his discourse: 'A little dance step would be in pace here … no … not pace … step … pace … in place!' (41). He is keenly aware of the fact that his language faculties are slipping away, and he describes this unsettling experience using imagery that implies that the loss of language represents the loss of personhood and is to him akin to death itself. Here the experience of the mind (losing words) is compared with the potentially lethal experience of the body (losing blood):

> I seem to lose words *like another person loses blood. …* [A] kind of seasickness in my mind, it seems. Under this life stirs another life in which all times, names and places whirl about topsy-turvy and *in which I no longer exist as a person.* (54; my italics)

The narrative suggests that language not only allows him to make sense of his world, to name and place objects that surround him, but that the loss of his language faculties means that he is no longer able to place himself, as a person, in relation to the objects themselves. The sea imagery highlights the chaos that the loss of language causes in his mind. As Maarten loses his language and memory, he also loses the means of experiencing himself as a distinct and coherent person with a narrative identity of his own. Significantly, the first-person pronoun is dropped more and more often as the narrative progresses or is replaced by the second-person pronoun 'you,' the third-person pronoun 'he' or finally the impersonal 'it' (111ff). The dissociation from his body is suggested by the way he continues to perceive his hands and feet, but without experiencing them as part of his body: 'Hands and feet it must have … eyes open and shut: same place … eyes open and shut and open again: same place' (122). This passage evokes Maarten's apparent frustration with the monotony of his situation, his wish to be some place or even some*one* else. He has lost all sense of identity and identification with his body parts as well as the cognitive capacities to understand his situation. The evocative language, using fragmented syntax and monotonous structures, as well as the personal pronoun 'it' - which is more painful to us than it might be to Maarten at this stage of his disease - allows the reader to feel both *with* and *for* him.[25] Interestingly, despite the technique of fragmentation and the emphasis on Maarten's dissociation from his body, the fact that Maarten remains the centre of consciousness and perception, the being that realises that he is in the 'same place,' paradoxically highlights his continuing identity; showing that very 'base' cognitive functions might be sufficient to accord personhood to a subject. In any case, the reader continues to see him as a character, a 'person' in whom we are interested and with whom we empathise.[26]

The narrative also speaks to current personhood debates in other ways. Since the reader is aware of the thought processes that form the context to Maarten's utterances, the reader can still make sense of the little language Maarten is able to use in conversation. The narrative technique here is that of monitoring the distribution of *fabula* details. For instance, Maarten's answer to the question how he is feeling makes perfect sense to the reader because we are familiar with Maarten's peculiar experience of gravity: his feeling that he is losing substance (being 'scooped empty,' 122) and his fear of drifting away (114). However, his response is likely to be categorized as nonsensical by his caregivers:

> Question: 'How are you feeling?' A question that can be answered. Wait a moment. Wave briefly with those hands. Like this. Only very briefly. Quickly grab hold of the wood again. Wait a moment. 'Not enough gravity!' (115)

The ethical significance of this account lies in its suggestion that the enigmatic utterances of people with dementia might indeed make sense in the affected person's life experience and should not be entirely disregarded.[27]

Interestingly, Maarten still sees language as the means to counter the experience of losing oneself:

> Words, that's what provides energy. A human being should be made of words. Totally. It's so obvious. (At last something of worth again, supply of words there must be, that's what can save the situation, stories, supply, import of stories). (116)

Earlier in the narrative Maarten had already decided to invent his reality once he lost the memories that allowed him to make sense of his life (59). For instance, he is forced to reconstruct (or rather invent) 'memories' when looking at photos with a care-giver because he is neither able to recognize Vera, his wife, in the photograph nor able to remember the exact circumstances in which it was taken (101). Language also represents the only means for action once his bodily functions degenerate: '(You see, when you use the right words something always happens)' (116) or 'only in language can I still undertake anything' (123). To some extent, however, Maarten becomes weary of the inadequacy of language to express his experience: 'At least pinching still causes a slight pain … an event … using the choke but where has the engine gone … nothing but metaphors, boy … nothing but metaphors' (124).

So while Maarten sees his language faculties slowly deteriorate and at times experiences language as insufficient, language and narrative are instrumental for him in maintaining a sense of identity. Losing language means losing himself, which possibly represents the most painful aspect of his struggle with dementia. Narrative, or what linguists refer to as confabulation,[28] can to a certain degree counter this effect. The narrative as a whole also clearly maintains the identity of Maarten as a character. Until the end, the sustained inside view of his consciousness allows us to read *Out of Mind* as the narrative of a person, no matter how 'out of mind' this person may seem: the apparently nonsensical utterances by people with dementia should not be disregarded but might necessitate (re)constructing a context for their utterances that differs from the apparent context at hand. However, while autobiographies and verbal accounts by people with dementia suggest that aphasia is indeed a particularly troubling symptom, the view that the capacity to use language and to formulate one's life-narrative is what accords people the status of persons is, I believe, based on reductionist concepts of personhood. J. Bernlef's novel works against such concepts, even though narrative fiction, which uses language as its means to construct meaning, usually runs the risk of reaffirming the primacy of language over other aspects of personhood, identity, humanity.[29]

Surprisingly, the nature imagery that closes the novel suggests a positive outlook on dementia. From the start, the weather mirrors Maarten's condition. Just like the winter mist outside, a mist hangs over his more recent memories. Maarten's assessment of the weather might be read as a bleak description of what is in store for him: 'there is nothing in the distance except a black hole. Not even a light anywhere' (9). What do we make then of the ending of the novel in which Vera's voice tells a very attentive Maarten that 'there is a glass again … glass you can see through … outside … into the woods and the spring that is almost beginning' (130)? We associate spring with renewed life and hope. How can there be a metaphorical spring in dementia? Is not the future of people with dementia indeed a 'black hole' devoid of meaning and, as is often suggested, devoid of personhood? Taking this view, one might read the last page of *Out of Mind* as cruelly ironic. However, the tone of this passage is hopeful. Maarten takes pleasure in listening to the whispering voice that tells him about life outside. The literal ravages his dementia has wrought on his old house have been repaired: one can again see through the window he broke. If the motif of seepage - the breaking of barriers and windows, sinking, leaking and bleeding - has evoked the threat that dementia poses to the coherence of the person, the final image of repair suggests restitution of an enduring quality of selfhood. Maarten is apparently beyond the stage of being troubled by attempts to make sense of his world. He believes himself back in the safety of his mother's arms. He regresses to very early childhood, re-experiencing the reassuring feeling that someone will take care of him: 'she carries you … I carry you little boy of mine … the whole long frightening night I will carry you until it is light again' (129). While the loss of 'knowledge' - both memories and language - is depicted as an excruciatingly painful experience, it ultimately seems to offer a respite. Maarten seems to have left his personal darkness behind, possibly experiencing a certain serenity in his last stages of dementia, which might indeed represent a form of spring after the winter of dementia.[30]

4. *Still Alice*: An Inside View of Early-Onset Alzheimer's

Lisa Genova's novel *Still Alice* (2007) combines recent insights into the neurology of Alzheimer's disease with an attempt to portray the effect of neuronal decline from an inside perspective.[31] Nearly the entire narrative is focalized through Alice, the protagonist, but the voice is that of a third-person narrator. The use of focalization can be seen as a means of offering an imaginative insight into how Alice's mind works, an attempt at mirroring the workings of a deteriorating mind. As in *Out of Mind*, the symptoms form part of the narrative. As Alice's thoughts begin to circle around themselves, the narrative also circles, creating an almost verbatim repetition of its parts. And yet, briefed by the blurb and the prologue, the reader has a better awareness than the experiencing protagonist of what is happening. This very often leads to dramatic irony rather than parallel experience. While Alice, for example, attributes certain minor difficulties to her stressful life, the reader can immediately file these as first indicators of her disease. This instance of dramatic irony raises the reader's interest in the plot ('When will Alice find out the truth?'), and potentially also the reader's emotional engagement with the protagonist, as we know what the narrative has 'in store' for her.

The use of Alice as a focal character highlights her psychological reactions to what she experiences. Frequently, the emotional impact of an experience is rendered in italics and in her own words - as at the moment of diagnosis of probable Alzheimer's disease (70)[32], her interview with her boss during which she is progressively stripped of her responsibilities at Harvard as a teacher and a research scientist (118ff), or when she forgets how to make the Christmas pudding she has made since she was a little girl (65). Confined to her perspective, the reader can see situations through her eyes and understand how her declining cognitive faculties distort her perception of reality - this technique might have a consciousness-raising effect, heightening our sensitivity towards people with dementia in our own lives. It registers Alice's humiliation, her fear and her frustration and the particularly painful *awareness* of all her losses. The knowledge she has of her own decline only exacerbates the pain she experiences. Finally, as in *Out of Mind*, this inside perspective also mimetically depicts the growing dissociation Alice feels from her 'self': her sense of becoming 'less and less human' as she loses the ability to use language (270), her disinterestedness in things that concern her and her lack of emotional involvement in decisions she formerly felt strongly about (264).

Arguably, seeing the world through Alice's eyes allows for a greater amount of emotional engagement and empathy. We can feel both *with* and *for* Alice.[33] The double perspective of seeing with but also knowing more than the protagonist allows for the reader to engage with the Other while remaining aware of his or her own perspective. This awareness of our status as witnesses calls for an ethical engagement with the demented Other. We are offered a certain degree of (imaginative) insight into what it feels like to have dementia, and yet we are the non-demented other(s) ready to identify also with Alice's family, friends and colleagues. Thus, we are offered an insight into how 'our' behaviour is perceived, critically at times, by the person with dementia.

Apart from focalization, the novel uses a number of techniques to address the complex issue of personality loss in dementia. Both the first and the second part of the novel have neurological prologues that present what has happened or will happen on the neurological level, at the same time setting the scene for what Alice will experience due to the neuronal loss occurring in her brain. While these prologues give a relatively accurate account of state-of-the-art neurological explanations for Alzheimer's disease, their language is highly metaphorical. The neurons are personified and come to stand symbolically for the person experiencing the disease. Thus, the prologue introduces the central theme of *Still Alice*: the relationship between mind and self, brain functioning and identity. While Alice's sense of self resides primarily in her extraordinary mental capacities, the onset of Alzheimer's will force her to contemplate alternative aspects of self and identity, such as may be saved from the 'onslaught' (117) of disease. As the narrative progresses and Alzheimer's takes its toll, both the reader and Alice come to recognize that previous criteria of self-worth have to be re-thought (187-88).

The question of self-awareness is central to a reading of *Still Alice*. Aside from the loss of one's mental faculties and the disorientation that this entails, the high degree of self-awareness of decline, especially in early-onset Alzheimer's patients, makes this disease particularly painful. Like Maarten,

Alice is at times simultaneously aware and unaware of the incongruence of certain situations, such as her inability to resolve the logical conflicts she experiences due to hallucinations. Alone at home, she suddenly fails to recognize the floor rug as such and thinks that there is a black hole in the middle of the corridor with the mail hovering over the void. Like Maarten, she tries to make sense of the situation ('Had John [her husband] hired a contractor?' 206). She is aware that her perception is wrong but cannot resolve it: '*Floating mail. My brain is fried*' (207-208). When she finally recognizes the black hole as her 'black hallway rug' that has 'been there for years' (211), she is overcome by a wave of fury and humiliation.

As her disease progresses, Alice finds it more and more difficult to be sure of anything: time of day, place and even her own identity. She begins to read her environment for clues to what she has been doing: while her memory is severely impaired, her rational, meaning-making faculties are still intact (144). Her scientific approach also mirrors a certain amount of detachment she is developing towards her own self, while the simile of a fragile membrane about to be shattered is reminiscent of the imagery in *Out of Mind*: 'Her sense of Alice - what she knew and understood, what she liked and disliked, how she felt and perceived - was also like a soap bubble, ever higher in the sky and more difficult to identify, with nothing but the thinnest membrane protecting it from popping into thinner air' (242). To a certain extent, this waning of interest in things that concern her seems to provide Alice with a degree of relief and tranquillity, comparable to Maarten's sense of safety and belonging at the end of *Out of Mind*. Similarly, the ending of *Still Alice* stresses the importance of physical contact and human relations, for instance with her daughters, no matter that she is no longer able to recognize them as such.

In contrast to *Out of Mind,* the experience of stigmatization is a central aspect of *Still Alice.* Alice begins to develop Alzheimer's in the middle of her career and has to deal with a high degree of discrepancy between what her environment expects of her and what she will still be able to accomplish in the future. Confronted with the diagnosis, Alice already foresees how Alzheimer's disease might lead to stigmatization: 'Alice expected to be outcast. Even the well-intentioned and educated tended to keep a fearful distance from the mentally ill. She didn't want to become someone people avoided and feared' (118). Although ashamed of these thoughts, she would willingly trade Alzheimer's for cancer: 'With cancer she'd have something that she could fight. ... Her family and the community at Harvard would rally behind her battle and consider it noble. And even if defeated in the end, she'd be able to look them *knowingly* in the eye and say good-bye before she left' (117, my italics). Here, the particular pain of dementia is seen as located in the loss of memories and of the ability to recognize one's loved ones and be recognizable to them. Significantly, this part of the novel is introduced by the second neurological prologue that symbolically depicts the effects of loneliness and stigmatization. It seems to suggest that communication with others and the capacity to act and be treated as a full person is vital for the person with dementia. Inability to connect meaningfully to others will hasten the progress of decline; the loss of a meaningful occupation as well as of nurturing relationships may actually *cause* the death of the person.[34] The prologue introduces the themes and topics of the second part of the novel: Alice's struggle with losing her job (and therefore part of her identity), her abandonment and stigmatization by her colleagues, and the role relationships play in her remaining sense of self.

Stigmatization arises, on the one hand, from other people's fears and prejudices, and on the other hand from the affected person's inappropriate behaviour. Various examples highlight the extent to which Alice is ostracised by her colleagues. They cut off contact with her; the chair next to Alice remains empty at a meeting: 'She looked at everyone not looking at her. About fifty people crowded into the room, people she'd known for many years, people she'd thought of as family' (185). The insight that follows echoes Burke's moral concern with how we as a society treat people with mental illnesses:[35] 'Facing her meant facing her mental frailty and the unavoidable thought that, in the blink of an eye, it could happen to them. Facing her was scary. So for the most part . . . they didn't' (185). Focalizing this situation through Alice highlights the hurt such behaviour inflicts. The situation sits uncomfortably with the reader who might recognize his or her own conduct in similar circumstances. The reader identifies with her colleagues' guilt and uneasiness at not knowing how to react, while simultaneously empathizing with Alice.

Alice's reaction to this snub is an impulse to fight for her rights and self-respect, but her intent is diminished to the same degree as her short-term memory is flawed. The narrative successfully demonstrates the tragedy of her impaired memory through repetition, in both the story and the narrative discourse. Alice realizes a mistake in the experimental design that is presented during a seminar. Her valuable criticism and everybody's reaction to it enormously boosts her shaken self-esteem:

> She felt victorious and a little smug. The fact that she had Alzheimer's didn't mean that she was no longer capable of thinking analytically. The fact that she had Alzheimer's didn't mean that she didn't deserve to sit in that room among them. The fact that she had Alzheimer's didn't mean that she no longer deserved to be heard. (186)

However, only shortly afterwards Alice has already forgotten that she has voiced the same observation about the design and repeats it. The very different reaction - everybody is obviously embarrassed and Alice cannot understand why they ignore her comment - hurts her acutely:

> It was a valid point . . . Alice was sure of it. Yet no one else seemed to see it. She looked at everyone not looking at her. Their body language suggested embarrassment and dread. … The fact that she had Alzheimer's didn't mean she couldn't think analytically. The fact that she had Alzheimer's didn't mean she didn't know what she was talking about. (187)

This passage attempts to imaginatively answer the question what it feels like for people with dementia to try to make sense of their environment and fail, to be simultaneously aware and unaware of their impaired capacities. It is the degree of awareness that seems to make this situation so hurtful. Alice has not yet reached a state of 'mere oblivion' (as envisaged by Shakespeare's Jacques as the last stage of a person's life[36]) that might offer a reprieve from pain (if such a stage is ever reached during our life, even in advanced dementia), but she can no longer decode her colleagues' reaction; she therefore experiences their behaviour as starkly unjust and painful. The stylistic device of verbatim repetition has the potential of increasing the reader's empathy and understanding of the particular plight of Alzheimer's disease.

Finally, the novel addresses the difficult topic of suicide in dementia and with it the complex ethical issue of what makes a life a 'good life,' a life worth living and protecting. *Still Alice* questions the decisions the non-demented person may make for her prospective demented self. It suggests that cognitive capacities are not the only thing that makes us who we are and that no clear boundary exists between 'self' and 'loss of self.' This too is largely an effect of focalization and an array of devices through which the third-person narrative makes the reader see what remains obscure to the focal character herself.

When she is confronted with her diagnosis, Alice's thoughts soon turn to suicide (78). The question arises as to where the cut-off line for a meaningful existence can be drawn. It is significant that Alice hatches her suicide plan during one of her 'ice-cream moments,' on a 'day not to be wasted sitting in an office, especially if you had Alzheimer's' (115). Thus her suicide plan and the *carpe diem* motif are intertwined as well as contrasted from the start. Enjoying a giant ice cream, she reflects on what is important to her and what she wants in the future. Her reasoning is entirely rational: 'She didn't want to be here . . . when the burdens, both emotional and financial, grossly outweighed any benefit of sticking around' (116).

Although many activities she loves do indeed depend on an intact memory and intact language capacities, physical and emotional pleasures need not be tainted by the loss of these abilities. It is ironic that the things Alice decides are worth living for do not involve a large degree of higher cognitive functioning: holding her grandchild in her arms, seeing her children, enjoying more 'sunny, seventy-degree days and ice-cream cones' (118) are what qualifies. Yet the criteria she devises to test whether she has passed the point of living a meaningful life are entirely based on a functioning memory: '*1. What month is it? 2. Where do you live? Where is your office? When is Anna's birthday? How many children do you have?*' (119). She instructs herself to act on the suicide plan in the 'Butterfly' file on her computer should she be unable to answer any of these questions. But how does knowing the exact location or address of one's office, a symbol of her former 'intellectual brilliance' that she has just decided 'she was willing to live without' (119), reflect whether she is still capable of enjoying the physical closeness of her grandchild? Alice's questions reflect her incapacity at this point to imagine what it will be like once her dementia progresses. Her perspective is thus similar to an outsider's perspective and her rational reasoning expresses the detachment she feels in respect to her future self. After devising this plan, she concludes 'that there were a lot of potential problems with this design, that it was by no means foolproof. She just hoped she opened 'Butterfly' before she became that fool' (119-20). Her trope of people with dementia as 'fools' can be read as an ironic witticism, but it highlights her outside perspective viewing rationality and self-awareness as paramount qualities of a person. Simultaneously, the use of the word 'fools' draws attention to the traditional function of jesters (in Shakespearian drama) in critiquing society and societal practices.

Alice's self-devised questions to test her mental state reappear at intervals, allowing the reader to assess her decline as her answers become less detailed or correct. When this happens, however, she is no longer able to recognize her answers as wrong: her suicide plan is, indeed, flawed (226). Later stumbling over the 'Butterfly' file by chance and reading the letter to herself, she is no longer capable of following her own suicide instructions. She no longer knows how to print them out, and in the space of going upstairs to take the sleeping pills she forgets her intentions (272-73). The narrative suggests that her incapacity to follow through with her suicide is a good thing. Although one might experience a sense of frustration with Alice, who is trying to accomplish something but fails, the chapter that immediately precedes her stumbling over the 'Butterfly' file stresses the fact that Alice has not yet passed the point of enjoying an ice cream cone, the warmth of the sun or her husband's presence. John, her husband, asks her the exact questions she typed into her BlackBerry, making the reader suspect that he might be aware of Alice's suicide plan. At this stage, Alice is unable to answer these questions but her reasoning is yet intact (she attempts to deduce the answers). She also makes a strong point that this knowledge is irrelevant to her: that she does not need to know where her office is because she no longer goes there. In this context, the way John poses his final question suggests that he is actually asking her whether she still wants to be alive: '"Alice, do you still want to be here?' His eyebrows bent into a serious shape and the creases next to his eyes deepened. This question was important to him' (267-68). Alice is happy to be able to answer this question confidently: "Yes, I like sitting here with you. And I'm not done yet" (268). Although referring to her ice cream, the passage suggests that there are many things for Alice still to enjoy, such as holding John's warm hand. She thus inadvertently answers his deeper question: she is happy to enjoy this moment with him. Why should she want to die? The internal focalization thus invites us to contrast her former conceptions of a meaningful life with her developing experience of life and to draw our own conclusions.

If *Out of Mind* represents the type of illness narrative that could be described as a 'chaos narrative,'[37] *Still Alice* might best be described as a 'quest narrative'[38] in that it depicts the spiritual growth that the experience of disease potentially leads to. Alice learns to live productively with her disease. She founds a support group for early-onset Alzheimer's patients. In her speech at an Alzheimer's conference, she raises fundamental questions of identity and criticizes society's response to this disease: 'Being diagnosed with Alzheimer's is like being branded with a scarlet *A*. … But I am not what I say or what I do or what I remember. I am fundamentally more than that' (252). She concludes her speech with an appeal to the audience demanding respect for and empowerment of people with Alzheimer's (253). She has learned something from her illness experience that is worth passing on to others. The novel stresses the importance of relationships and the attempt to enjoy every moment for itself as what can be set in opposition to this devastating disease. This *carpe diem* motif runs like a thread throughout the narrative.

Yet Alzheimer's takes its toll. Alice has not reached a safe place from which she can reflect on her experience and share her insights. The story and Alzheimer's progress continue, partly subverting a comfortable reading of her story as a quest narrative.[39]

The fact that *Still Alice* ends well before the onset of the last stages of dementia can be seen either as its strength or as its weakness. On the one hand, one might criticise the author for evasion; on the other, one might praise her for emphasising the continued potential for development in the relationships between people with and without dementia. Genova highlights what frequently persists even in the last stages of dementia: the emotional and sensual aspects of relationships that do not depend on higher-order cognitive functioning.

5. Conclusion

While many fictional and non-fictional accounts focus on the care-giver's point of view or employ dementia for their own structural ends, *Out of Mind* by J. Bernlef and *Still Alice* by Lisa Genova represent the condition from the sufferer's perspective. In Bernlef's novel the perspective of a narrator with a slowly progressing dementia entails the narrative's re-enactment of his mental deterioration, giving the reader a sense of the experience of the progress of his disease; we struggle to understand the narrative as the narrator struggles to understand his world. This parallel activity has the potential of leading us to a fuller imaginative immersion in the experience of dementia. At the same time, narrative devices, such as the use of brackets, allow us to disengage from the narrator and, as it were, enter into dialogue with the author behind him. The imagery, furthermore, not only invites new ways of seeing how a person with dementia might feel or perceive things but also suggests an almost positive view of the very last stage of dementia. However, the conflict between the role of the *narrator*, who has to communicate his story with at least a minimal coherence, and the experience of the narrator as *character*, who is losing any sense of coherence and his capacity to communicate, limits the reader's empathetic view of his experience.

This effect is forestalled in *Still Alice*: through focalization we receive an inside view of dementia filtered through a self-effacing third person narrator. As in *Out of Mind*, the symptoms of dementia form part of the narrative. We are presented with Alice's restricted world view and experience her symptoms with her, through her eyes, her mind and emotions. Through the use of such techniques as repetition the workings of both the protagonist's deteriorating mind and the minds of the people around her are suggested to the reader.

The narratives show that the sufferer's awareness of his or her cognitive decline and the struggle to come to terms with it is what makes dementia such a devastating and painful disease. *Still Alice*, in particular, highlights the humiliation people with dementia experience due to stigmatization. At the same time the novels brings into high relief the redemptive qualities of love and care-giving, as the emotional capacities of the sufferers are shown to persist even when 'recognition' of the loved ones - on a linguistic or intellectual level - is no longer possible. They also suggest that the loss of knowledge in terms of memory and self-awareness, though initially excruciatingly painful, might offer some form of relief from emotional pain in the final stages of dementia.

The inside view of Alzheimer's patients that these novel offer have the power to engage us in a discussion about what we consider to be a good life; they can raise our consciousness of what it might feel like to suffer from this disease; and they can hold up a mirror to our thoughts, attitudes and behaviour that potentially aggravate the pain of the sufferer. The pain of another is essentially unknowable, but narrative fiction has its ways (focalization, metaphoric language, dramatic irony, conditions for parallel experience) to bring us closer to an understanding of what it may be like, and to show that the demented Others are similar to us, and that they have inner lives of their own that demand the respect that we owe to any human being.

Notes

[1] Patrick Fox, 'From Senility to Alzheimer's Disease: The Rise of the Alzheimer's Disease Movement,' *Millbank Quarterly* 1 (1989): 58-102.
[2] Ecclesiastes 1:18.
[3] Cf. Arthur W. Kleinman, *The Illness Narratives: Suffering, Healing, and the Human Condition* (New York: Basic Books, 1988), 18-26, 159. Erving Goffman, *Stigma: Notes on the Management of Spoiled Identity* (Englewood Cliffs: Prentice-Hall, 1963).
[4] See Tom Kitwood and Kathleen Bredin, 'Towards a Theory of Dementia Care: Personhood and Well-Being,' *Ageing and Society* 12 (1992): 269-87.
[5] Lucy Burke, 'The Poetry of Dementia: Art, Ethics, and Alzheimer's Disease in Tony Harrison's *Black Daisies for the Bride*,' *Journal of Literary Disability* 1 (2007a): 65.
[6] Dorrit Cohn, *Transparent Minds: Narrative Modes for Presenting Consciousness in Fiction* (Princeton: Princeton University Press, 1978), 5-6.
[7] This novel was originally published in Dutch in 1984 as *Hersenschimmen* under the pseudonym J. Bernlef and first translated into English in 1988 (my parenthetic references pertain to this edition). It greatly contributed to its author's (Hendrik Jan Marsman's) fame and has since been adapted to the cinema and stage.
[8] Cf. Arthur W. Frank, *The Wounded Storyteller: Body, Illness, and Ethics* (Chicago: University of Chicago Press, 1995). Cf. Arthur Kleinman, *The Illness Narratives*, xiii-xiv.
[9] Cf. Arthur W. Frank, *The Wounded Storyteller*, 7-10.
[10] Ibid., 13.
[11] Cf. Christine Bryden, *Dancing with Dementia: My Story of Living Positively with Dementia* (London: Jessica Kingsley Publishers, 2005); Thomas DeBaggio, *Losing My Mind: An Intimate Look at Life with Alzheimer's* (New York: The Free Press, 2002); Cary Henderson, *Partial View: An Alzheimer's Journal*, ed. Jackie Henderson Main, Ruth D. Henderson and Nancy Andrews (Dallas: Southern Methodist University Press, 1998); Diane Friel McGowin, *Living in the Labyrinth: A Personal Journey Through the Maze of Alzheimer's* (New York: Delta, 1994 [1993]).
[12] Lucy Burke, 'Alzheimer's Disease: Personhood and First Person Testimony,' paper presented at CDSRN. (2007b): 1. http://www.cdsrn.org.uk/Burke_CDSRN_2007.pdf, viewed November 15, 2009.

[13] Käte Hamburger, *The Logic of Literature*, trans. Marilynn J. Rose (Bloomington: Indiana University Press, 1993 [1973]).
[14] Cf. amongst others, Harriet Scott Chessman, *Someone Not Really Her Mother* (New York: Plume, 2004); Debra Dean, *The Madonnas of Leningrad* (London: Harper Perennial, 2006); Patrick Gale, *Rough Music* (London: Harper Collins, 2000); Michael Ignatieff, *Scar Tissue* (London: Vintage, 1993); Amy Tan, *The Bonesetter's Daughter* (New York: Ballantine Books, 2001); Marcia Willett, *The Children's Hour* (London: Bantam Press, 2003).
[15] For other uses of dementia as locus of social criticism cf. Margaret Forster, *Have the Men Had Enough?* (London: Penguin, 1989); John Irving, *The Cider House Rules* (London: Black Swan, 1985).
[16] Another example of a narrator suffering from dementia is found in Mordechai Richler's *Barney's Version* (1997); although the question of memory is essential to the novel's themes, the representation of the symptoms of dementia is relatively marginal. A review of the numerous insane narrators, afflicted by mental diseases other than dementia, is beyond the scope of this article.
[17] Leona Toker, *Eloquent Reticence: Withholding Information in Fictional Narrative* (Lexington: University Press of Kentucky, 1993), 4.
[18] Ibid.
[19] Uri Margolin, 'Of What Is Past, Is Passing, or to Come: Temporality, Aspectuality, Modality, and the Nature of Literary Narrative,' in *Narratologies: New Perspectives on Narrative Analysis*, ed. David Herman (Columbus: Ohio State University Press, 1999), 142-66.
[20] Cf. Wayne C. Booth, *The Rhetoric of Fiction* (Chicago: University of Chicago Press, 1983 [1961]), 71-76.
[21] The foregrounding of the narrative as a textual construct could be seen as fulfilling an ethical function. It reminds the reader that what she is reading is the author's attempt to imagine what it is like to experience dementia, thereby inviting the reader to problematise the truth value of this account. Although the marketing of the novel *as a novel* already brackets the expectations of 'truth-value,' disrupting an immersive reading experience in this way highlights this issue, calling the reader's attention to the risk of effacing the Other by writing her story for her.
[22] Agnosia is an inability to recognize objects, faces, sound or smells due to a neurological disorder. It is one of the symptoms of dementia.
[23] The term 'theory of mind,' originally coined in 1978 by Premarck and Woodruff in 'Does the Chimpanzee Have a Theory of Mind?' *Behavioral and Brain Sciences* 1 (1978): 555-57, has been taken up by psychology, especially developmental psychology, anthropology, linguistics, psychiatry, medicine, cognitive science, neuroscience, philosophy of mind and even literary

studies. Some issues raised are when and how theory of mind develops in children, whether impaired theory of mind is the underlying cause of autistic and other developmental or cognitive disorders or even whether theory of mind is actually an accurate description of how we understand other persons' thoughts, feelings and behaviour - on the latter point cf. Matthew Ratcliffe, *Rethinking Commonsense Psychology: A Critique of Folk Psychology, Theory of Mind and Simulation.* (Basingstoke: Palgrave Macmillan, 2007). Work on literature and theory of mind includes, among others, Lisa Zunshine, *Why We Read Fiction: Theory of Mind and the Novel* (Columbus: Ohio State University Press, 2006) and recently *Theory of Mind and Literature*, edited by Paula Leverage, et al. (West Lafayette: Purdue University Press, 2011).

[24] Pia C. Kontos, 'Embodied Selfhood: An Ethnographic Exploration of Alzheimer's Disease,' in *Thinking About Dementia: Culture, Loss, and the Anthropology of Senility*, ed. Annette Leibing and Lawrence Cohen, (Piscataway: Rutgers University Press, 2006), 195-217.

[25] Cf. D. W. Harding, 'Psychological Processes in the Reading of Fiction,' *British Journal of Aesthetics* 2 (1962): 145.

[26] Cf. Suzanne Keen, *Empathy and the Novel* (Oxford: Oxford University Press, 2007), 68-69.

[27] Compare a similar scene in *Scar Tissue* by Michael Ignatieff (London: Vintage, 1993), 156-57. This novel is written from the perspective of the caregiver who can only speculate about whether his mother's utterances have any meaning at all.

[28] Linda Örulv and Lars-Christer Hydén, 'Confabulation: Sense-Making, Self-Making and World-Making in Dementia,' *Discourse Studies* 8 (2006): 647-73.

[29] In *Rethinking Commonsense Psychology*, Ratcliffe points out the importance of gestures and facial expressions, amongst others things, in understanding others. Although he would certainly not negate the importance of language for human understanding, he does draw attention to the fact that not all thinking and all understanding is necessarily verbal. This might open up new ways of understanding others, especially those suffering from the last stages of dementia.

[30] For a more explicit discussion of the relation of knowledge and pain, and whether the loss of knowledge might ultimately decrease pain, see *Scar Tissue* by Michael Ignatieff (1993). In this fictional memoir, dementia and amyotrophic lateral sclerosis (ALS), a neurodegenerative disease that first entails the loss of body functions while cognitive functions remain intact, are contrasted with each other by the philosopher-narrator.

[31] The author holds a Ph.D. in neuroscience, allowing her an understanding of the neuropathology of dementia, while her grandmother's dementia sparked

her interest in understanding what it is like for a person to experience this disease. She was in contact with the Alzheimer's association and discussed the experience of Alzheimer's with those afflicted. She was also in contact with Christine Bryden (formerly Boden), an early-onset Alzheimer's patient, who has published two autobiographical accounts of her experience of living with Alzheimer's.

[32] The parenthetic references in this section are to Lisa Genova, *Still Alice* (London: Simon and Schuster, 2007).

[33] Harding, 'Psychological Processes,' 145.

[34] For the effect of social factors on dementia cf. Tom Kitwood 'The Dialectics of Dementia: with Particular Reference to Alzheimer's Disease,' *Ageing and Society* 10 (1990): 177-96 (where Kitwood speaks of a 'malignant social psychology' as a definite influence on and even potential cause of the development of dementia); Kitwood and Bredin, 'Towards a Theory of Dementia Care,' 269-87; and Steven R. Sabat and Rom Harré, 'The Construction and Deconstruction of Self in Alzheimer's Disease,' *Ageing and Society* 12 (1992): 443-61.

[35] Burke, 'The Poetry of Dementia' and 'Alzheimer's Disease.'

[36] William Shakespeare, *As You Like It*, Act 2, vii, 166.

[37] Cf. Frank, *Wounded Storyteller*, 97-114.

[38] Cf. Ibid., 115-36.

[39] Although Frank's validation of the ill person's point of view as well as the importance he accords to the act of witnessing can easily be endorsed, his injunction to tell a 'good story' as the right way to rise to the challenges of illness is problematic, especially for a person with dementia, as it 'promotes a specific model of the self as an agentic, authentic, autonomous storyteller; as someone with unique insight into an essentially private and emotionally rich inner world; as someone who possesses a drive for storytelling, and whose stories reflect and (re)affirm a sense of enduring, individual identity'; Angela Woods, 'The Limits of Narrative: Provocations for the Medical Humanities,' *Journal of Medical Humanities* 37 (2011): 74.

Bibliography

Bernlef, J. *Out of Mind.* Translated by Adrienne Dixon. London: Faber and Faber, 1988 [1984].

Booth, Wayne C. *The Rhetoric of Fiction.* Chicago: University of Chicago Press, 1983 [1961].

Bryden, Christine. *Dancing with Dementia: My Story of Living Positively with Dementia.* London: Jessica Kingsley, 2005.

Burke, Lucy. 'Alzheimer's Disease: Personhood and First Person Testimony,' Paper held at CDSRN (2007b). <http://www.cdsrn.org.uk/ Burke_CDSRN_2007.pdf>. Viewed November 15, 2009.

———. 'The Poetry of Dementia: Art, Ethics, and Alzheimer's Disease in Tony Harrison's *Black Daisies for the Bride.*' *Journal of Literary Disability* 1 (2007a): 61-73.

Chessman, Harriet Scott. *Someone Not Really Her Mother.* New York: Plume, 2004.

Cohn, Dorrit. *Transparent Minds: Narrative Modes for Presenting Consciousness in Fiction.* Princeton: Princeton University Press, 1978.

Dean, Debra. *The Madonnas of Leningrad.* London: Harper Perennial, 2006.

DeBaggio, Thomas. *Losing My Mind: An Intimate Look at Life with Alzheimer's.* New York: The Free Press, 2002.

Forster, Margaret. *Have the Men Had Enough?* London: Penguin Books, 1989.

Fox, Patrick. 'From Senility to Alzheimer's Disease: The Rise of the Alzheimer's Disease Movement.' *Millbank Quarterly* 1 (1989): 58-102.

Frank, Arthur W. *The Wounded Storyteller: Body, Illness, and Ethics.* Chicago: University of Chicago Press, 1995.

Franzen, Jonathan. *The Corrections.* New York: Picador, 2001.

Gale, Patrick. *Rough Music.* London: Harper Collins, 2000.

Genova, Lisa. *Still Alice.* London: Simon and Schuster, 2007.

Goffman, Erving. *Stigma: Notes on the Management of Spoiled Identity.* Englewood Cliffs, NJ: Prentice-Hall, 1963.

Grant, Linda. *Remind Me Who I Am, Again*. London: Granta Books, 1998.

Harding, D. W. 'Psychological Processes in the Reading of Fiction,' *British Journal of Aesthetics* 2 (1962): 133-47.

Hamburger, Käte. *The Logic of Literature*. Translated by Marilynn J. Rose. Bloomington: Indiana University Press, 1993 [1973].

Henderson, Cary. *Partial View: An Alzheimer's Journal*. Edited by Jackie Henderson Main, Ruth D. Henderson and Nancy Andrews. Dallas: Southern Methodist University Press, 1998.

Ignatieff, Michael. *Scar Tissue*. London: Vintage, 1993.

Irving, John. *The Cider House Rules*. London: Black Swan, 1985.

Keen, Suzanne. *Empathy and the Novel*. Oxford: Oxford University Press, 2007.

Kleinman, Arthur. *The Illness Narratives: Suffering, Healing, and the Human Condition*. New York: Basic Books, 1988.

Kitwood, Tom. 'The Dialectics of Dementia: with Particular Reference to Alzheimer's Disease.' *Ageing and Society* 10 (1990): 177-96.

Kitwood, Tom and Kathleen Bredin. 'Towards a Theory of Dementia Care: Personhood and Well-being.' *Ageing and Society* 12 (1992): 269-87.

Kontos, Pia C. 'Embodied Selfhood: An Ethnographic Exploration of Alzheimer's Disease.' In *Thinking About Dementia: Culture, Loss, and the Anthropology of Senility*, edited by Annette Leibing and Lawrence Cohen, 195-217. Piscataway: Rutgers University Press, 2006.

Margolin, Uri. 'Of What Is Past, Is Passing, or to Come: Temporality, Aspectuality, Modality, and the Nature of Literary Narrative.' In *Narratologies: New Perspectives on Narrative Analysis*, edited by David Herman, 142-66. Columbus: Ohio State University Press, 1999.

McGowin, Diane Friel. *Living in the Labyrinth: A Personal Journey through the Maze of Alzheimer's*. New York: Delta, 1994 [1993].

Örulv, Linda, and Lars-Christer Hydén. 'Confabulation: Sense-Making, Self-Making and World-Making in Dementia.' *Discourse Studies* 8 (2006): 647-73.

Premack, D. G. and G. Woodruff. 'Does the Chimpanzee Have a Theory of Mind?' *Behavioral and Brain Sciences* 1 (1978): 515-26.

Ratcliffe, Matthew. *Rethinking Commonsense Psychology: A Critique of Folk Psychology, Theory of Mind and Simulation.* Basingstoke: Palgrave Macmillan, 2007.

Richler, Mordechai. *Barney's Version.* Toronto: Knopf Canada, 1997.

Sabat, Steven R. and Rom Harré. 'The Construction and Deconstruction of Self in Alzheimer's Disease.' *Ageing and Society* 12 (1992): 443-61.

Shakespeare, William. *As You Like It* [1598/1623]. Edited by Juliet Dusinberre. London: The Arden Shakespeare, 2006.

Small, Jeff A., Kathy Geldart, Gloria Gutman and Mary Ann Clarke Scott. 'The Discourse of Self in Dementia.' *Ageing and Society* 18 (1998): 291-316.

Sparks, Nicholas. *The Notebook.* London: Sphere, 2008 [1996].

Suter, Martin. *Small World.* Zürich: Diogenes Verlag, 1997.

Tan, Amy. *The Bonesetter's Daughter.* New York: Ballantine Books, 2001.

Theory of Mind and Literature, edited by Paula Leverage, Howard Mancing, Richard Schweickert and Jennifer Marston William. West Lafayette: Purdue University Press, 2011.

Toker, Leona. *Eloquent Reticence: Withholding Information in Fictional Narrative.* Lexington: University Press of Kentucky, 1993.

Willett, Marcia. *The Children's Hour.* London: Bantam Press, 2003.

Woods, Angela. 'The Limits of Narrative: Provocations for the Medical Humanities.' *Journal of Medical Humanities* 37 (2011): 73-78.

Zunshine, Lisa. *Why We Read Fiction: Theory of Mind and the Novel*. Columbus, Ohio: Ohio State University Press, 2006.

Fending Off Pain: David Grossman's Labyrinth of Language

Nourit Melcer-Padon

Abstract
The protagonists of Grossman's *To the End of the Land* (*Ishha Borachat miBesorah*) are bound to one another by their linguistic inventiveness. For more than thirty years, they expand their special vocabulary and build on it, using language as a device to fortify what they believe to be their private, secluded shelter. Yet contrary to their wishes, the protagonists' idiolect does not constitute an exclusively private language. Their lexical inventiveness relies on the basic array of tools offered by Modern Hebrew grammar and world-building. Thus, their inventions are intelligible to a reasonably educated speaker of Hebrew. Some of these inventions follow the precise patterns of naïve creativity of many toddlers as they grapple with Hebrew morphology and word-formation. The protagonists' 'language capsule' proves to be another prison, suffocating them from within as reality does from without. Ora, the main female protagonist, eventually rebels against the two male protagonists' cerebral over-use of language, which represses femininity and the emotive side of their experience. Viscerally sensing the power of words, Ora runs away in an effort to avoid hearing the announcement of her son's death - as if this could keep him alive. Yet it is precisely language, as a means of communication rather than separation, which may be the key to some form of hope in the future, and a better alternative in negotiating pain.

Key Words: Israel, war, announcement, Hebrew word formation, idiolect, landscape, private language, escape, mental prison, communication.

*****

The first chapter of *To the End of the Land* (2008) begins in 1967. While the Six Day War is being waged, three teenagers, two boys and a girl, are confined to a world of their own. Within the state of isolation Israelis experienced in a country at war with all of its neighbours, they are further enclosed by hospital walls, the only patients left in an infectious-disease ward. No one is allowed to visit them for fear of contagion, and they are completely cut off from the world. Not only are they running a high fever, which confuses their sense of time, but the windows are covered because of the black-out, turning days into indefinite stretches of time, almost indistinguishable from nights. Left in the hands of a hostile Arab nurse, the protagonists are further subjected to Egyptian radio propaganda in Hebrew, announcing the purported advancement of the Egyptian army and the Israeli defeat. The actual, unprecedented victory of the Israeli army, and the euphoria that followed it, is thus not part of their experience. Instead, they are caught up in the complicated friendship that is being forged between them, a friendship that continues throughout the novel.

The next chapter is set in 2002. The three protagonists are middle aged, and Israel has changed too. The confident triumphant state of 1967 has undergone the traumatic experience of the 1973 Yom Kippur War. The protagonists have been directly affected by the political upheavals of the country. Avram, one of the men, was a POW in Egypt in 1973, and this became the determining event for all three protagonists in the following years. Although their private tragedy is one among innumerable similar tragedies many Israelis faced, its effect on them is their increased separation from their society. Instead of seeking assistance outside their circle, they become even more enclosed among themselves, perpetuating a state of isolation similar to that of 1967. The unusual relationship between Ora, the female protagonist, and the two men, Avram and Ilan, entraps them further in the need for secrecy.

The confines of their little group are demarcated by the seemingly private language of the protagonists, made of private neologisms and lexical games. 'Their' language proved quite effective in bringing Avram out of the coma he was in due to the torture he had been subjected to in Egypt. Nevertheless, the novelty of their use of the language, which captivated them in 1967, has faded by 2002. By this point, their language has become one more factor which pressurizes them from inside their capsule, adding to the pressure of the difficult reality without. The last pages of the novel indicate that language can provide a form of solace for a fated loss. Used as a means of communication with others, rather than as a device of exclusion and separation, language can both contain the memory of a dead loved one and maintain this memory as an integral part of life.

1. The Three Word Title

Grossman's novel was given the title *To the End of the Land* in its English version.[1] The title in Hebrew is a three-word one: *אשה בורחת מבשורה* (*Ishah Borachat miBesorah*) - literally, 'A Woman in Flight from an Announcement.'

The Hebrew title is related to the plot: Ora runs away from her house, and travels to the farthest northern part of Israel. The reason for this flight is that her younger son, Ofer, has rejoined his army unit in order to participate in a major operation. Instead of waiting for her son at home with a warm meal, Ora convinces herself that if she is absent, the army officers who inform families that their sons have been killed in battle will not be able to find her, and so their announcement will not be delivered and therefore its message will not materialise.

Yet Grossman's choice of the three words rewards closer attention. אשה (*ishah*) is 'a woman,' carrying the indefinite article 'a,' rather than 'the woman.' This non-specificity extends the meaning of 'woman' to encompass not only this character but also a more general presence of feminine feelings and features in all the characters of the novel. Grossman carries his protagonists' denial of femininity and of their emotive side to tragic extremes. The language he uses, the dialogues, the scenes, even the body language, all signal suppression of natural feelings. As a result, his protagonists are confined to a cold, cerebral over-consciousness. The discourse of the text, the repetitions of ideas and the use of the various dramatic personae all participate in crushing the essence of existence, motherhood. The most natural of female attributes is thus stifled and repressed. Moreover, Ora's stream of consciousness contains and conveys many more voices than her own. This strategy, which uses various discursive levels of the text in relation to one character, allows Ora's voice to take over the narrative and become the focal point of the readers' attention. This strategy also enhances the poignancy of the threat to a society that puts femininity in jeopardy.

Ora is a woman in flight: בורחת (*borachat*) means 'running away from.' Read as a verb or as an adjective,[2] the word suggests two possible interpretations: Ora is in a constant state of flight throughout the fictional present, yet an attempted flight into denial can also be seen as an inherent, pre-existing feature of this 'collective' Israeli woman, perhaps pointing to the existential state of Israelis, especially as parents.[3]

The word 'announcement' in the title is also indefinite: it is 'an' announcement rather than 'the' particular announcement. The word בשורה (*besorah*) can be a good announcement, as in *besorot tovot*, good news, usually used in the plural form. Less frequently, it can also refer to a bad announcement, such as *besorat iyov*, (announcement made to Job).[4] The word *besorah* can also be translated as annunciation, especially in religious terms, and more often than not reveals good news.[5] The image that naturally springs to mind is that of the announcement of the birth of a child, either to the Old Testament Sarah or to the New Testament Mary. Yet instead of joy and pride, the birth of Ora's two children, by Ilan and by Avram, generates alienation and discord among their parents. Staged against a precarious political background, the boys receive a bleak welcome from their respective fathers. Moreover, each of the fathers, in turn, stifles Ora's maternal feelings: one father leaves the house shortly after the baby's birth; the other demands an abortion and, when the child is born, wants nothing to do with him. Yet above all, natural parental instincts are subdued by the fathers' overpowering use of language, as shall be discussed further on: the feminine in the men and in the woman alike is repressed by the cerebral. The word *besorah* cannot but invoke the joyful announcement of the birth of a child, yet in collocation with 'in flight' such an expectation is supplanted by a fear of the announcement of the child's death.[6] The announcement that Ora dreads exists as a potential. If and when realized, it will take the shape of a ritual complete with its own vocabulary and grammar. The procedure of the announcement of the death of a soldier is well known in the Israeli context. Notifications are delivered to the next of kin personally, by several trained officers. The notification is a text that is performed orally, and can take place at all hours of night or day, since according to the Jewish tradition, the dead must be buried as soon as possible. Envisioning the arrival of these officers at her door, Ora runs away from this text, from the words whose articulation will confirm her worst fears. She is running away from something which already exists by virtue of its potentiality. Like a hypochondriac who is convinced he has the symptoms of an illness he is reading about, Ora is imprisoned within her fears of hearing the announcement that she, like every member of Israeli society, has witnessed delivered to others.

Her response is her own alternative ritual, a ritual which dictates that she will stay away from her house as long as the operation takes place.[7] She forces Avram, Ofer's biological father, to come along on a hiking trip that she had originally planned to go on with her son. She rules that they will not listen to the radio or talk to anyone they might meet about the news so as not to hear any details of the operation. Ora's flight is a kind of magical pact she tries to make with destiny: as long as she cannot be found to receive the announcement, her son's life will be safeguarded. Clearly, destiny is not bound by such a contract.

One may be reminded here of the paradox of Schroedinger's cat: two options are theoretically possible 'at the same time,' so long as one does not open the cat's box to ascertain which of them is actual. From Ora's perspective, Ofer is alive as long as she does not receive the announcement of his death. Nevertheless, despite her efforts to create an alternative reality, in which her actions can safeguard her son, the threat to Ofer's life exists even there, within her 'closed' system, from the moment he was conceived. This is driven home when she and Avram sleep together, towards the end of the novel and recall their promises to each other:

> And we will always, always be together? Ora asks Avram, echoing Avram's promise to her in a telegram he sent her for her twentieth birthday. Until death do us connect, he completed without a second thought the sentence he had written then. And there, at that moment, Avram felt that Ofer is in danger. … You felt it? [Ora] whispered in his ear in terror, you felt it, right? Avram breathed mutely into her hair. Her body was covered with cold sweat. Think about

> him, she whispered and hugged him with her entire body until she put him in her, think about him in me. (615)

In desperation, Ora and Avram reenact Ofer's conception. Yet death is inherently present at the moment of conception. Avram's words have 'opened the box' of Ora's alternative reality, reintroducing doubt. A few pages later, Avram asks to see Ofer's picture for the first time, and

> Ora closes her eyes, she sees people standing on both sides of the street that leads to her house. Some of them have already entered the yard, some stand on the steps that lead to her door. They await her in silence, their faces lowered. Waiting for her to pass between them and enter her house. So that it will be possible to start, the words pass through her. (629)

Ora refers to the beginning of the delivery of the dreaded announcement, as though once Avram has 're-birthed' Ofer with her, and seen the child, Ofer is once again open to the threat of death, without the deceptive protection of her invented reality.

2. A Prison-House of Language

Ora temporarily disconnects from home, from her phone and from the news. Yet she is caught in a double bind. She is as entrapped by the geography of the land as she is by its language: the confines of Israel are clearly delineated by its hostile neighbouring countries, and its entire length can be negotiated in a few days' walk. No sooner has Ora reached the 'end' of the land in the north, than she turns around again and heads back home, where the news, whether good or bad, will await her. Land and language are intertwined along the hiking trail: Ora and Avram pass by places which project textual, biblical allusions. In addition, they inevitably come across monuments erected along the way, bearing inscriptions memorializing soldiers killed in action. The land is thus inscribed by the telling of its history. The one cohesive factor of the Zionist project in the land of Israel is the fact that the language unifying all the people who live in Israel is Hebrew, whether they are Jews or Arabs, secular or religious, native-born or new immigrants from many diasporas. The commemorating inscriptions mentioned in the novel are a tangible proof of this, since they are written in Hebrew, and memorialise soldiers of various backgrounds, Jewish, Bedouin or Druze. The connection between the land, its language and its inhabitants is also clear in the depiction of the protagonists. If things exist in their being verbally performed, then Ora can only exist in Hebrew and in Israel. As Avram thinks but refrains from saying to Ora, 'Only here, in this landscape, in the rocks, the cyclamens, in Hebrew, in this sun, does she have a meaning' (411).

The novel suggests that running away is in itself a state of captivity, because it is futile. Ora's attempt to distance herself from the knowledge of Ofer's death is a hopeless effort to escape a maze. The walls of the maze that surround her are rendered by a mixture of internal and external focalisations, a mesh of consciousnesses - Avram's, Ora's and the narrator's, at times almost indistinguish-able from each other. Ora's consciousness, focused on her flight, is inflated till it seems to take over the entire space of the novel, enclosing Avram and the readers. The identification readers may feel towards Ora engulfs them from the start in a collective yearning to escape the announcement.

Except for the case of the letters that Avram wrote to Ora in their youth, there are no quotation marks in over 600 pages of what reads like a constant dialogue. The breaking up and mixing of points of view, flashbacks, internal dialogue and external details, as well as the use of direct and free indirect speech, create the sense that the entire novel is an expression of Ora's consciousness. In the following passage, for instance, Ora and Avram are resting after a hard climb on their hiking trail. Ora is telling Avram about Ofer, who at the age of four discovered where meat comes from and became a vegetarian:

> Ora?
> Where was I?
> That you saw what kind of kid he is.
> Then I said to Ofer, that it's nothing, meat. I said in the most banal voice, this is nothing special, meat. You know, the same as we eat almost every day, meat.
> *And she sees:* the tiny, meager Ofer, her delicate Ofer, starts to jump from foot to foot, as he always used to do when he was perplexed or scared - *she rises and demonstrates to Avram* - or he would pull again and again on his left ear, like this, or he would walk to the sides, there and back, quickly.
> *Avram doesn't stop looking at her. She comes back and sits in front of him with a sigh. Her soul goes out to that Ofer.*
> And I stuck my head deep in the fridge and tried to avoid him, from the look he had, but he did not relent, and asked from whom did they take this meat.
> And you should know that he really liked meat then, beef and poultry. Aside from that he ate nearly nothing, but meat balls and schnitzels and hamburgers he did like. A real predator he was then, which made Ilan very glad, and me

> too somehow.
> What?
> That he liked meat, I don't know, a primary satisfaction. You understand that don't you?
> But I am a vegetarian now.
> So that's it, *she cries out,* I noticed yesterday, at the Moshav, you didn't touch
> Three years already.
> But why?
> No reason. I felt like cleaning up. *But his eyes are punctiliously stuck on his fingertips.* Well, you remember, there was already another time that I didn't eat meat for a few years.
> When he came back from the POW jail, *of course she remembers.* (306, italics mine)

The italicised words represent the omniscient narrator's voice, which intervenes in Ora and Avram's dialogue and provides information about the protagonists' physical movements, as well as insights into Ora's thoughts. In the case of '*And she sees,*' the word 'And' at the beginning of the sentence gives the reader the illusion that it follows a discourse by the same voice, continuing something this voice said before. Yet this 'And' refers to a continuation of the mental picture Ora has at that moment of Ofer at the age of four. The second 'And,' in the sentence beginning with 'And I stuck my head deep in the fridge,' pertains to the continuation of Ora's direct speech rather than of her thought. In a similar manner, 'of course she remembers' could be either the omniscient narrator's comment or an expression of her thoughts, in free indirect discourse. The narrator's voice is mingled with Ora's consciousness in such a way as to make it irrelevant whether it is her voice or not, since in any case the narrative focus is hers. Another kind of such a mingling occurs a little later in this same scene. The omniscient narrator provides a description of Ora and Avram's actions in the present tense, combined with barely noticeable reported speech, in which the verbs are in the past tense:

> She drinks water from a bottle, rinsing her face. Handing him the bottle, and he, without thinking, empties it over his head. *And his face immediately closed, locked up,* like that - she shows. (310)

The beginning of the sentence 'And his face immediately closed' can confuse the reader into thinking that the 'he' to whom the face belongs is the same as in the previous sentence, Avram, whereas Ora is still talking about

Ofer, as she did before drinking. Even if one notices the change in tenses to the past, denoting a reported action, the fact that the reporting clause 'she shows' follows rather than precedes the first clause allows the assumption that 'And his face immediately closed, locked up' refers to Avram rather than to Ora's recollection of Ofer. The 'And' in this case records Ora's voice, mingling Ofer and Avram into one 'he,' as she endeavours to do all along. On the level of the plot, this corresponds to Ora's constant effort to bring father and son closer together, to make Avram assume his role as a parent. Grossman thus takes advantage of the possible ambiguity between Free Indirect Discourse and Free Direct Speech[8] to efface the voice of the narrator in favour of that of the protagonist.

Two pages later (312), Grossman uses the word 'and' as a deictic element in the text, linking Ora's thoughts and her speech as though she spoke her thoughts out loud, placing these thoughts on the same textual level as the omniscient narrator's comments regarding her movements. In other cases, the mingling of voices involves Ora's thoughts and Avram's thoughts (249-50), or a mingling between their thoughts and their speech (248). In another instance (212), the reader experi-ences Avram's speech as part of Ora's speech, although the narrative is that of Avram's thoughts and memories. The resulting overall impression is that the entire narrative is Ora's.[9] The mingling of voices into one narrative, achieved by merging FID and FDS and by deictic elements in the text, brings to the fore another kind of blending, namely between the protagonists' experiences of pain. The common nature of each protagonist's ordeal, enmeshed in the pain of others, is thus highlighted. This is especially poignant, since this narrative is juxtaposed to Ora's self-centeredness. Engulfed by her own fears, Ora does not realise they are not only hers. Just as she ignored other parents who had brought their sons to Ofer's unit's meeting point and barely listened to the account of a mother of three soldiers on the radio, she is now incapable of registering what Avram is telling her. Not only is Avram also worried about Ofer, but his strategy in dealing with his feelings is similar to Ora's: his renewed vegetarianism is his own 'pact' with destiny, like Ora's flight (307). It will take Ora the entire length of the novel to begin to recognise that the pain experienced by others is very similar to her own.

Grossman's use of language is subtle and sensitive in other ways as well, and in keeping with the times in which the novel is set and with the identity of each speaker. Thus, the language the protagonists use in 1967 includes the 1960s' slang and alludes to the books teenagers read in those years. The Arab driver's Hebrew reflects Arabic vocabulary and pronunciation (134-35), and a Jewish Yemenite's speech (199-207) is likewise faithfully rendered. Grossman also uses appropriate military jargon to render conversations Ora has with her sons during their military service (112-15).[10]

Like Avram, Grossman's third-person narrator uses playful word games, based on metaphors, alliterations and derivations: his use of language is thus blended with the protagonists' language. Language thus emerges as a common prison-house throughout the novel.

Words are weapons, part of the arsenal of emotional power games that the characters play with each other. The novel begins with the sentence: 'Hey, you, [be] quiet!' (7) - Avram's effort to silence Ora's singing, which is how they start talking to each other. Their dialogue makes it clear that, of the two, Avram is the more talented user of Hebrew. He is witty; he constructs new words and invents word games. Ora knows, before she even speaks, that Avram will deride her rhyming efforts to popular tunes which won her schoolmates' admiration. She senses the danger of self effacement in being drawn to Avram and his language:

> Maybe she should be careful, because she suddenly felt that she was in a place that was dangerous for her, at the brink of his larynx, and in another moment his suction power will completely draw her in, and when she is ejected from there, she will start talking exactly like him, with his jokes, and his witticisms and flowery phrases and all his antics. (79)

Though Ora feels the threat to her very being, she needs Avram to be able to understand herself and her dreams. Even though Avram is angry at her for repeatedly waking him at night, Ora needs him to help her understand what song she was singing in her sleep, a clue to her recurrent dream of Ada (8), her best friend until she died in a car accident two years before the novel begins. Thanks to his linguistic capacities, Avram replaces Ada for Ora. Ora's relationship with Ada was also based on word games: the two girls used to communicate in class through comic notes; they read the same books and tried to translate their favourite book to Esperanto, so the whole world would appreciate it; together they created the 'almanac of protected words' and wrote a learned exegesis of *Kofiko*, a children's book about a naughty monkey (28-30). Ora feels it was her relationship with Ada that prepared her for Avram: 'if it hadn't been for Ada, she wouldn't have known at all that it is possible, it is allowed, for two people to be so close' (30). In the almost daily letters Avram wrote Ora for six years after their first meeting, he included limericks, quotes, and parts of sketches he wrote for plays and stories, complete with footnotes. Ora reads Avram's letters, and feels an 'almost physical longing for Ada,' though she also feels as if she were betraying Ada by becoming close with Avram (373). At the same time, it is only to Avram that Ora can confess how much she misses Ada (374), and it is to Avram that Ora confides, by letter, her most intimate thoughts (374). Ada was a young writer: when Ora learns that Avram's every moment is likewise spent writing, the information 'closes in on her . . . the words descended on her like a vulture on its pray' (60). The web in which Avram entraps Ora is thus made of words and of his capacity to use them both orally and in writing.

Avram, for his part, is grateful to Ora for every letter she writes him. In Hebrew, this gratitude is enhanced: he is 'אסיר תודה' (*asir todah*), which literally means 'a prisoner of his gratitude to her,' and he is grateful for every part of the alphabet she sends him, every 'אות' (*ot*), which means both 'a letter of the alphabet' and 'a sign' (374). Avram successfully uses words to woo her. Yet he too needs Ora to understand himself and what he is planning to write. 'You,' Avram tells Ora, 'disclosed to me what I had invented' (52). Later on, Ora blames Avram and Ilan for being too verbal. Avram retorts that if he played so much with words, it 'was all because of you, for you' (365). Thus, for Avram, Ora and Ilan, language becomes a cohesive and formative force but also a stifling and imprisoning one.

Over the thirty years of their friendship, the use of 'Avram's' words' becomes the characteristic trait of these three protagonists. Ilan marries Ora, and they have a son, Adam. Before Adam is born, Ilan tells Ora that he will not be able to love a baby until it starts to talk (403). For him too, language is central. When Ilan becomes the father of both Adam and Ofer, he transmits what he knows to have been Avram's love of the language to the children as well. Avram once said to Ilan that if he ever had a child, he would give him every new word, and it would be 'like a covenant' between them (353). The Hebrew term for covenant is ברית מילה (*brit milah*). The word ברית (*brit*) means covenant, and the word מילה (*milah*) has two meanings: 'a word' and 'circumcision.' Teaching a child to speak, for Avram, is akin to God's gift of a covenant with His people, a pact of fidelity.

The relationship of the father to the child is therefore predominantly a verbal one. Ilan welcomes the newborn baby home by posting a humorous page on the bedroom door, a page Ora finds to be 'packed with words, too many words' (222). The mother is the one who is silenced, stifled. Ora, like Ilan, suffers because of Avram's fate as a POW, and grieves the ruin of his life and of their friendship. Nevertheless, Adam's birth fills her with joy and renewed hope. 'I felt that the entire world was completely changed as soon as Adam was born . . . a new dimension was added . . . to everything and every person in the world' (220-21). Yet when they drive home from the hospital with the baby, Ilan is so quiet that Ora is compelled to keep quiet too. 'Suddenly I couldn't get a word out of my mouth. Even when I wanted to talk I couldn't. I felt completely strangled, as though someone was holding me by the throat, and that was you' (221), she explains to Avram, years later. Sandwiched between the two men, Ora is smothered and cannot express her feelings or enjoy her motherhood.[11] 'There was a kind of mad circle around both of us,' Ora explains, 'and all my instincts, the natural ones, as though – listen, I don't know where I was then. It was as though I didn't exist' (242).

After a timid effort at leading a normal life with Ora and Adam, Ilan's guilty feelings towards Avram drive him out of the house. Ilan only returns to live with Ora when he learns that Ora has become pregnant with Avram's son, Ofer. Ofer receives a better welcome than Adam did from Ilan, yet his biological father has tried to convince Ora to have an abortion. She refused, but Avram wanted nothing to do with her or the child. Ofer was born into silence and secrecy, raised as Ilan's son - since Avram insists that the child should know nothing about him. Ora takes advantage of the moments after Ofer's birth, when she is alone with the baby, to tell him for the first and last time the whole truth about his two fathers and her relationship with them (295).

Contrary to Ora's silence, Ilan's return to the family, after a three-year absence, entails an avalanche of words. In his attempt to 'fix' Adam, who had been silent for most of the years he was alone with his mother, Ilan submits Adam to what Ora terms as 'a soldier's basic training of speech.' Ora blames Ilan for repossessing the child within his delineated territory (365-66), and of trying to create with Adam a substitute partner to Avram, with whom he could enjoy the possibility to shine and 'besmarten'[12] (להבריק ולהשתנן) (*l'havrik ul'hishtanen*, 367). Copying Avram, Ilan plays with words, inventing nicknames for Adam, 'a pretty-braying donkey' or 'an angry-browed cat' (400). Ora is far from happy with Ilan's zeal, and regards what he does to Adam as experiments on a human being. Adam complies with his newly acquired father's whims, soon inventing his own words. Yet once he masters language, its overdose crushes him. At first he simply talks all the time, blabbering on, 'as though his subconscious were completely open to us,' says Ora (401). The situation worsens when Ofer is born, and Adam senses that Ilan has betrayed him again, giving Avram's son all his fatherly attention. Adam's retaliation is carried out with the same weapon that Ilan has provided. For months, the child speaks in rhymes, frightening himself when he cannot stop (406-407).

Language *is* Avram. Language is the distinctive trait of the 'old' Avram as opposed to the POW Avram. Avram feels that he actually died when the Egyptian soldiers buried him alive, and declares that he wants nothing to do with life, that he is 'finished with words' (283). His denial of language is all the more poignant since words have a physical dimension for him: he 'tasted the name 'Ora' in his mouth when he said it' (76); he savours the words he hears (16, 28, 47, 153, 616). Avram tells Ora that in order to write, he must understand any character he invents from its body, from besmearing himself with its meat and saliva and milk, in order to 'feel the texture of its muscles and tendons. … Everything he writes must be alive and tangible and physical to him' (282-83). When Ora wants to revive Avram, to bring him back to consciousness at the hospital in 1973, after he is returned from Egypt, she reads aloud the letters he sent her before the war (371).

Despite Ilan's apprehension, her stratagem works: Avram comes out of his coma (380-81).

Avram's inventiveness with language apparently stems from the same source as his immature behaviour with Ora.[13] When they were teenagers, incapable of becoming physically involved with Ora, Avram had wheeled Ilan into her room. Ilan proved to be a successful substitute, and the one who eventually married Ora. Years later Avram seems stuck at a childish stage with language, as immature as his sexual approaches. As a teenager, he planned to write a symphony solely for human voices (50-51). Grossman makes sure that the allusion to Jean Cocteau, the *enfant terrible* of the French avant-garde theatre, and his work *La Voix Humaine*, is not lost on his readers: Avram later admits that he is an eternal child who refuses to grow up (186).[14]

Avram's playful word games are typical of Hebrew-speaking children who are learning the morphology of the language through trial and error.[15] Children form word derivations and conjugate verbs after their own fashion, yet the results are words which can be explained by the rules of the Hebrew morphological system. Avram uses the morphological system at will, but never changes its rules or its set of possibilities. Rather, he makes use of what the system offers any linguistically creative Hebrew speaker. Among the options Avram deploys are using a higher register than is expected in a specific context, alluding to idioms by alliteration, using existing roots in verbal slots left unused by Hebrew, deriving verbs from nouns according to the word-formation regularities, applying the diminutive or the dual to nouns which officially do not take it, inventing nouns by using existing nominal forms which carry a specific semantic content (thus inventing a colour or a tool or a place). All this can be seen in children in the early phases of acquiring active language proficiency and in creative uses of Hebrew, as indeed can also be seen in the narrator's own playfulness with the language. Here are some examples of Avram's neologisms. להתאדש (*lehit'adesh*, 373), 'to become apathetic' - a verb created by using an existing root, א.ד.ש. (*a.d.sh*). משוקקים אותו (*meshokekim oto*, 174), 'make him crave [something],' a verb created by using an existing root, ש.ק.ק. (*sh.k.k.*) in a 'free slot' in the table of Modern Hebrew verbal forms. סדיים (*sadayim*, 261), Avram's term for Ora's bra, a dual form of סד (*sad*), 'pillar' or 'support,' i.e. 'two pillars,' playing on 'שדיים' (*shadayim*), 'breasts.' מלקיקה (*malkikah*, 262), a verb meaning 'I lick' in an erotic scene, created from an existing root, ל.ק.ק. (*l.k.k.*) in a causative 'free slot' of verbal forms, erotically stronger than the existing *melakeket*, 'licks.' לזאב אותו (*leza'ev oto*, 334), 'to wolf him,' a verb created from a noun, a known word-formation device in colloquial Hebrew. מרעמים (*mir'amim*, 372), the word Avram creates for 'telegram' on the basis of *ra'am* ('thunder'), instead of the word *mivraq*, created from the root *b.r. q.* (ב.ר.ק.) which also forms the word 'lightning.' Avram's use of language is contagious: beside Ora and others, the omniscient narrator seems to be caught up in it as well. Grossman thus blurs the lines between the protagonists and the narrator, luring his readers to share their playful linguistic prison-house.

A week into the trail, Ora and Avram meet a stranger who asks them if they are 'doing the trail.' They do not understand what he means, and he explains: 'the Israel Trail,' and points to the 'blue-white-orange marking on one of the rocks.'[16] Ora realizes, to her great annoyance, that 'the humble and intimate trail, along which she and Avram had been walking alone for a week already, has a name, and she [is] immediately robbed of something' (318). Ora's feelings reflect the protagonists' delusion. While Ora believes they were walking along a trail all their own, they have actually been walking along the mapped national trail. Similarly, the protagonists' use of the Hebrew language gives them the illusion that they have created a private language, distinct from everyone else's, yet what they see as a private barrier which distinguishes them from the rest, and protects them in their cocoon, actually belongs to the public domain. Not even Avram's invented words make up a new language, since his inventiveness is merely an application of existing morphological possibilities: the reader of Hebrew instantly understands what Avram's odd-looking combinations mean and can classify them as witty, clever or crafty. The private language invented and inflicted on the three protagonists by Avram is but an enhancement of the standard Hebrew lexicon.

3. The Language of Performance

Ora has already experienced the fateful power of words: she is the one who was forced to draw a piece of paper with a man's name out of a hat in 1973. Although she could not know it at the time, this random lottery decided which of the two men was to become a POW and which was to be spared. In 2002, she is determined to keep her son alive. This must be done by fending off the fateful production of words in the shape of an announcement, which must not be physically voiced. She feels Ofer within her, calling to her again and again, in different voices and at different ages, claiming her for himself. She realizes she must not only constantly think about him, but talk about him incessantly to whoever she meets, 'even to the trees and the stones and the thorns, and say his name out loud and in her heart again and again and again . . . because he needs her now to simply *exist*' (182). Ora tells Avram everything she can about Ofer, 'such small stories,' she apologizes, 'but from story to story, from word to word, baby Ofer resounds to her too, and is moulded into a child' (351). Ora's words recreate Ofer for Avram, in the same way that she wants Ofer's clothes to allow Avram to 'guess [Ofer] . . . his height, width, size. … [I]f she really makes an effort . . . she could pull and deliver from the depth of his backpack his very self as well, Ofer . . . and she kneads her child from the cloths' (315-16). Ora talks her child, and writes him in her diary, reduced to repeatedly writing his name as she has repeatedly said it out loud, in her frantic effort to prevent his death.[17]

The most interesting aspect of the use of language in the novel is thus its performative function and the magical power words have on the protagonists.[18] Avram is alive as long as his vocabulary is in use; and Ora believes that saying Ofer's name repeatedly, and talking about him with his father, will safeguard him. She discovers that writing about him in her diary even allows her to feel that she no longer needs to run: as long as she can write about Ofer, he is safe (258). The daughter of Holocaust survivors, Ora obeyed their decree. She did not visit Ada's parents after Ada died, nor talked about her: 'it is best this way, one doesn't have to talk about everything,' she parroted her parents' words to Avram in 1967 (33). Ora was taught that not talking about something painful makes it less present, yet Ada's linguistic disappearance from her life added to the pain of her physical disappearance. 'No one in class speaks about her anymore, never, two years . . . as-though-she-ne-ver-e-xis-ted-at-all,' Ora laments to Avram, rhythmically banging her head against the hospital wall (34). No such fate will be inflicted on Ofer, if it depends on her.

The private shelter that endless witticisms seem to give Ilan and Avram prove ineffective in protecting them from the horrors of war, both in Avram's case in 1973, and in Ofer's case in 2002. Moreover, their artificial cocoon stifles not only Ora's motherly instincts but the feminine in themselves as well. Instead of providing the three protagonists with a safe haven, their language created an additional pressure chamber within the shared realities of their country.

At the end of the novel, Ora vexes Avram and claims he does not know Ofer, for 'who is Ofer to you? Ofer is just words to you' (628). Yet Avram is now sufficiently restored to his previous self and can help Ora by the only means at his disposal, verbally. Although all Avram knows of Ofer are the words Ora has used, he can now talk of his son and give him back to his mother. Just as Avram needed Ora to explain to him the script he proposed to write in the hospital in 1967, she now needs him to explain to her that they both need Ofer: 'we are holding him together, between us, all the time' (630). Yet the Ofer Avram sees in his mind is sleeping, and Ora is afraid that it means he is already dead.

Superstitiously, Ora begins to think that she may have been wrong all along, and that trying to protect Ofer by talking about him with Avram could have had the opposite effect. She does not understand the inner workings of her own ritual. Her only motivation was to keep Ofer alive by avoiding the words that would *make* him dead. The futility of her ritual of escape is proved to her as soon as Ofer's probable death enters her consciousness. Until now, her memories were 'filled with life' and at the same time 'filled Ofer with life, far away' (284). From this moment on, she needs Avram to remember her, their common story and Ofer. She asks Avram to remember 'everything . . . from the beginning, from when we knew each other, and the war there was then, and how we met in the isolation ward, and the second war, and what happened to you, and Ilan, and me, and everything that happened, yes?' (631). By remembering, Avram will continue both her and Ofer's existence, and maybe 'in the end,' as she tells Avram, 'you will remember everything . . . [and] we will beget a book from this' (523). Ofer's existence, like Ora's, now depends on being remembered and on their story being told. Language becomes a tool for consolation and for a measure of redemption.

4. The Consolation of Language

Ora has fled from the verbal performance of the death of her son, from the language which would make her fear come true. Yet language does not only kill: it can also revive and keep a person's memory alive. Along the hike, Ora brings Avram back to life once again, in the same way she did when he returned from the Egyptian prison. As in 1973, Ora now revives Avram by talking to him, forcing him out of his stupor. Together, they give birth to Ofer once more, in words rather than in the flesh. They will 'raise' Ofer again, keeping him alive, at least in their memory.

The hiking trip also allows Ora to rediscover writing. She used to be her family's writer, documenting the holidays despite Ilan's and her sons' indifference. On this trip, her writing is an endeavour to reconnect to herself. Nonetheless, what Ora writes in her notebook contains only factual details and is devoid of emotions. She describes Ofer's delivery, and recalls how she used 'Avram's' language to talk to the newborn baby, so that he would hear his 'father-tongue' (297) from the start, especially since language was going to be Ofer's only contact with his biological father. Ofer's birth is seen through Avram's language and Ilan's witticisms. What is blatantly missing in Ora's written recollection is her own cooing over her newborn baby. Conspicuous in its absence is an expression of an emotion, which one could expect from a personal diary.

The doctor whom Ora and Avram meet along the trail takes Ora's forgotten notebook, and continues writing his own thoughts precisely where she left off, his handwriting looking like a masculine version of her own (424). A widower, the doctor has already received an announcement similar to the one Ora is trying to flee. He has already understood there was no escape from knowing the death of his beloved wife. When Ora recovers the notebook, she too continues to write in the blank lines the doctor has left on the page (507). In the end, it does not matter who the narrator of the story is or who owns the narrative: at the end of the novel Grossman's own author's note appears in italics, a cursive graphically identical to the italics used for the doctor's and Ora's entries in her diary, adding a third to their mutually complementary entries. The tragic loss of Grossman's own son is thereby made an integral part of the novel. Grossman started writing the novel towards the end of his older son's military service, and during his younger son's military service. He admits that he had 'the feeling - or more accurately the wish - that the book [he] was writing would protect' his son (633). Like his protagonist, Grossman tried to interfere in the workings of fate - in vain.

Of all the people walking along the trail, it is a paediatrician who finds the notebook, a man whose profession is to examine and heal small babies or children who do not yet possess a spoken language. Ora's body language made it clear to the doctor that she was distressed even before he read her journal. Ora's own reaction to seeing the figure of the doctor produces an intellectual association to Giacometti, while Avram blocks the path, creating a physical buffer between Ora and the doctor, as though unwilling to allow Ora out of his grip (317). The short meeting with the doctor could not create a change in the protagonists' cerebral attitude towards themselves and their reality. Yet the doctor's ensuing intervention in Ora's writing plants the seeds for a different apprehension of reality, one which may legitimize the expression of long repressed feelings.

The doctor is not ashamed to walk with his wife's sunglasses. He demonstrates the possibility of keeping a balance between femininity and inner self on the one hand and the necessity of finding a way to negotiate life's hardships on the other. The doctor is a healer, of body and soul, and he points out the way to use language to the best advantage. Instead of allowing it to separate an individual from the rest of society, language should be used to connect with others, and with the inner parts of one's self. Through the conversations the doctor entertains with other hikers, he can keep communication lines open not only with living people but also with his dead wife. She was the one who instructed him to ask each person he met two questions that were bound to start a conversation, thus maintaining connection to other people. Despite her initial anger at the doctor's invasion of her diary, Ora is 'sucked into' his accounts of his meetings with various people (426) as well as his own handling of his grief (433). The diary becomes a healing medium for her, showing her that she is not alone in her pain. The balance the doctor manages to keep between his grief and his present life, between the different parts of his inner self and people around him, is a higher linguistic achievement language than the protagonists' private idiom. The hope a novelist[19] can provide for his readers is that imagination, sensitivity and the turmoils of the soul can find an outlet in a different language that unites instead of dividing.

Notes

[1] All the references to Grossman's text are to the Hebrew edition, David Grossman, *Ishah Borachat miBesorah* (Benei Brak: HaKibbutz HaMeuchad, 2008). The translations are mine, because the published translation omits passages of the Hebrew text. The English title of the published version points at a symbolic and existential meaning: though Ora travels as far as the borders of the country allow, she is forced to realise the futility of her endeavour. At the end of the novel, Ora lies on a rock, feeling underneath her the cold stone and 'the entire mountain, gigantic and condensed and infinite' (632). No matter how far Ora goes, as long as she is alive, she is doomed to live within the confines of the land.

[2] The Hebrew *borachat* is a verb in the Present tense (in English, the equivalent can be either Present Simple or Present Continuous). The same word can be read as a Present Participle, and, as such, adjectival - what Lewis Glinert calls a 'verb-shaped adjective' of the kind that 'share the same patterns as present tense verbs'; see *The Grammar of Modern Hebrew* (Cambridge: Cambridge University Press, 1989), 485.

[3] In an interview with Manuel Carcassonne, entitled 'David Grossman: Death is a Way of Life,' given to *Magazine Littéraire*, Grossman referred to Israel as 'a whole country that lives death as a routine. I [Grossman] don't want to separate the private from the collective, the individual from the general. Every time I send my children to school, I worry whether they will return alive.' *Magazine Littéraire* 427 (2004): 86 (my translation).

[4] In his entry on the word *basar*, Eliezer Ben Yehuda translates the word into German as 'eine Botschaft bringen' and to English as 'announcer; to announce.' In this and in the next entry, *besorah*, Ben Yehuda gives many biblical references, mostly meaning good tidings (*A Complete Dictionary of Ancient and Modern Hebrew* [Jerusalem: Ben Yehuda Publishing, 1948], 2: 646-47). Regarding *besorah* as 'Job's announcement,' see Avraham Even Shoshan, *Even Shoshan Dictionary: Renewed and Updated for the Year 2000* (Tel Aviv: Hamilon Hahadash Publishing, 2003), 1: 215.

[5] Ora says to Avram, 'Just remember, that sometimes a bad announcement can be a very good one you didn't understand, and what may have once been a bad announcement, can be overturned in time into a good announcement, maybe the best one you need' (322). These words, at about the middle of the novel, provide an ironic juxtaposition to the announcement Ora is running away from throughout the novel, namely the announcement of her son's death in an army operation.

[6] Yael Feldman suggests that 'Ora is Mary's anti-type,' since she rejects the proposition that her son Ofer 'will be offered up along with all the other

tender human sacrifices' (*Glory and Agony: Isaac's Sacrifice and National Narrative* [Stanford: Stanford University Press, 2010], 317). I think that Grossman's use of the word *besorah* (announcement) rather than other words he could have chosen, such as *khadashot, yediot, hoda'ah, yediah* (various ways of saying 'news,' also playing with the meaning of 'knowledge') indicates the tragic existential *Angst* that must be faced by parents in a country at war, where the birth of a male child already involves the threat to his life.

[7] In his speech upon receiving the Peace Prize at the Frankfurt Book Fair (October 2010), Grossman noted that while factual reality cannot be changed, the way to deal with it can. Within days of his own son's death in a military action, Grossman had been back at his desk: 'I discovered,' he said, 'that writing was the best way for me to fight arbitrariness . . . and the feeling of being at its mercy like a helpless victim.' Instead of being entrapped in a language that has become overdetermined, loaded, and closed, a writer (and his characters) can try to forge a different language, opening more hopeful horizons. Grossman's speech was reported in Annika Breidthardt's article, 'Grossman Wins German Peace Prize,' Article upon Grossman's receipt of the Peace Prize at the Frankfurt Book Fair <http://m.iol.co.za/article/view/s/11/a/25949>, viewed on February 22, 2012.

[8] Anna Jaubert lists other interesting examples of ambiguity between FID and FDS; see 'Le discours indirect libre. Dire et montrer: approche pragmatique,' in *Le style indirect libre et ses contexts*, ed. Sylvie Mellet and Marcel Vuillaume (Amsterdam: Rodopi, 2000), 62-64.

[9] While FID, as a stylistic device, is often used to present a character in a comic or ironic light, Grossman's use of FID in this novel is devoid of such intentions towards Ora. *Pace* Louise Flavin's statement that FID is 'a means of controlling the reader's sense of distance from characters' 'Free Indirect Discourse and the Clever Heroine of *Emma*,' *Persuasions* 13 (December 16, 1991), <http://www.jasna.org/persuasions/printed/number13/flavin.htm>, viewed on December 15, 2010. Grossman's use of this device intensifies the reader's sympathy towards Ora. Moreover, several passages in Grossman's novel can illustrate Reiko Ikeo's observation that 'the omniscient narrator's intervention into the character's memory' sometimes 'gives the segment more credibility.' See 'Unambiguous Free Indirect Discourse? A Comparison between "Straightforward" Free Indirect Speech and Thought Presentation and Cases Ambiguous with Narration,' *Language and Literature* 16 (2007): 384.

[10] In rendering soldiers' speech on several occasions, Grossman depicts their linguistic playfulness, especially in their use of acronyms. One example is Ofer and Adam's macabre interpretation of an accepted army acronym, which

shocks Ora (307). Yet, as opposed to Avram's language, which gives the three main protagonists the illusion of exclusivity, Ofer and Adam use the language shared by the soldiers of their generation. As Raphael Nir explains, 'acronyms as a phenomenon are common in armies in general and in the IDF in particular.' *Modern Hebrew Lexical Formations* (Kfar Saba: Open University Press, 1993), 229 (Hebrew). Nir explains further that 'slang speakers are aware of the fact that they use expressions which are outside the normative, "respectable" language, and they do so in order to emphasize a trendy behavior or as a sign of belonging to a specific social circle. ... The members of the group use words from the general slang, but dot their speech with a sort of code of cipher-words which are known to the members of the group. In this, closed groups such as the military stand out particularly.' 'Introduction: The Song of the Simple Person,' in *The Hebrew Slang Dictionary*, ed. Rubik Rosenthal (Jerusalem: Keter, 2005), 2: vii (Hebrew; my translations).

[11] In her article about works by Grossman and Castel-Bloom, Smadar Shiffman claims that 'it takes a female writer to portray the dreadful relationships between Politics and Motherhood, between the social expectations from a mother and the madness it takes to raise sons in our part of the world . . . it takes a woman writer to fully uncover, from the mother's perspective, the cruel implications of these demands.' 'Motherhood under Zionism,' *Hebrew Studies* 44 (2003): 139, 144. Yet Grossman proves that a male writer can also convincingly convey an Israeli mother's perspective, her feelings and her thoughts regarding her relationship with her son under the constraints of reality.

[12] The original Hebrew text includes many such neologisms. The translators to Spanish and to Catalan chose to invent words in order to reflect the character of the novel's lexicon: Grossman's use of Hebrew morphological patterns of inflection and derivation to invent words. David Grossman, *La Vida Entera*, trans. Ana María Bejarano (Barcelona: Lumen, 2010) and David Grossman, *Tota una vida*, trans. Roser Lluch (Barcelona: Edicions 62, 2010).

[13] In her article about David Grossman's *The Book of Internal Grammar*, Rachel Feldhay Brenner also points to a connection between the immaturity of the protagonist and his creation of a private code, consisting of 'words that he considers totally his own.' 'Unsealing the Letters: The Making of an Artist in David Grossman's *The Book of Internal Grammar*,' *Critique* 40 (1999): 208.

[14] Aharon, the protagonist of Grossman's novel *The Book of Internal Grammar*, also refuses to grow up, both physically and emotionally.

[15] Avram is pleased to discover, through Ora's recollections, his son's inventiveness with words (307). Ofer's playfulness with word-formation

occurs at the age of four, the 'accepted' age for such games.

[16] Each hiking trail has a distinctive three-colour mark (in this case blue-white-orange), which is painted on rocks along the trail, to assist hikers. About the Israel National Trail, see <http://www.israelnationaltrail.com/>, viewed on December 15, 2010.

[17] Ora is neither an 'aggressively invasive' nor an 'absent' mother as Smadar Shiffman claims all of Grossman's mothers are ('Motherhood under Zionism,' 147-48). Even in her flight, Ora is not absent from Ofer's life. Not only was she very much present in Ofer's upbringing, but her choice of flight as a way of dealing with the danger he faces tightens the mother-son relationship on both spiritual and ritual levels.

[18] Avidov Lipsker writes that, like Nathan Alterman before him, Grossman puts in motion the devices of the perseverance of the living body: walking and talking. In an effort to both sustain and safeguard life, hiking the Israel trail is an expression of the faith in the magical power of walking, a ritual of deep conviction that the walking rhythm is a basic element of life. Grossman's characters' constant speech, according to Lipsker, both represses and arouses fears. He identifies a theme of 'daily talk ritual' that has a life of its own. The obsessive ritual Ora engages in through her walk does not protect her from pain but merely outlines it. Lipsker goes on to claim that Ora is the most complete embodiment of Grossman's language, confirming the collective language in which he lives; see '*To the End of the Land* by David Grossman: Perseus's Shield and the Mining Project.' *Alpa'yim: A Multidisciplinary Publication for Contemporary Thought and Literature* 33 (2009): 260-69 (Hebrew).

[19] In her analysis of another novel by Grossman, *See under Love*, Johanna Baum points to 'the possibility of healing through artistic endeavour.' 'A Literary Analysis of Traumatic Neurosis in Israeli Society: David Grossman's *See under Love*,' in *Other Voices* 2 (February 2000). <http://www.othervoices.org/2.1/baum/seeunderlove.php>, viewed on March 25, 2012.

Bibliography

Baum, Johanna. 'A Literary Analysis of Traumatic Neurosis in Israeli Society: David Grossman's *See under Love*.' *Other Voices* 2 (February 2000). <http://www.othervoices.org/2.1/baum/seeunderlove.php>. Viewed on March 25, 2012.

Ben Yehuda, Eliezer. *A Complete Dictionary of Ancient and Modern Hebrew*. Jerusalem: Ben Yehuda Publishing, 1948 (Hebrew).

Breidthardt, Annika. 'Grossman Wins German Peace Prize.' <http://m.iol.co.za/article/view/s/11/a/25949>. Viewed on February 22, 2012.

Brenner, Rachel Feldhay. '"Unsealing the Letters": The Making of an Artist in David Grossman's *The Book of Internal Grammar*.' *Critique* 40 (1999): 203-14.

Carcassonne, Manuel. Interview with David Grossman. 'David Grossman: Death is a Way of Life.' *Magazine Littéraire* 427 (2004): 86-87.

Even Shoshan, Avraham. *Even Shoshan Dictionary: Renewed and Updated for the Year 2000*. Israel: Hamilon Hahadash Publishing, 2003 (Hebrew).

Feldman, Yael S. *Glory and Agony: Isaac's Sacrifice and National Narrative*. Stanford: Stanford University Press, 2010.

Flavin, Louise. 'Free Indirect Discourse and the Clever Heroine of *Emma*.' *Persuasions* 13. Jane Austin Society of North America, December 16, 1991. <http://www.jasna.org/persuasions/printed/number13/flavin.htm>. Viewed on December 15, 2010.

Glinert, Lewis. *The Grammar of Modern Hebrew*. Cambridge: Cambridge University Press, 1989.

Grossman, David. *Ishah Borachat miBesorah* [*To the End of the Land*]. Benei Brak: HaKibbutz HaMeuchad, 2008 (Hebrew).

Ikeo, Reiko. 'Unambiguous Free Indirect Discourse? A Comparison between Straightforward Free Indirect Speech and Thought Presentation and Cases Ambiguous with Narration.' *Language and Literature* 16 (2007): 367-87.

Jaubert, Anna. 'Le discours indirect libre. Dire et montrer: approche pragmatique.' In *Le style indirect libre et ses contexts*, edited by Sylvia Mellet and Marcel Vuillaume, 49-69. Amsterdam: Rodopi, 2000.

Lipsker, Avidov. '*To the End of the Land* by David Grossman: Perseus's Shield and the Mining Project.' *Alpa'yim: A Multidisciplinary Publication for Contemporary Thought and Literature* 33 (2009): 260-69 (Hebrew).

Nir, Raphael. 'Introduction: The Song of the Simple Person.' In *The Hebrew Slang Dictionary*, 2 vols, edited by Rubik Rosenthal. Jerusalem: Keter, 2005: 2: 7 (Hebrew).

———. *Modern Hebrew Lexical Formations*. Israel: Open University, 1993 (Hebrew).

Shiffman, Smadar. 'Motherhood under Zionism.' *Hebrew Studies* 44 (2003): 139-56.

The Israel National Trail. <http://www.israelnationaltrail.com/>. Viewed December 10, 2010.

Part VI

IMAGES: RECIDIVISM OR HOPE?

Tangled Complicities: Extracting Knowledge from Images of Abu Ghraib

Rebecca A. Adelman

Abstract
Since their release in April 2004, photographs of torture at Abu Ghraib have become sites of intense scholarly inquiry. This paper considers the ethics of such academic spectatorship. I begin with an account of the intellectual and affective pleasures that might inhere in this research so intimately predicated on others' pain. I then use this framework to problematize the language of obligation that many American academics invoke to explain their motivation for working on the Abu Ghraib photos and the related claims of epistemic authority they make over them. Subsequently, I analyze specific scholarly reactions to Abu Ghraib, key texts that utilize photos from the prison. Next, I attend directly to the practice of reproducing the images in academic publications, which I contend is far more ethically complex than it might appear, particularly because it often rests on a questionable claim of ownership over the photos. I conclude by exploring alternate approaches to the Abu Ghraib images that might allow us to engage them without reanimating the violences they depict, work that necessarily begins with a self-reflexive acknowledgment of the power differential through which American academics view them and an honest reckoning with the rewards derived from that looking.

Key Words: Torture, spectatorship, Abu Ghraib, photography, knowledge production, academic ethics.

*****

In an effort to distinguish sight from the other senses, Susan Sontag makes a deceptively simple observation, noting that sight is unique because 'sight can be turned off (we have lids on our eyes, we do not have doors on our ears).'[1] Of course, there are times when those eyelids do not operate fast enough, leaving us exposed to scenes that we never intended or wanted to see. But in the lucky instances when we can choose, when we deliberately look toward something and fix our eyes upon it willingly, it is because there is a pleasure in doing so: the aesthetic pleasure of immersing ourselves in a piece of art, or the scopophilic pleasure of gazing at an attractive body, or the emotional pleasure of beholding a snapshot of a loved one. Commercially-produced images are generated with pleasure in mind; they are designed for profit and meant to please their viewers, to cultivate a desire and then to satisfy it visually. And so we, as spectators, eagerly keep our eyes open in darkened movie theatres, before magazines full of glossy advertisements, crowded around a friend's digital camera. Here, I am interested in a different kind of looking and a different kind of pleasure. I focus on *academic* spectatorship, the ways that we watch conference paper PowerPoint presentations, or engage with images reproduced in others' articles and monographs, or scrutinize pictures in the process of producing our own scholarship. Academic spectatorship is different from other kinds of looking, but also contiguous with them, in that it gratifies. The dividend of pleasure that it promises might be intellectual rather than emotional or physical (though these three can coexist), but it is a pleasure - even when the work is hard or the pictures unpleasant - nonetheless.

Certainly, academic spectatorship - as in the analysis of a difficult photograph, the exegesis of a mystifying work of art, or the mapping of gazes in film - is vitally important. At its best, it can produce valuable knowledge about images, the contexts out of which they emerge, and their social and political consequences. Ethically, academic looking can be neutral or unproblematic, perhaps even wholly good. But things get much murkier when that scholarly looking takes suffering as its object, and I want to ask whether the production of knowledge, even valuable knowledge, is an adequate offset for the harms that might be done or abetted in the process. Toward that end, in this essay, I explore the confluences of knowledge and pain in academic discourses around the photographs of torture from the converted prison at Abu Ghraib.

To contextualize these questions, I begin with a consideration of Patricia Yaeger's discussion of 'academic melancholy' and the recent intellectual fashion-ability of studying phenomena like pain, suffering and trauma; the incisive critique she offers provides the foundation for my methodology in this article. From there, I provide a general overview of academic discourse on the Abu Ghraib photographs and the various visualities that Western, particularly American, scholars have created around them. With that framework in place, I turn to specific examples, attending to the ways the images are reproduced and circulated, and the kinds of claims scholars make about them, both descriptive and prescriptive. Then, drawing on insights from postcolonial theory and political philosophy, I offer a critique of this discourse and the practices of knowledge extraction and production that it entails. Finally, focusing directly on the ethics of spectatorship, I ask whether (and how) it might be possible to engage these images without reproducing the violences that constitute them.

1. On the Visual 'Pleasures of Academic Melancholy'

In 'Consuming Trauma: Or, The Pleasures of Merely Circulating,' Patricia Yaeger provides a meta-commentary on the contemporary fascination with and emphasis on trauma in the academy. Focusing on what she describes as the 'pleasures of academic melancholy,' Yaeger offers an ethical and political critique of these intellectual indulgences.[2] She argues that academic concern with injury often and paradoxically occludes the material circumstances surrounding it, while also providing scholars with pleasures that are intellectual, affective, and possibly even sensual. Ultimately, for Yaeger, the problem with this variety of intellectual masochism is that it can function to 'jolt us out of pathos,'[3] perhaps because our own suffering quickly distracts us from that of the others with whom we were initially concerned.

Yaeger's argument has been instructive for me in my efforts to make sense of the intensity of the discursive production around the images released from Abu Ghraib, and seems especially apposite for questions of spectatorship in particular, as a process to which pleasure, in a variety of forms, is intrinsic. At least in American visual culture studies, the intellectual frisson ignited by the photographs is by far the most intense of any to date in the Global War on Terror. Here, there is no shortage of pathos; the scholarship is often vigorous, almost electrified, saturated with feeling. In this paper, as I consider the discursive proliferation around the images, I build on Yaeger's intervention by considering where that upwelling of feeling gets directed and how it is subsequently interpreted.

My goal in this essay is not to decode the scenes from Abu Ghraib; my interest lies elsewhere, in the pervasive academic temptation to narrate, interpret and extract knowledge from them. Instead of partaking in this spectatorship, I seek to interrogate it, to provide a reading of the discourse *but not of the images themselves*. But I do so accompanied by the awkward fact that I myself have not always been as careful as I should have been in my own engagements with images of others who are suffering, wounded, dying, dead or made vulnerable by the camera. And so I try to navigate between the two visual injustices that Georges Didi-Huberman cites in his staggering book, *Images in Spite of All: Four Photographs from Auschwitz.* Didi-Huberman observes that when confronted with images of horror, viewers tend to ask 'too much' or 'too little' of them.[4] Expecting that photographs ought to reveal absolutely everything and serve as transparent and comprehensive representations dooms them to inadequacy. Alternately, treating them as mere documentary records obscures all of the other ways they might matter and deprives them of their full ontological significance. In either case, whether viewers are too critical or too condescending, they overlook the phenomenology of the photographs' creation and consumption. I am particularly interested in the latter, and so want to explore the precise mechanisms by which the photographs from Abu Ghraib are made to yield the knowledge they seem to contain.

My argument about the Abu Ghraib has a specific ambit: academic spectatorship.[5] Ethical questions about journalism and Abu Ghraib, for example, are worthy of consideration but beyond the scope of this paper. Journalists and academics have distinct responsibilities, and consequently employ the images differently. The photographs in question were not taken in a journalistic endeavour to expose the abuse of Iraqi prisoners by American military personnel at Abu Ghraib; they were taken by those personnel as part of that abuse.[6] Journalists like Seymour Hersh and filmmakers like Errol Morris, for example, have used them in an effort to expose the systematic nature of that abuse. Academic commentators might want to join in that intervention, but their (our) work has a different temporality. It refers to a harm that has already been done and made public, and relies for its impact upon already-familiar images. I do not mean to suggest that journalistic treatments of Abu Ghraib should not be subject to critical examination. Nor do I argue that scholars should not write and speak about Abu Ghraib. My objective is make explicit the ethical complexities inherent in doing so. My intention in this essay is not to impugn the morals or motivations of the authors of that voluminous body of work, but rather to consider the ways in which these images are employed in the processes of extracting knowledge from them and translating that knowledge into material for scholarly consumption.

2. Claiming Authority over the Abu Ghraib Photographs

The Abu Ghraib images first appeared before the American public on April 28, 2004, when they were aired on the news program *60 Minutes II*. Almost immediately, they became iconic, particularly for the anti-war Left. The photographs were a hyper-visible sign of what those activists opposed, and seemed to have the potential to justify their dissent and clarify its stakes in a post-9/11 discursive climate where opposition to the war was still widely regarded as unpatriotic and consequently untenable. Within that movement's academic quarters, the photos spawned a distinct subgenre of writing: the analysis of the torture image. Suddenly, torture (this torture in particular) was a topic about which nearly everyone had something to say. Outside of the academy, the events at Abu Ghraib and their photographic legacy rapidly slipped into what Julie Gerk Hernandez described as an 'epistemological void' of forgetfulness and unconcern.[7] Into this bottomless pit, scholars - myself included - flung an endless supply of words in an effort to participate in the processes of interpreting the photographs and deciphering their meanings.

In some ways, this is an echo of the compulsion that David Simpson sensed among scholars in the immediate aftermath of September 11, 2001. After the attacks, Simpson detected a pervasive urge among academics to speak about what had happened. He recalls that academics were compelled to talk about it, even if we were not sure what to say, 'as if it were a moral duty that each of us should speak,' prompted by what he describes as a 'need to register awareness of some sort' and to make that awareness known to various interlocutors.[8] Likewise after Abu Ghraib. The outpouring was impassioned and trans-disciplinary. Abu Ghraib gave American scholars license to reclaim some of the discursive freedom that had been eroded after September 11, making it seem reasonable and indeed urgent to resume critique of the state and its practices. That this opportunity was purchased through the suffering of others signals that scholarship on Abu Ghraib was vexed from the outset.

Despite this, academic engagement with Abu Ghraib and its visual archive is important, politically and civically. Outside of the academy, the photos quickly 'disappeared down the memory hole,'[9] and both the government and the general public seemed eager to forget what they had seen. This easy amnesia has long been a common reaction among American spectators to others' tragedy. In her analysis of the linkages between U.S. citizenship and mediated witnessing of others' suffering, Carrie A. Rentschler suggests that we are often perplexed by emotionally provocative images because we 'have not been taught how to transform feeling into action' in confrontation with atrocity.[10] It is uncomfortable, perhaps, to have all that affective energy but lack a means or direction to channel it - easier just to let it recede and then turn to something else. And so while public attention meandered away from the torture photos, scholars remained vigilant, trying to reawaken that initial outrage and recapture its potential to galvanize sustained and meaningful opposition to U.S. policy.

Reproducing the photos may have seemed like a logical way to do that. An emphasis on their terrible corporeality, amplified with descriptions of and commentary about what they depicted, was a way to assert that something objectionable and indeed criminal had taken place. It was a way to refute the sophistry of those who sought to downplay what the photographs depicted, who compared it to hazing and so suggested that it was not a serious transgression or who quibbled that it was not technically torture because it was not the infliction of physical punishment to elicit information during interrogation. Against this, the photos were the most obvious and compelling evidence that something was amiss.[11] They clearly showed agents of the United States wantonly, gleefully violating international law. Article 3 of the Third Geneva Convention on the treatment of prisoners of war, adopted August 12, 1949, expressly prohibits not only the torture of enemies during interrogation but all other forms of 'violence to life and person.' The photos seemed to testify to such violence more eloquently than anything else.

And so it was taken for granted that the images ought to be recirculated. Stephen Eisenman encapsulates this imperative to reproduce and explicate the images at the outset of *The Abu Ghraib Effect*. He contends that '[a]ny effort to uncover and thereby weaken the Abu Ghraib effect will require careful attention to some disturbing photographs; there is simply no alternative.'[12] David Simpson makes a similar claim: 'We must argue for more pictures, and more words to go with them, to offer the dead and the dying, all of them, alternatives to the frames so far imposed upon and around them.'[13] These exhortations are premised on the belief that sight will lead uncomplicatedly to the outcome of eroding public support for (or at least ambivalence about) torture, but no one has specified how, precisely, this transmogrification will occur.

Notwithstanding this vagueness, academic discourse on the Abu Ghraib photos is exacting in its language of obligation. Many commentators on the photos assert that the weighty visual burden of torture must simply be shouldered: by them, by their readers and by the American public at large. This duty is often cast as penance, a way of atoning for not having done enough to pre-empt that torture in the first place. In this way, the scholar volunteers to visually self-inflict a measure of pain (channelled through knowledge) in response to that which is depicted in the photographs, using them as a hinge for this potentially comforting reallocation of suffering and blame.

Different writers have taken up this felt responsibility in different ways. Some have focused on grim specifics, while others preferred abstract analysis. Some treatments fixate on the physicality of the scenes, the various accoutrements of torture - underwear, an MRE box, permanent markers, wires, a leash - and seize on small details. Others engage the images indirectly, reading them as signs and symptoms of a much larger pathology. Many articles extrapolate from the images to develop theories about the vapidness of contemporary American culture,[14] or the state, or the military as a whole.[15] Searching for causal explanations, authors have attributed the torture to everything from video games to homophobia in the American military. The signifier of the tortured detainee has proven capacious enough to accommodate all sorts of truths. And always, in the routes that lead to these various conclusions, there is a tropism toward the pictures. In the process, the very same images that seem to defy description or even comprehension are recast as limitless troves of information and secrets waiting to be revealed. And so the academy has been prolific, recycling the images into articles and books (and lines on CVs), writing and writing in an effort to uncover these facts, to determine definitively why the pictures were taken, who is guilty, what they really show.

Scholars undertake that work motivated by a variety of hopes: to clarify that what transpired at Abu Ghraib was indeed torture, to alert the public to the systematic nature of it, to document the suffering that resulted from it, to inspire Americans to care about it, to offer a rebuttal to those (especially politicians and public figures) who deemed it to be insignificant, to explain why it happened, to keep it from ever happening again. Unquestionably, these are admirable reasons to research and to publish. And the urgency of this mission might explain why so many have something to say, no matter their training, discipline or specialty. They are licensed to speak by the sheer fact of their anguished spectatorship and, in the case of American academics, from their association with the state responsible for what they saw. Citizenship, in this instance, is understood as a set of visual rights (to have access to the photographs, to be able to reproduce them, to be able to speak and write freely about them) and obligations (to look at and think about the photographs and to encourage others to do the same).

Consequently, many pieces include reproductions of the images, though not all of them engage the images in the same way. Some use them as visual exhibits, situating them directly as objects of analysis and making extensive reference to the photographs accompanying the text. Alternately, others use them as illustrations or embellishments, offering very little analysis of the images, but rather allowing them to speak (show?) for themselves. However, I suggest that the decision to reproduce the images is not as straightforward as it might seem. Circumstances conspire to make it easy: the sense of a right to do so makes it seem justifiable, the feeling of an obligation to do so makes it seem necessary, and the fact that the images are in the public domain because they were taken by on-duty U.S. military personnel makes it (seem) cheap.[16] But all of these privileges are contingent; they depend upon the prioritization of the claims of the American spectator above all else.

3. Visions of Abu Ghraib

Less than a month after the photos were first publicized, on May 23, 2004, Susan Sontag published 'Regarding the Torture of Others ' in *The New York Times Magazine*. In it, she argued for the inextricability of the horror of the deeds from the fact of their being photographed. Accordingly, she compared the Abu Ghraib photos to lynching souvenirs and pornography,[17] as other instances in which violence and the visual blur together. Sontag further linked the practice of torture at Abu Ghraib to Bush administration foreign policy, and suggested that the act of photographing it is basically contiguous with the larger digital-age phenomena of visually documenting and circulating the minutiae of one's everyday life.

The adduced photographs, which depict the banalisation, normalisation, and sexualisation of violence, provide evidence for these claims. Parenthetically, it is worth noting that not all readers encounter them in the same way, as this groundbreaking and oft-cited essay currently exists in multiple formats. The original version, which would have gone out in print to the magazine's paid subscribers, is richly illustrated with the photographs that made headlines the previous month. Alternately, the text of the essay is available free online through the *Times*' website, but this version contains no pictures,[18] just a list of the captions from the photos that appeared in the print edition. Here, the price of the subscription buys access to the regenerated images and also to a particularly constituted spectatorial community.

Whether one re-views the pictures alongside Sontag's analysis or not, her arguments still illustrate the myriad conditions of possibility for what happened at Abu Ghraib. However, in the necessary process of distributing accountability, they risk re-centering American subjects and so overlooking those whose suffering is rendered in the photographs. Criticizing the tepid expressions of 'disgust' at the images by President Bush and Secretary of State Rice, Sontag calls it an 'insult.'[19] But she goes on to specify not that this woefully inadequate response is an affront to the prisoners themselves, but rather to 'one's historical and moral sense,'[20] with 'one' presumably being the American condescended to by her dissembling government. A similar dynamic is operative in her now-famous and controversial contention that 'the photographs are us,'[21] i.e. all Americans. This identity is manifested literally when the photographs depict actual Americans like Spc. Lynndie England and Spc. Charles Graner and indirectly when the photographs visualize the consequences of state 'counterterrorist' policy. But they are crucially and primarily of others, who despite being hypervisible also risk being eclipsed in the inward turn to self-examination.

Ultimately, Sontag contends that the photographs were 'necessary to get our leaders to acknowledge that they had a problem on their hands,'[22] succeeding where previous reports and warnings of abuse had failed.[23] This is no doubt true. But that truth coexists alongside a question that has so far remained unasked, about the ease with which the tortured bodies depicted in these photographs were transformed into things they never consented to be, including instruments of political enlightenment for the very people whose leaders authorized the torture they document.

The Retort collective, in the polemical *Afflicted Powers: Capital and Spectacle in a New Age of War*, makes a claim akin to Sontag's, arguing that the Abu Ghraib photographs had the potential to be a course of shock therapy for the state that 'was entrapped in its own apparatus of clichés.'[24] Arguing that 9/11 was an insuperable 'image-defeat' for the spectacular state, Retort theorizes the subsequent Global War on Terror as a mission for spectacular redress of that embarrassment. In their analysis, the Abu Ghraib photographs threatened to undermine that endeavour by compounding the hypervisible, hypervisual American humiliation of the collapse of the World Trade Center towers by exposing the cravenness of American military power. They write, '[t]he Towers keep falling, and now they are joined by the imagery of Abu Ghraib' in the loop of American failures endlessly replayed.[25]

In a gesture presumably meant to accelerate the demise of the spectacular American empire, the frontispiece of the book is the so-called

'Gilligan' image of the wired detainee perched atop the MRE box. The book, which is printed on heavy, high-gloss paper and also includes other potentially unpalatable images, implies that the decision to reproduce the photo is an affront to the sensibilities of the mainstream media and the machinations of the administration. According to such logic, reprinting it is a radical act and a visual intervention.

The apparently uncritical reproduction of the image is striking to me in a book that is otherwise so analytically meticulous. As a frontispiece, the image is distant from the text, and because it lacks a caption, readers have no guidance on how to interpret it. It is meant to be consumed and perhaps to lure readers who might not otherwise be interested. The glossy and full-colour reproduction is strangely lavish, visually sumptuous; it invites us to interpret the unhedged image as a victory and to consume it with relish for that reason. I am concerned that such a form of spectatorship goes beyond the political *Schadenfreude* provoked in many members of the anti-war Left whenever things went wrong in the Global War on Terror;[26] that morbid and muted happiness was understandable, if not justifiable, in light of the very limited space for dissent in the months and years after September 11. Satisfaction in the face of Abu Ghraib bleeds into a far more dangerous insouciance that accepts scenes like this in exchange for the promise of a spectacular state defeat to come.

In his 2006 *Radical History Review* article 'Invisible Empire: Visual Culture, Embodied Spectacle,' Nicholas Mirzoeff evaluates the photographs' effects differently. Contrary to Retort, who saw in them a tremendous potential, Mirzoeff notes that the scandal following their release was little more than a flash in the pan, barely registering in the 2004 election.[27] For Mirzoeff, this is proof that '[w]hat was seen was assented to.'[28] Mirzoeff offers two interventions in his article, which is an exploration of visuality under conditions of globalization and 'permanent war.' First, he argues that the behaviors depicted in the images of the torturers are part of a larger effort by the administration to portray Arabs as 'sodomitical.'[29] Second, he makes a broader claim about visual freedom and its importance in and for political participation.

Accordingly, the article reproduces images liberally: sometimes blurred or pixellated, but everywhere, interrupting the flow of sentences and paragraphs, occupying large portions of the page, utterly intrusive. Mirzoeff engages directly and ekphrastically with the photographs, attending to and analyzing the details of the scenes they depict. He concludes the paper with a claim for the 'right to look,' including a bulleted list of what this liberty might entail. Mirzoeff argues that this should include the rights 'to be seen by the common as a counter to the possibility of being disappeared by governments' and 'to know when one is under surveillance.' His list prioritizes visibility, calling for transparency for governments and corporations and for a 'right to visual self-representation' for individuals.[30]

I suggest an addition to the list: in tandem with a call for freedom from surveillance, the right to be left visually alone - not to have your picture taken while you are tortured, obviously, but perhaps also to have some say over the terms by which those images of you are recirculated. Like many rights claims, such an assertion might impinge on the freedoms of others, specifically those who seek to reproduce such images, even when their choice to do so seems obligatory, excusable, or beneficial.

4. 'Insults and Public Curiosity'

By their nature, the Abu Ghraib photos place those who seek to see and engage them in a complicated position vis-à-vis international law, which is often the very thing that their most ambitious critics want to restore. Article 13 of the Third Geneva Convention on the treatment of prisoners of war dictates that 'prisoners of war must at all times be protected, particularly against acts of violence or intimidation and against insults and public curiosity.'[31] The spirit of the 'public curiosity' clause has been extended to prohibit exploitative or degrading media access to prisoners of war. For this reason, and also because it functioned to make the humiliation of the abuse more acute, photographing the torture 'was itself a form of torture.' [32] Can the good intentions of those who would reproduce the photos ameliorate this fundamental wrong? And when we reproduce them, to what extent are we abetted by and entangled in the logic that partially enabled the torture itself: that it did not technically contravene international law because the victims were not technically prisoners of war, but merely 'enemy combatants'?

Now that the photographs have been taken, knowing that the torture cannot be undone, what are the ethics of circulating them? This is a question of ends and means. Unless one knows that the people depicted in the pictures agree to their replication and circulation in every instance, the choice to reproduce the images either presumes the consent of the photographed or implies that the needs of the spectators trump those of the subjects. Asking this question about ethics requires an interrogation of the ostensible goodness of academic curiosity and a serious evaluation of the benefits it yields. After all, torture itself almost always has an epistemic justification. Intelligence-gathering is the most common rationalization for torture, a practice with a precedent in Roman law, in which information given under the duress of torture could be used to fortify otherwise questionable evidence.[33] Although there is sharp disagreement in the intelligence community about the efficacy of torture for eliciting valuable information, there seems to be no such scepticism about the informational value of the images of torture on the part of those who analyze them professionally. What new evidence do now-familiar torture photos promise to reveal under scrutiny that we as scholarly witnesses could not have otherwise obtained? It is safe to assume that most of the academics who take up the images already oppose torture, and so what else is there to prove by looking at them?

At some point, it seems, scholars came to an agreement about the status of the photographs (and, by extension, the people they depict) and our entitlement to them. This entitlement papers over the contradictions inherent in scholarship on these images. It makes the act of recirculating the photographs and thus reiterating part of the harm that they do seem necessary for preventing future instances of the harm that they depict. Reflecting on Abu Ghraib, Dora Apel notes that 'torture images do not inherently produce their own undoing - it depends on us.'[34] In light of the state's repressive tendencies toward images of death and violence in general, David Simpson reasons that

> [w]e will never know whether we are indeed already numb, or need to numb ourselves, when faced with images of death and duress unless we see them. Only then will we know whether we can pass from seeing them to feeling them, and from feeling them to acting on those feelings.[35]

This logic has become axiomatic.

Similarly, W. J. T. Mitchell urges persistence in the effort to extract meaning from the photographs:

> What I am suggesting . . . is that there is something more to be learned from these pictures than the story of what happened at Abu Ghraib, and who is to blame for it. These images were, after all, paid for with the tax dollars of American citizens. We own them, and must own up to what they tell us about who we are, and what we are becoming.[36]

Although his reference to tax dollars reminds American readers of our shared culpability for these acts of torture, it also implies that the images are 'ours' to do with as we wish, a privilege bought with our (now besmirched) citizenship. How much, precisely, do we believe ourselves to have purchased in this bizarre commodity exchange? From whom did we buy the pictures? And what does this possession grant us? If these questions seem absurd, that is perhaps because we have pre-determined that these photographs are rightfully ours. If they seem trivial, that is perhaps because we have calculated that the good use to which we might put them matters more than the circumstances in which they were created. In this accounting, it is expedient to overlook the cost that we externalize to others when we go about performing the presumed duty, implied by our citizenship, to look at difficult images.

Ultimately, there are two problems with the presumption of ownership over the images: this proprietary logic threatens to erase the subjectivity of the people in the photos, and might also vindicate the practices of the state that authorized torturing them. Firstly, I am concerned by the prevalence of the first-person in these exhortations. There is someone missing in this emphasis on the 'we' and the 'us,' and in the effort to claim what is ours. Indeed, the assertive language of ownership suggests an awareness that they might once have belonged to someone else. Certainly, I am not arguing that they ought to be property of the state, or of the soldiers who created them. I do wonder whether the people depicted in them might have some kind of relevant claim to the images that is overshadowed in the clamour to begin opposing torture by using them. The vast majority of scholars have refused to speak on behalf of the soldiers whose actions are recorded for this gloomy posterity; some have ventured partial exoneration by blaming their superiors or the military itself, but the consensus for the most part is that what they did is inexcusable. Agreed. But what logic authorizes so many academics to speak on behalf of the tortured, or to use them as the signs of our own feelings of guilt and shame? Gayatri Spivak's canonical assertion that the subaltern cannot, by definition of either term, speak may be useful here.[37] No matter how hard or carefully researchers work to sift meaning from the photographs, we cannot capture knowledge about their subjects' interiority; the photographs leave them both hypervisible and mute, and no one has yet figured out how to correct for that.[38]

And so we tend to insert our own voices into that caesura, as if to compensate for the silence of the photographs with a garrulous assertion of our own culpability. Timothy Kaufman-Osborn offers a lucid critique of the assertion, common to the American anti-War Left, that all Americans are guilty of the torture that transpired at Abu Ghraib. He writes, '[w]ithin the context of the contemporary security state, when it is said that torture is committed "in our name," it is no longer clear in what sense "we" may be said to be authors of that abuse' because state power is so consolidated and so far removed from the will of the people.[39] He continues, 'however unwittingly, when the Left affirms collective accountability for Abu Ghraib and like crimes, it proves complicitous in perpetuating the very regimes it seeks to criticize,' legitimizing them with the implication that they reflect some kind of popular sovereignty.[40]

Moreover, by claiming ownership of the contraband images for which 'we' are purportedly accountable, we deny their fundamental illegality, and provide their creators with a larger and more attentive audience than they could have reached alone. Jasbir Puar has argued that for the torture photographers, the act of sending the photographs was (sexually) gratifying in itself because 'dissemination is the ultimate form of territorial coverage and conquest.'[41] Reframing them, no matter how critically, does not automatically defuse that circuit. To endorse Kaufman-Osborn's position is not to eschew responsibility. Rather, it requires everyone to be more conscientious in their assignations of blame and more precise about the extent of their involvement.

5. A Partial Surrender

In offering my critique, I am not advocating censorship, but hoping to think through the complicities that enable our scholarship. In academic contexts, the claim for public ownership of the Abu Ghraib images often shades into a defence of academic freedom. But what, precisely, is permitted by that invocation? And what constraints, if any, might we be willing to accept in deference to (rather than in trade for, as if there could be such an even exchange) the suffering of others? Below, I explore some different ways of approaching and relating to the pictures. I am seeking possible methods for engaging the images without reanimating the violences they depict; avenues for being self-reflexive about them without being self-centered; modes of attending to the intricacies of our connections to the regimes that authorize the abuse without vindicating them; and frameworks for acknowledging our intellectual and affective responses without ever suggesting an equivalence between that angst and the suffering documented in the images.

This necessitates an acknowledgment of the differential of power through which American academics relate to the others depicted in the photographs. One of the ways Edward Said defined Orientalism is as a 'flexible *positional* superiority, which puts the Westerner in a whole series of possible relationships with the Orient without ever losing him the upper hand.'[42] Said's contention suggests to me that even the purest of intentions expressed in the desire to write on the side of justice and to condemn torture (just like feelings of pity[43] or shame) can only privilege the Westerner, who demonstrates his sentience and ethical superiority by confessing to and demonstrating penitence for a wrong. In the U.S., this effect is redoubled by pervasive discourses of American exceptionalism. Donald E. Pease has recently demonstrated that the 'fantasy' of American exceptionalism 'permitted U.S. citizens to achieve their national identity through the disavowal of U.S. imperialism,' even as the state pursued precisely imperial objectives abroad.[44] In this way, the American citizen's condemnation of detainee abuse can only ever reaffirm the utterly disingenuous myth that, by definition, Americans do not torture.

Relatedly, academics must figure out a way to account for and document the atrocities committed at Abu Ghraib, and the pain that resulted, without reducing the afflicted people to mere victims of torture, who can thus never appear as full subjects. Excessive emphasis on the pain of the other 'splits the subaltern into ruined bodies and dismembered demanding voices,'[45] and so reifies their dissimilarity from the subjects who speak on their behalf and reduces them again to the status of objects. For Rosalind C. Morris, part of what distinguishes the events that took place at Abu Ghraib was the way they visualized 'the violent demand that the other perform his submission to violation as a source of satisfaction,' which she perceived in the scenes where detainees were forced to simulate their own sexual pleasure for the camera.[46] When the satisfaction of academic curiosities is contingent upon a meticulous recounting of the details of the suffering captured in these pictures, scholarship risks reproducing this debasement. Even the most careful toting up of abuses will never amount to full recognition of the subject in pain. Instead, it merely forces the photographed person to ventriloquize the answers to our questions, while the muteness of the photograph seems to suggest that they have no objection to doing so, nothing to say for themselves.

Counterintuitively, as a rhetorical strategy, a shift in focus off the detainees' suffering might also help to generate more effective critiques of the regimes we wish to undermine. It is tempting to seek redress by elucidating the precise harms that took place before the camera so as to make them seem more real. But some, like Julie Gerk Hernandez, have argued that it was the very obscenity of the images, their apparently extraordinary or unthinkable nature, which made it possible for the government to disavow them.[47] Because the scenes seemed fundamentally incompatible with fantasies about America and its conduct, more lurid detail makes it easier to deny the connections between what happened at the prison and the ideologies and practices of the nation-state and its operatives.

This reorientation might yield a tactical benefit, and also has the potential to make an ethical repair. Attending less to the specifics (many of which are by now well-known) might mean less speaking for others and so less replication of Orientalism and its effects. In *Torture and the Twilight of Empire*, Marnia Lazreg argues for the importance of an inviolable and internationally-recognized 'right to silence' as a prophylaxis against torture.[48] If everyone agreed that no one should ever be forced to speak, then intelligence-gathering torture would be out of the question. John Limon, in his essay on shame and Abu Ghraib, seems to recognize the importance of adapting such a protection to scholarly inquiry, relinquishing a portion of his discursive authority:

> I want to say as little as possible about the military and civilian torturers at Abu Ghraib and their victims. Above all I want to avoid the unearned frisson an academic latecomer to this material can offer his readers, with a

> practised rhetoric of voyeuristic repugnance, partisan disinterest, and deadpan outrage.[49]

Extending this right to visual representations of torture would be a first step toward returning authority over the images to those who are debased within them.

Such a partial surrender might require ceding some epistemic privilege and acknowledging that there might be things that no one will ever be able to know about the photographs: about the circumstances surrounding their creation and about the people, living and dead, pictured within them. Wendy Kozol, in her discussion of a family collection of photos and personal effects from an uncle's time in World War II, directly acknowledges the 'unanswerability' of the questions she poses about the images and objects, so as to 'explore this unknowability in relation to the various kinds of violence that hover over this archive.'[50] To accept a similar uncertainty in the face of Abu Ghraib is to entertain the possibility that some things might exceed our capacity to know them; what is really at stake for us when we feel the need to be absolutely, definitively right about the Abu Ghraib photos?

One way of answering this question is to be explicit about the kinds of knowledge we seek to produce about the images. Much of the discourse on the Abu Ghraib photographs is redundant. Visually, it tends to focus on just a handful of photographs out of the many hundreds that exist, like the hooded man atop the box of MREs or the man on the floor at the end of a leash. It is analytically monotonous as well, as in the repeated comparisons to lynching spectacles and the emphasis on the sexualized nature of the torture. The recurrence of these analyses might be an indication of their accuracy or astuteness. It might also indicate that there is a motivation here other than the production of new knowledge, some sort of need that we want our work to gratify. This sort of investment might result in more impassioned scholarship, but it also involves exacting something from the photographs, expecting the people represented within them to perform a service for us, even if only to act as screens, even if we do all the work for them.

The remedy for this is not to assume the mantle of suffering for ourselves. There may be a presumption operative in some of this discourse that there is an obligation on the part of the well-meaning Westerner to suffer the pain of visually confronting these realities in order to intervene on behalf of the others thus depicted. This is problematic not only because it assumes some kind of equivalence between the two forms of suffering, but also because in the context of Orientalism, the suffering of the Westerner will always matter and signify more than that of her other. This is not to say that we ought to perform stoicism if we are not feeling stoic. Likewise, there is no concrete or tangible benefit - though there may be some political ones - to performing discomfort if we do not feel any. An alternative to affective colonization is what Dominic LaCapra describes as 'empathic unsettlement.'[51] Unlike spuriously claiming to identify with another's suffering or opportunistically seeking to appropriate it, adopting a position of empathic unsettlement allows one to register that suffering and articulate awareness of it while recognizing and avowing an unbridgeable distance from it. This orientation has the potential to result in a more nuanced and candid approach to the photographs, and so to generate narrower but more substantive scholarly accounts of their significance.

This also means refusing to employ the pictures as a litmus test for our own humanity by using them to experiment with our capacity for empathy and then taking the results either as evidence of moral success or failure. That is simply too much for the photographs to bear. Neither does it reveal anything meaningful. There is, after all, a long history in America of staging the confrontation with another's suffering as a demonstration of one's own fitness for citizenship.' Liberal national culture,' Lauren Berlant writes, 'has long hailed citizens through scenes of empathic identification with less fortunate others, risking the unending reverberations of publicized violence to deliver a sense of generalized moral propriety to the privileged.' Our responses, she continues, start to seem like 'expressions of one's true capacity for attachment to other humans rather than … effects of pedagogy.'[52] Here, Berlant offers a reminder that Americans are always being taught how to deal with the knowledge of another's pain as part of their citizenship, and that this education is primarily self-serving. Merely being realistic and honest about one's reactions to the Abu Ghraib photographs is not sufficient, and it can be counterproductive if it devolves into self-absorption under the guise of critical self-reflexivity. But this kind of candour is necessary for any effort to begin reconciling our ethical obligations and our intellectual agendas.

All of this work might begin by explicitly locating ourselves as spectators. Kozol maintains that when looking at images of violence, the motive of 'ascertain[ing] the "facts" of atrocities in the assumption that there is a better truth behind the image' is ethically inadequate.[53] Rather than wringing meaning from photographs of suffering, often captured in dubious situations, she argues that academics ought to focus on the dynamics of our own spectatorship, its conditions of possibility and political implications. Being critically aware of our image-consumption is a way to be specific about our agency in this situation, and is distinct from blanket assumptions of blame and guilt. It enables us to account for the essentially visual nature of these connections to torture and the tortured, and might also attune us to the visual pleasures and rewards that we seek when we assert them.

Acknowledging our own pleasure might also militate against overstating our own pain or its significance. What if we were all to reflect on the needs that these images fulfil for us? Many assert that reproducing them is necessary to illustrate the extent of the harm done. And it is possible that the sight of this suffering might arouse compassion. But in the commentary on images from Abu Ghraib, this is often subordinated to, and eventually erased by, a kind of spectatorial self-pity, a meditation on the wound that resulted from the encounter with the images and all the betrayals they seemed to suggest. Rentschler argues that an emphasis on spectatorial suffering precludes recognition of spectatorial 'accountability ' for the violences thus depicted.[54] Including torture photos in an article or book might reflect a wish to make amends, but does not address culpability in any substantive way. The focus on visual discomfort, the pain that is provoked by this new and graphically illustrated knowledge, deflects questions of ethical and political responsibility. In the academic context, it also obscures the professional rewards that we as scholars can reap from our confrontation with it, and the wage of rather more refined but no less intense pleasures that can be earned through that labour.[55]

Notes

[1] Susan Sontag, *Regarding the Pain of Others* (New York: Farrar, Straus and Giroux, 2003), 118.

[2] Patricia Yaeger, 'Consuming Trauma; or, the Pleasures of Merely Circulating,' in *Extremities: Trauma, Testimony, and Community*, ed. Nancy K. Miller and Jason Tougaw (Urbana: University of Illinois Press, 2002), 29.

[3] Ibid., 44.

[4] George Didi-Huberman, *Images in Spite of All: Four Photographs from Auschwitz*, trans. Shane B. Ellis (Chicago: University of Chicago Press, 2008), 32-33.

[5] It might also be modified and extended to encompass certain activist appropri-ations of these images. For example, my initial interest in the afterlives of the Abu Ghraib photos was piqued when I received an especially tasteless invitation to an anti-war poetry reading that included a large reproduction of the 'Gilligan' image apparently meant to entice me to attend. Though I was sympathetic to the cause, I was concerned about the ease with which the sponsoring organization transformed this document of torture into the centerpiece of its marketing campaign.

[6] In her interview with Errol Morris that appears in the film *Standard Operating Procedure*, Spc. Sabrina Harman claimed that she had taken the photographs in an effort to create visual 'proof' of what was happening at Abu Ghraib because it seemed so unbelievable. In May 2005, Harman was sentenced to six months in prison for her role in the abuse at Abu Ghraib (including her orchestration of the scene captured in the 'Gilligan' photo of the man atop the MRE box) and discharged from the Army.

[7] Julie Gerk Hernandez, 'The Tortured Body, the Photograph, and the U.S. War on Terror,' *CLCWeb: Comparative Literature and Culture* 9 (2007): 1-11.
[8] David Simpson, *9/11: The Culture of Commemoration* (Chicago: The University of Chicago Press, 2006), 13.
[9] W. J. T. Mitchell, 'Cloning Terror: The War of Images 2001-2004,' in *The Life and Death of Images: Ethics and Aesthetics*, ed. Diarmuid Costello and Dominic Willsdon (Ithaca: Cornell University Press, 2008), 197.
[10] She continues, importantly, 'being a spectator of others' suffering trains us how to imagine ourselves as the victims of the violence we witness, or feel relieved that "it wasn't me"' (Carrie A. Rentschler, 'Witnessing: US Citizenship and the Vicarious Experience of Suffering,' *Media, Culture & Society* 26 [2004], 300).
[11] In many ways, they still are. For example, it was later revealed that agents from the Central Intelligence Agency (CIA) had destroyed videos that recorded the waterboarding of Abu Zubaydah, a member of Al-Qaeda, during interrogation.
[12] Stephen F. Eisenman, *The Abu Ghraib Effect* (London: Reaktion Books, 2007), 9.
[13] Simpson, *9/11*, 116.
[14] See, for example, Kelly Oliver, 'Innocence, Perversion, and Abu Ghraib,' *Philosophy Today* 19 (2007): 343-56.
[15] See, for example, Elizabeth L. Hillman, 'Guarding Women: Abu Ghraib and Military Sexual Culture,' in *One of the Guys: Women as Aggressors and Torturers*, ed. Tara McKelvey (Emeryville, CA: Seal Press, 2007), 111-23; Lila Rajiva, 'The Military Made Me Do It: Double Standards and Psychic Injuries at Abu Ghraib,' Ibid., 217-28.
[16] When reproducing the photos, many authors and curators opt to credit the news sources that published them; on the politics of this at the 'Inconvenient Evidence' exhibit curated by Brian Wallis at the International Center for Photography, see Judith Butler, *Frames of War: When Is Life Grievable*? (London: Verso, 2009), 95-96. The logic behind this, presumably, is that it deflects publicity off of the torturer-*cum*-photographers that took them while also recognizing the courageous decision of the news organizations to make them public. Insofar as it prevents the photographers from benefiting from the pictures, this strikes me as a reasonable solution. At the same time, I am concerned that it also risks distracting us from the (suffering of the) people pictured in the photographs, whose names are unknown or unfamiliar, by drawing our attention to the American newspapers instead.
[17] Both of these comparisons are by now commonplace, though they have been subject to a great deal of debate. Few scholars quibble with their

relevance or the parallels between these visual phenomena, but there is disagreement about the specific similarities between them (e.g., Laura Frost, 'Photography/Pornography/ Torture: The Politics of Seeing Abu Ghraib,' in *One of the Guys: Women as Aggressors and Torturers*, ed. Tara McKelvey, 135-44).

[18] For a time, the online article contained one picture, of an empty corridor at the prison, entitled 'Between Tortures.' I accessed that version in the winter of 2008, though I am not sure how long it was available.

[19] Susan Sontag, 'Regarding the Torture of Others,' *The New York Times Magazine* (May 23, 2004), <http://www.nytimes.com/2004/05/23/magazine/23PRISONS.html>, paragraph 17, viewed on February 19, 2008.

[20] Ibid.

[21] Ibid., paragraph 8.

[22] Ibid., paragraph 20.

[23] Jasbir Puar reiterates this: 'the photos and their circulatory modalities double as representation and information, as the representation of information, and the only information taken seriously and validated by corporate media sources' (Jasbir K. Puar, 'On Torture: Abu Ghraib,' *Radical History Review* 93 [2005], 32).

[24] Retort (Iain Boal, T. J. Clark, Joseph Matthews, Michael Watts), *Afflicted Powers: Capital and Spectacle in a New Age of War* (London: Verso, 2005), 23.

[25] Ibid., 35.

[26] Martin Jay, *Refractions of Violence* (New York: Routledge, 2003), 185.

[27] Rosalind C. Morris makes a related observation, attributing the rapid fizzling-out of the scandal to the lack of subsequent images released after the first batch. She writes, 'the news photograph has a short half-life and fades quickly' (Rosalind C. Morris, 'The War Drive: Image Files Corrupted,' *Social Text* 91 [2007], 103).

[28] Nicholas Mirzoeff, 'Invisible Empire: Visual Culture, Embodied Spectacle,' *Radical History Review* 95 (2006): 35.

[29] Similarly, Alphonso Lingis argues that the sexualized torture organized at Abu Ghraib and depicted in the photos was 'staged as specifically Muslim degradation' (Lingis, 'The Effects of the Pictures,' *Journal of Visual Culture*, 5 [2006], 85.)

[30] Mirzoeff, 'Invisible Empire,' 40-41.

[31] International Committee of the Red Cross (ICRC), 'Convention (III) Relative to the Treatment of Prisoners of War. Geneva, 12 August 1949, 2005,' <http://www.icrc.org/ihl.nsf/FULL/375?OpenDocument>, viewed on June 15, 2011.

[32] Wendy Kozol and Rebecca DeCola, 'Remapping the War on Terrorism: "U.S. Internationalism" and Transnational Citizenship,' in *Rethinking Global Security: Media, Popular Culture, and the 'War on Terror*, ed. Andrew Martin and Patrice Petro (New Brunswick: Rutgers University Press, 2006), 179. Grajeda calls the use of the camera in this context 'cultural terrorism' (Tony Grajeda, 'Picturing Torture: Gulf Wars Past and Present,' in *Rethinking Global Security*, ed. Andrew Martin and Patrice Petro, 229).
[33] Jerome H. Skolnick, 'On Controlling Torture,' in *Punishment and Social Control*, ed. Thomas G. Bloomberg and Stanley Cohen (New York: Aldine de Gruyter, 2003), 216.
[34] Dora Apel, 'Torture Culture: Lynching Photographs and the Images of Abu Ghraib,' *Art Journal* 64 (2005): 100.
[35] Simpson, *9/11*, 115.
[36] Mitchell, 'Cloning Terror,' 206.
[37] Gayatri Chakravorty Spivak, 'Can the Subaltern Speak?' in *The Postcolonial Studies Reader*, ed. Bill Ashcroft, Garrett Griffiths and Helen Tiffin (New York: Routledge, 1995), 24-29.
[38] In 2004, *The Washington Post* published translations of sworn statements from detainees at Abu Ghraib. This compilation provides a view into their experiences, but an intensely mediated one. In their statements, many of the detainees report that the guards used cameras as part of the abuse; none grant permission for those photos to be reproduced, <http://www.washingtonpost.com/wpsrv/world/iraq/abughraib/swornstatements042104.html>, viewed on December 6, 2011.
[39] Timothy V. Kaufman-Osborn, '"We Are All Torturers Now": Accountability After Abu Ghraib,' *Theory & Event* 11 (2008): <http://muse.jhu.edu/login?uri=/journals/theory_and_event/v011/11.2.kaufman-osborn.html>, viewed on June 20, 2011.
[40] Ibid.
[41] Puar, 'On Torture,' 31-32.
[42] Edward Said, *Orientalism* (New York: Random House, 1978), 25.
[43] Kurasawa's analysis of 'humanitarian visuality' in 'Perilous Light' is a useful model for mapping the vexed relationships between power, distance, sight and sympathy (Fuyuki Kurasawa, 'Perilous Light: On the Visual Representation of Distant Suffering.' Lecture, The Institute of Political Economy, Carleton University, March 28, 2008, <http://culturalshifts.com/archives/320>), viewed on April 12, 2008.
[44] Donald E. Pease, *The New American Exceptionalism* (Minneapolis: University of Minnesota Press, 2009), 20.

[45] Lauren Berlant, 'Uncle Sam Needs a Wife: Citizenship and Denegation,' in *Visual Worlds*, ed. John R. Hall, Blake Stimson and Lisa Tamiris Baker (New York: Routledge, 2005), 37.
[46] Rosalind C. Morris, 'The War Drive: Image Files Corrupted,' *Social Text* 91 (2007): 107.
[47] Hernandez, 'The Tortured Body,' 10.
[48] Marnia Lazreg, *Torture and the Twilight of Empire: From Algiers to Baghdad, Human Rights and Crimes against Humanity* (Princeton: Princeton University Press, 2008), 259.
[49] John Limon, 'The Shame of Abu Ghraib,' *Critical Inquiry* 33 (2007): 554.
[50] Wendy Kozol, 'Battlefield Souvenirs and Ethical Spectatorship' (paper present-ed at Feeling Photography Conference at the University of Toronto, October 17, 2009).
[51] Dominic LaCapra, *History and Its Limits: Human, Animal, Violence* (Ithaca: Cornell University Press, 2009), 65-66.
[52] Berlant, 'Uncle Sam Needs a Wife,' 32.
[53] Kozol, 'Battlefield Souvenirs.'
[54] Rentschler, 'Witnessing,' 301.
[55] I have benefited tremendously from the insights, guidance, and support of colleagues and mentors throughout my work on this project. The participants at the 'Knowledge and Pain' conference offered perspicacious feedback on an early draft of this paper. Jason Loviglio helped me think through the political and ethical complexities of academic freedom. For their early support of this inquiry and so much else, I remain deeply grateful to Ruby C. Tapia, Philip Armstrong, and Maurice Stevens.

Bibliography

Apel, Dora. 'Torture Culture: Lynching Photographs and the Images of Abu Ghraib.' *Art Journal* 64 (2005): 88-100.

Barkan, Elazar. 'The Worst is Yet to Come: Abu Ghraib and the Politics of Not Apologizing.' In *Taking Wrongs Seriously: Apologies and Reconciliation*, edited by Elazar Barkan and Alexander Kern, 311-30. Stanford: Stanford University Press, 2006.

Berlant, Lauren. 'Uncle Sam Needs a Wife: Citizenship and Denegation.' In *Visual Worlds*, edited by John R. Hall, Blake Stimson and Lisa Tamiris Baker, 15-44. New York: Routledge, 2005.

Butler, Judith. *Frames of War: When Is Life Grievable*? London: Verso, 2009.

Didi-Huberman, Georges. *Images in Spite of All: Four Photographs from Auschwitz*. Translated by Shane B. Ellis. Chicago: University of Chicago Press, 2008.

Eisenman, Stephen F. *The Abu Ghraib Effect*. London: Reaktion Books, 2007.

Frost, Laura. 'Photography/Pornography/Torture: The Politics of Seeing Abu Ghraib.' In *One of the Guys: Women as Aggressors and Torturers*, edited by Tara McKelvey, 135-44. Emeryville, CA: Seal Press, 2007.

Grajeda, Tony. 'Picturing Torture: Gulf Wars Past and Present.' In *Rethinking Global Security: Media, Popular Culture, and the 'War on Terror*, edited by Andrew Martin and Patrice Petro, 206-35. New Brunswick: Rutgers University Press, 2006.

Hernandez, Julie Gerk. 'The Tortured Body, the Photograph, and the U.S. War on Terror.' *CLCWeb: Comparative Literature and Culture* 9 (2007): 1-11.

Hillman, Elizabeth L. 'Guarding Women: Abu Ghraib and Military Sexual Culture.' In *One of the Guys: Women as Aggressors and Torturers*, edited by Tara McKelvey, 111-23. Emeryville, CA: Seal Press, 2007.

International Committee of the Red Cross (ICRC). 'Convention (III) Relative to the Treatment of Prisoners of War. Geneva, 12 August 1949,' 2005. <http://www.icrc.org/ihl.nsf/FULL/375?OpenDocument>, viewed on June 15, 2011.

Jay, Martin. *Refractions of Violence*. New York: Routledge, 2003.

Kaufman-Osborn, Timothy V. '"We Are All Torturers Now": Accountability after Abu Ghraib.' *Theory & Event*, 11 (2008). <http://muse.jhu.edu/login?uri=/journals /theory_and_event/v011/11.2.kaufman-osborn.html>, viewed on June 20, 2011.

Kozol, Wendy and Rebecca DeCola. 'Remapping the War on Terrorism: "U.S. Internationalism" and Transnational Citizenship.' In *Rethinking Global Security: Media, Popular Culture, and the 'War on Terror*, edited by Andrew Martin and Patrice Petro, 179-205. New Brunswick: Rutgers University Press, 2006.

Kurasawa, Fuyuki. 'Perilous Light: On the Visual Representation of Distant Suffering.' Lecture, The Institute of Political Economy, Carleton University, March 28, 2008. <http://culturalshifts.com/archives/320>. Viewed on April 12, 2008.

LaCapra, Dominic. *History and Its Limits: Human, Animal, Violence*. Ithaca: Cornell University Press, 2009.

Lazreg, Marnia. *Torture and the Twilight of Empire: From Algiers to Baghdad*. Human Rights and Crimes Against Humanity. Princeton: Princeton University Press, 2008.

Limon, John. 'The Shame of Abu Ghraib.' *Critical Inquiry* 33 (2007): 543-72.

Lingis, Alphonso. 'The Effects of the Pictures.' *Journal of Visual Culture* 5 (2006): 83-86.

Mirzoeff, Nicholas. 'Invisible Empire: Visual Culture, Embodied Spectacle.' *Radical History Review* 95 (2006): 21-44.

Mitchell, W. J. T. 'Cloning Terror: The War of Images 2001-2004.' In *The Life and Death of Images: Ethics and Aesthetics*, edited by Diarmuid Costello and Dominic Willsdon, 179-207. Ithaca: Cornell University Press, 2008.

Morris, Rosalind C. 'The War Drive: Image Files Corrupted.' *Social Text* 91 (2007): 103-42.

Oliver, Kelly. 'Innocence, Perversion, and Abu Ghraib.' *Philosophy Today* 19 (2007): 343-56.

Pease, Donald E. *The New American Exceptionalism*. Minneapolis: University of Minnesota Press, 2009.

Puar, Jasbir K. 'On Torture: Abu Ghraib.' *Radical History Review* 93 (2005): 13-38.

Rajiva, Lila. 'The Military Made Me Do It: Double Standards and Psychic Injuries at Abu Ghraib.' In *One of the Guys: Women as Aggressors and Torturers*, edited by Tara McKelvey, 217-28. Emeryville, CA: Seal Press, 2007.

Rentschler, Carrie A. 'Witnessing: US Citizenship and the Vicarious Experience of Suffering.' *Media, Culture & Society* 26 (2004): 296-304.

Retort (Iain Boal, T. J. Clark, Joseph Matthews and Michael Watts). *Afflicted Powers: Capital and Spectacle in a New Age of War*. London: Verso, 2005.

Said, Edward. *Orientalism*. New York: Random House, 1978.

Simpson, David. *9/11: The Culture of Commemoration*. Chicago: The University of Chicago Press, 2006.

Skolnick, Jerome H. 'On Controlling Torture.' In *Punishment and Social Control*, edited by Thomas G. Bloomberg and Stanley Cohen, 213-29. New York: Aldine de Gruyter, 2003.

Sontag, Susan. *Regarding the Pain of Others*. New York: Farrar, Straus and Giroux, 2003.

———. 'Regarding the Torture of Others.' *The New York Times Magazine*, May 23, 2004. <http://www.nytimes.com/2004/05/23/magazine/23PRISONS.html>. Viewed on February 19, 2008.

Spivak, Gayatri Chakravorty. 'Can the Subaltern Speak?' In *The Postcolonial Studies Reader*, edited by Bill Ashcroft, Garrett Griffiths, and Helen Tiffin, 24-29. New York: Routledge, 1995.

Standard Operating Procedure. Directed by Errol Morris. New York: Sony Pictures Classics, 2008.

'Sworn Statements by Abu Ghraib Detainees.' *The Washington Post*, 2004. <http://www.washingtonpost.com/wpsrv/world/iraq/abughraib/swornstatements042104.html>. Viewed on December 6, 2011.

Yaeger, Patricia, 'Consuming Trauma; or, the Pleasures of Merely Circulating.' In *Extremities: Trauma, Testimony, and Community*, edited by Nancy K. Miller and Jason Tougaw, 25-51. Urbana: University of Illinois Press, 2002.

'Sorting through My Grief and Putting It into Boxes': Comics and Pain

Ariela Freedman

Abstract
Comics may seem like the last place to think seriously about pain. But in recent years both artists and critics have increasingly turned towards the representation of pain, illness and trauma through the medium. The turn of graphic narrative, journalism and memoir, towards the representation of pain and trauma in history and private life has significant aesthetic, narrative and therapeutic implications and should be understood in medium-specific terms. My primary concern in this essay is a palpable shift in the representation of pain that occurs in the 1970s and that has a significant effect on both the content and form of comics. Comics after the 1970s mobilised a historically dense and sophisticated vocabulary for pain language, both synaesthetic and defined as much through its absences and exclusions as through what it represents. I want to suggest that contemporary comics transform the pain-language developed through the medium in accordance with discursive possibilities of pain, its overflow of our usual modalities of representation, and serve as new and ethically powerful modes of testimony.

Key Words: Autobiography, comics, graphic memoir, illness, pain language, Spiegelman, David Small, trauma.

*****

> 'You learned the concept pain when you learned language.'
> - Wittgenstein, *Philosophical Investigations*[1]

Comics may seem like the last place to think seriously about pain. But in recent years both artists and critics have increasingly turned towards the representation of pain, illness and trauma through the medium. *Maus I* and *II*, Art Spiegelman's Pulitzer-winning two-volume book on the Holocaust, is still the best-known work of comics testimonial, but many graphic memoirs and journalism have in recent years attempted to bear witness to personal and collective pain. Some of these books are situated at what Spiegelman calls the 'intersection of personal history and collective history';[2] these include Keiji Nakazawa's *Barefoot Gen,* Marjane Satrapi's *Persepolis* series, Joe Sacco's graphic war journalism in Bosnia and Palestine, Phillippe Stassen's *Deogratias*, and *The Photographer: Into War-Torn Afghanistan with Doctors Without Borders* by Guibert, Lefèvre and Lemercier. A number of texts follow Justin Green's memoir of Catholicism and OCD in *Binky Brown Meets the Holy Virgin Mary* in describing mental illness and childhood trauma; one of the most striking of these, Lynda's Barry's *One Hundred Demons* combines drawing with collage, in what Barry terms 'autobifictionalography,' in order to describe the tricky process of making story out of memory. There is also a growing body of work on illness: David B.'s autobiographical account of his brother's epilepsy in *Epileptic*, Brian Fies's *Mom's Cancer*, Harvey Pekar's *Our Cancer Year*, Marissa Acocella Marchetto's *Cancer Vixen,* Frederik Peeters's *Blue Pills: A Positive Love Story,* David Small's *Stitches* and the fictive but semi-autobiographical *It's a Bird*, written by Steven T. Seagle and drawn by Teddy Kristiansen, which strikingly juxtaposes the genre of superhero comics with a memoir of Huntington's Disease. Indeed, there are now too many substantial works of this kind to be contained in any brief catalogue.

This flowering of creative work has been met with considerable critical interest. Not only have literary scholars and historians addressed the representation of trauma in comics, but what Ian Williams calls 'Graphic Medicine' has also garnered attention in the medical humanities and in the field of narrative medicine.[3] The turn of graphic narrative, journalism and memoir, towards the representation of pain and trauma in history and private life has significant aesthetic, narrative and therapeutic implications and needs to be understood in medium-specific terms. Pain frustrates and isolates in part because of its resistance to communicability; it cannot be adequately explained or displayed, and it resists absolute containment through either word or image. But because comics employ both word *and* image, they can try to bridge the internal and external representation of pain; they can tell pain and show it. Perhaps even more strikingly, they can demonstrate the gulf between what can be told and what can be shown through a deliberate dissonance between the panel's narration and its visual content. My primary concern in this essay is a palpable shift in the representation of pain that occurs in the 1970s and which has a significant effect on both the content and form of comics. Comics after the 1970s mobilised a historically dense and sophisticated vocabulary for pain language, both synaesthetic and defined as much through its absences and exclusions as through what it represents - what Spiegelman calls, in a nod to the framing conventions of comics panels, 'sorting through my grief and putting it into boxes.'[4] Spiegelman, Nakazawa, David B. and many others worked against the conventions of earlier comics to return pain and consequence to a genre that has specialized in the representation of a neutered imaginary violence. In using the genre of comics as a mode of (frequently autobiographical) attesting, they have resisted what Susan Sontag once termed the tendency of images to 'anesthetize'[5] and have explored new possibilities of representing pain in a manner that rejects the aesthetisation and trivilialisation of comic slapstick and epic even as they enlist familiar techniques and images in order to reinvent pain language for the medium. This article attempts to situate the representation of pain and trauma in comics, first by historically placing the reader, and, second, by exploring some of the medium-specific strategies that lend themselves to the representation of pain through a close reading of a recent graphic memoir, *Stitches*, by David Small. In doing so, I want to suggest that contemporary comics transform the pain-language developed through the medium in accordance with discursive possibilities that respond to what Scarry calls the 'unmaking'[6] power of pain, its overflow of our usual modalities of representation, and that serve as new and ethically powerful modes of testimony.

1. Ow: A Comic History of Pain

Comics are historically and conventionally associated with the humorous; thus the name 'comics,' or the older title, 'funnies.' Frequently, the 'funny' in the funnies has to do with the infliction and representation of physical and psychic pain. Comics begin here: the broken heart, the disappointment, the pratfall, the beating, the brick to the head, the caricatured grimace, the wail. This slapstick violence forms part of what in his *Lectures on Don Quixote* Nabokov calls 'our history of pain' - 'the banged heads and kicked groins and punched noses that are such delectable features of our movies and comics.'[7] Comics have a rich established pain vocabulary to draw upon, a lexicon of images, characters and situations that provide precedent and inspiration to later artists. In *Les Amours de M. Vieuxbois*, Rodolphe Töpffer (1839), frequently identified as the father of comics, depicts a protagonist repeatedly thwarted both in love and in his many attempts to take his own life. Töpffer's tragic-comic, melancholic narratives were copied and imitated by later artists; he imprinted the medium with his iconic intermingling of desire and suffering. George Herriman's newspaper strip *Krazy Kat* ran from 1913 to 1944 on the premise that its title character, Krazy Kat, is in love with Ignatz the mouse, who constantly schemes to throw bricks at his head; Krazy Kat sees these bricks as love tokens, and is disappointed when Ignatz's plans are thwarted (Figure 1).

The paradigm of a couple united by repetitive, comic violence without real pain or consequence is a powerful one in the medium. This violent, romantic duet is inherited by numerous interpreters in comics and animation: Hanna and Barbera's *Tom and Jerry*, Antonio Prohias's *Spy vs. Spy*, Charles Schultz's Charlie Brown and Lucy, and more recently, Chris Ware's Quimby the Mouse and Sparky the Cat Head. Laughing at these anthropomorphized animals and cartoon people, and this repeated, mechanistic, sadomasochistic compulsion - for Krazy Kat, to declare his love, for Ignatz, to throw the brick - requires something like what in his essay 'Laughter' Henri Bergson calls 'a momentary anaesthesia of the heart.'[8] We laugh, Bergson argues, in response to the involuntary and rigid quality grafted upon the living in the comic scene. 'The comic person is unconscious,' he writes, and is both mechanistic and material, giving the impression at once of 'something mechanical encrusted on something living'[9] and of 'a person embarrassed by his body.'[10] The early anthropomorphic creatures of comics seem human, animal and mechanical at once; they are distant enough for us to laugh at their pain.

Pain in comics first appears in a comedic and fantasy mode; it also develops into the spectacular violence of superhero comics.[11] Though in these comics the representation of pain was often not funny, it was aestheticised and melodramatic, and was folded into a practice of spectacle and consumption that precluded empathy with the victims. These comics also elaborated on the most obvious and familiar element of pain language in the medium: the iconic 'Ows' and 'Bangs,' used in earlier newspaper comics but now blown up into colourful, jagged-edged ejaculations so familiar that they can stand in on their own for an entire genre. Through typographic variation - modifying the size and style of the pictured words in the panel - comics establish a range of cries far broader than those used in conventional written English. Cries of pain in comics have a lability and creativity impossible to translate into another mode though these are frequently used for bombastic rather than realistic effect.[12] The non-words of comics' ejaculations are suggestively close to Scarry's description of pain as triggering the destruction of language, though it is true that unless they are used ironically or paradoxically, in comics these cries signify sublimed pain, a pain that is deliberately marked and enjoyed as unreal.

The slapstick mode of the funnies and the aestheticized violence of the superhero genre form an important background for the history of the language of pain in comics. Indeed, these foundational comics provided the basic language, symbols, scenarios and formal strategies for later artists to use and explore, and created reading conventions for a growing audience that now included many adult readers. Their representation of pain is more subtle and multivalent than this brief sketch can fairly represent. Later comics need to wrestle with the playful, humorous and shocking implications of their antecedents: one striking visual example is the unruly early cartoon characters that infiltrate Art Spiegelman's account of the attack on the World Trade Centers.[13] Comics as a medium is constituted through homage, parody and even theft, and the prominence of pain language is a dominant motif in these intertextual, cross-genre repetitions. Representations of pain in comics are consciously and necessarily juxtaposed with earlier iterations: they serve as palimpsests. These repetitions often work against the grain of their earlier iterations as they attempt to use fantasy conventions for serious and realist subject matter.

In the 1970s the scope, ambition and effect of comics pain-language changed as many artists abandoned the genre narratives of the comics workshops and newspaper strips and wrote autobiographical, painfully confessional work which was frequently self-published or published by artist's collectives, intended for adult readers and sold and marketed outside of comics shops. The aesthetic of these early, underground comics (or comix, as they were frequently entitled to designate themselves in view of their transgressive qualities) was frequently grotesque, in deliberate reaction to the stylized bodies of superheroes; the drawing style was inflected by neo-realism or expressionism rather than filtered through the clear lines and hyper-kinetic style of superhero comics; as opposed to the bright colours of newsstand comics, the drawing was usually black and white and relied heavily on chiaroscuro, zipatone, pointillism and cross-hatching to create a world of darkness and shadows; the characters were ordinary, or if they were exceptional, they were exceptions in terms of the depths of their neurosis. Frequently, these new comics told stories that had not previously been told in the comics medium, and had rarely been explored in any medium: struggles with mental illness, sexual obsession, political oppression, war, Holocaust. And the mental, physical and historical violence depicted in these comics was different: it was based on autobiography or acts of witnessing, it was depicted in a way that did not glamorise violence or render it humorous. It was meant to hurt.

The first long autobiographical comic, Justin Green's *Binky Brown Meets the Holy Virgin Mary* (1972), depicts Green's struggle with Catholicism and obsessive compulsive disorder or what the church called 'scrupulosity.' Green's alter-ego Binky Brown accidentally breaks an icon of the Virgin Mary as a child; he starts to suffer from obsessive thoughts, compulsive behaviours, and the belief that his penis and other extremities shoot unclean rays that defile his surroundings. Binky Brown opens with an ornate page titled 'A Confession to Readers' in gothic script. The panel is limned like a medieval manuscript, and shows the author, nude and suspended upside down, a sickle threateningly positioned between his legs, his hands tied behind his back, a pen gripped between his teeth beside a vial of ink labelled 'dad's blood,' a record-player blasting 'Ave Maria' beside him. Two obscene cherubs frolic in the upper left-hand corner, while a praying patron occupies a box to the lower right. The page exults in the heretical inversion of religious iconography and juxtaposes comics conventions with the artistic conventions of depicting martyrdom even as it appropriates the confessional mode as a form of artistic catharsis. 'O, my readers, the saga of Binky Brown is not intended solely for your entertainment, but also to purge myself of the compulsive neurosis which I have served since I officially left Catholicism on Halloween, 1968.' But the comic is intended to act not only as individual catharsis, but also as spur for the reader:

> My justification for undertaking this task is that many others are slaves to their neurosis. Maybe if they read about one neurotic's dilemma in easy-to-understand comic-book format these tormented folk will no longer see themselves as mere food-tubes living in isolation. If all we neurotics were together we would entwine the globe in a vast chain of common suffering - please don't think I'm an asshole. Amen.[14] (Figure 2)

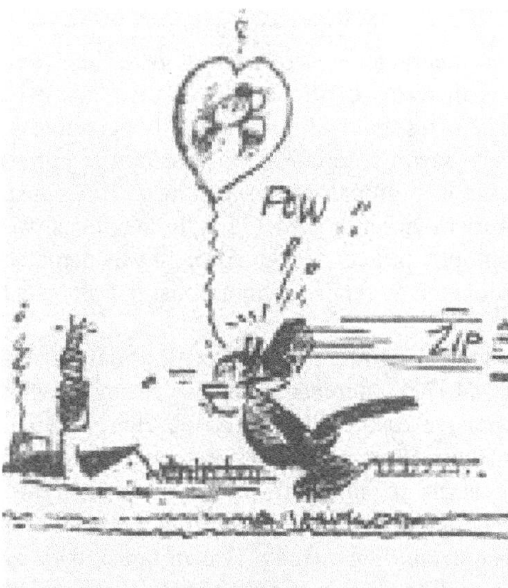

Fig. 1 George Herriman. *Krazy Kat.* Reprint in *Krazy Kat and Ignatz* (Fantagraphics Books, 2002)

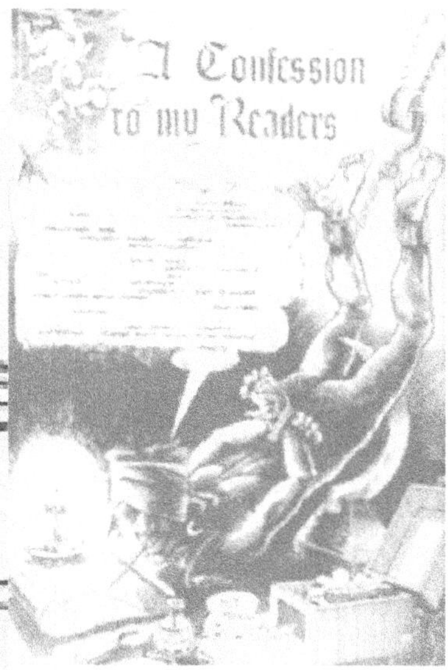

Fig. 2. Justin Green. Frontispiece to Binky Brown. *Binky Brown Sampler 10* © Justin Green

Despite the self-deprecatory, ironic tone of these remarks, Green's insistence on staging the spectacle of his suffering for the purposes of solidarity is serious. Even as the icon of the crucified Christ served to consolidate the community of Christians who were united through his martyrdom, Green turns himself into a latter-day saint speaking for the collective suffering of neurotics and providing a common catharsis, if not salvation, through autobiographical confession. Jared Gardner writes of the empathic possibilities of Green's work, riffing on the comics term 'bleed' which pertains to the extension of an image to the limits of the page: 'Only by allowing the past to bleed into history, fact to bleed into fiction, image into text, might we begin to allow our own pain to bleed into the other, and more urgently, the pain of the other to bleed into ourselves.' He continues, 'there is no body of work that is better suited to the task than that of graphic memoir, which began telling its own multimodal "autobifictionalographies" thirty-five years ago.'[15] Green, Art Spiegelman asserts in the Introduction to the *Binky Brown Sampler*, turned 'comic book boxes into intimate, secular confession booths.[16] Green's elevation as founder of the genre of confessional autobiographical comix has raised his own work to iconic status: the recent new edition published by McSweeney's Press is bound in an embossed hard cover and advertised by the canonizing accolades of other comics artists.

Just as Justin Green's *Binky Brown* galvanized Spiegelman, Spiegelman's *Maus* served as a powerful inspiration for subsequent artists; its audacity, historical rootedness, autobiographical reflexivity, narrative strategies and stylistic footprint can be found in most subsequent graphic narratives. *Maus* remains the most canonical attempt to tell a traumatic history through the comics medium. Indeed, the subtitle of the first volume - 'My Father Bleeds History' - suggests the embodied, material quality of the telling of history, as if it were the wound itself that spoke. Autobiography and testimony, the book speaks to a pain both personal and communal, passed on across a generational divide. Spiegelman's famous choice to draw the Jews as mice and the Nazis as cats, which imposed a speaking mask upon the act of testimony, was a device that freed him to represent what is nearly unseeable and unsayable; it spoke back both to Nazi caricatures of Jews as vermin and the established comics vocabulary of anthropomorphic animals including, of course, Mickey Mouse (the first three pages of *Maus* were published in 1973 in the underground comic *Funny Aminals*). The dark eyed, clear mouse faces serve as a staging point for empathy. The cartoon face acts as a blank slate, 'a vacuum into which our identity and awareness are pulled…an empty shell that we inhabit which enables us to travel in a different realm….When you look at a photo or a realistic drawing of a face you see it as the face of another but when you enter into the world of the cartoon you see yourself' (McCloud 36).[17] Spiegelman's mice are deliberately abstracted and simplified in order to facilitate readerly identification, but there is also a reflexive nod to the conventions and limitations of comics representation.[18] In his use of this conspicuously literal metaphor - the Nazis as cats, the Jews as mice - Spiegelman is also warning us of the dangers of caricature and its historical link to racialization.

Spiegelman does not just express what his father has seen, and the severe price of the Holocaust for a second generation; he also gives voice to the complication of attesting a collective experience and the tensions of doing so through comics. In chapter five of *Maus I*, Vladek describes a transport from Srodula to Auschwitz. Spiegelman juxtaposes Vladek's testimonial with a reimagining of the events; he grounds the narrative jointly in the past and present, and ties it to the speaker. In this panel, Vladek reports that the children who cried too loudly while waiting for the transport were thrown against a wall. This panel is darkly inked, in Spiegelman's stark black and white. The aggressor is anonymous, his back to us, but the victim is also obscured, deliberately cut off by the very devices of the comic - the panel border, the speech bubble. Spiegelman borrows the speed lines and the splatter of a comics language, but to totally different effect. Pain language is supplemented by what Mort Walker in *The Lexicon of Comicana* calls 'symbolia': a medium-specific shared set of symbols used to signify heat, motion, shock, pain. Symbolia quickly signify phenomena which are invisible or are difficult to represent, like smells, emotions, temperature or speed.[19] Part of the shock of this panel is in noticing Spiegelman's use of conventional cartoon symbolia - zip lines, which would often be used for far more innocent subject matter, and the speech bubble, subversively used to show the event and hide it from view. For Spiegelman it is important that the narration of the trauma through comics is possible, but it is also important that it should be difficult. He reminds us of his devices, and of the tenuous ethical status of his testimony. Spiegelman's signature combination of autobiography and testimonial, his brave use of a subject matter that had become auratic and untouchable and his subversive use of anthropomorphic animals and other comics conventions won broad acclaim and a cross-over audience. He helped create new possibilities for artists, publishers and audiences and laid the groundwork for later comics testimonials.

Outside of North America, artists had concurrently begun to do pioneering work in documenting trauma through the comics medium. In 1972-1973, Keiji Nakazawa serialized the first volume of Barefoot Gen (*Hadashi No Gen*) in the *manga* anthology *Weekly Shonen Jump (Shūkan Shōnen Jampu).* This autobiographical comic loosely documents Nakazawa's experiences as a child in Hiroshima when the atomic bomb was dropped. It reached an audience of millions in Japan and, like *Maus*, testified to a historical trauma that many chose to repress and forget. Project Gen, a non-profit, volunteer group of translators organized by the peace activists Masahari Oshima and Yukio Aki to bring Nakazawa's work to a wider audience, translated parts of the series into English, French, German, Italian, Portugese, Swedish, Norwegian, Indonesian, Tagalog and Esperanto[20] in order to promote nuclear disarmament. The translation into Esperanto is both surprising and appropriate: if Esperanto aspired to be a universal language then comics had a similar claim to cross cultural relevance. *Maus* and *Barefoot Gen* bore witness to two of the greatest traumas of the twentieth century; in doing so they not only demonstrated the possibilities of the medium for the representation of trauma, but also helped comics gain a broader audience and authority.

2. Ack: Pain and Loss of Voice in *Stitches*

But how does this highly charged medium facilitate the narration of painful history? What comics devices do artists use to give voice to experiences that have been suppressed and silenced? David Small's memoir *Stitches*, one of the most recent and powerful contributions to the narration of pain and illness through the medium of comics, thematises the problem of using comics to voice traumatic history. Small is an illustrator of children's books, and this is his first graphic memoir. In it, he tells the story of his childhood illnesses, his painfully dysfunctional family, the cancer that nobody told him he had, and the operation that severed his vocal chord and left him mute at the age of fourteen. This memoir is a drama of voicelessness: the story of a household in which the most important things were never said, of a family history full of secrets and gaps, of an illness that dare not speak its name, and a voice stolen and then finally restored through the medium of art. Through the comics medium, Small articulates the silences of his childhood, his literal and figurative loss of language, and his self-conscious creation of a language to respond to his early trauma.

The first element of language in comics is typography; we read not only words but also word-objects. Like many autobiographical comics artists, Small uses a lettering designed from his own handwriting in order to create an effect of realism, spontaneity and intimacy. In autobiographical comics, the custom, hand-written font becomes a signature of authenticity as the author writes himself. But writing oneself is the problem as well as the solution in this memoir. On the cover the author's name is put inside a speech bubble that is 'spoken' by the grandmother (Figure 3). The author's name is bracketed by white writing small enough that you need to hold the book closer to your eyes to make it legible: 'by my durn grandson' over the name, 'durnit…' under the name. These curses are the underwriting of Small's childhood, the scaffolding of his identity. Small is named and derided by other people; his challenge will be to name himself.

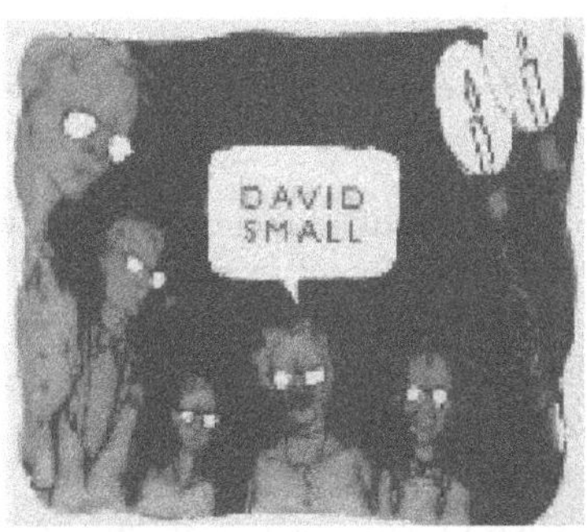

Fig. 3. David Small. Cover to *Stitches* © David Small

Small begins his memoir in deliberate and dallying silence. His first four pages unfold without a single speech bubble or piece of extra-diegetic narration, and takes us from the industrial Centre of Detroit to its tree-lined suburban streets into the open door of a generic home, up the stairs and to the narrator. The graphic form allows for these extended silences. As Small said in an interview, 'all the silence and the necessity for reading body language as a means of survival, those elements made the graphic form seem an appropriate medium for my tale.'[21] Small frequently uses what McCloud calls 'aspect-to-aspect transition,'[22] panels that show elements of a single scene in non-narrative sequence: the smokestacks, the dark streets, the open doorway, the subject presented from behind in profile, and then from the front. These sequences do not move the story forward: they slow it down and create mood, in this case contributing to a looming sense of threat. Small also deliberately restricts his palette to convey the chiaroscuro of his childhood, using brush and inkwash to emphasise a muted world of greys and shadows. In this atmospheric and loaded silence the first sound we hear is comics ejaculations that signify impact.

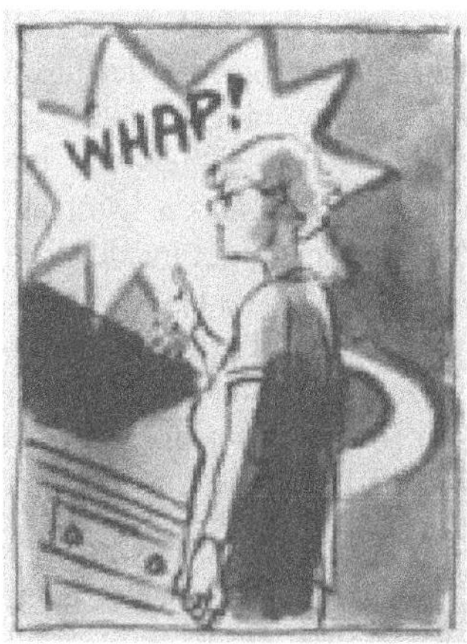

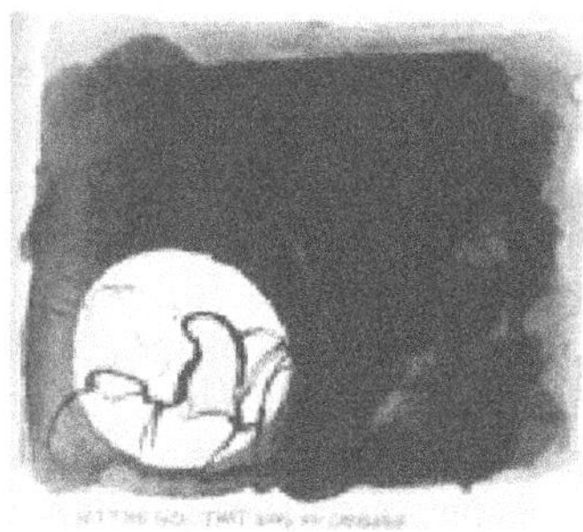

Fig. 4. Small, *Stitches* 15 (excerpt) Fig. 5. Small, *Stitches* 19 (excerpt)

Small's mother's repetitive, neurotic cough: the first of the alternate languages that his family has found in their painful silence (Figure 4). Our picture of her is preceded by her shadow, and the image of her coughing is unbordered, uncontained. The expression of the cough itself - 'knh!' - is darkly inked and assertive, while the repetitive 'whaps' of the slamming of cupboard doors are outlined in jagged comic bubbles frequently used in genre comics but here deployed to indicate the everyday aggression of kitchen sink tragedies. In Freud's words, these are the symptoms that chatter and ooze out at every pore. Small presents a catalogue of these alternate languages, his family's symptoms: his mother's cough and slamming of cupboards, the 'pocketa pocketa pocketa' of his father's punching bag, his brother's drums.

'Getting sick, that was my language,' the narrator comments, under a large, dark panel that dispenses with the frame, and reverses subject and ground, showing his child-self illuminated against a deep field of black (Figure 5). Pain becomes manifest not just in the subject but in the form of the drawing. Since comics relies as much on line and colour as it does on the content of word and image, pain can appear in a dissolving line, or in a panel suddenly densely cross-hatched and dark, or in a change of palette. As Thierry Groensteen and Scott McCloud have pointed out, the panel organizes not just space but also time in comics. Playing with panel conventions - which imply closure and exclusion as much as they frame the narrative - provides numerous opportunities for the representation of illness and trauma. Blowing a panel up, stretching it, extending or making it 'bleed' to the very edge of the page, can give emphasis, suggest significance, and provide a sense of time dilated, or even of timelessness. When the line of the panel is shaky and drawn by hand, it can contribute to a sense of anxiety; when the solid black line of the frame is broken, there is a break in the world being represented. Play with panel conventions lends itself to figurative and expressionistic usage: beyond the physical, it attempts to chart the psychic and emotional costs of pain. Though Small does not quite bleed the image off the page, the use of inkwash and the lack of a box makes the borders of the picture blurry and undefined, creating the effect of extended duration outside of conventional narrative time. The 'unresolved, lingering'[23] effect of these borderless panels is particularly effective in this memoir of illness and of a traumatic childhood. These borderless panels imply not a singular moment, but a repeated, habitual moment, and the lack of perimeters communicates their heightened emotive significance. They also seem frozen in time: not past, but present. These painful, recollected childhood moments are not over. In Beckett's memorable gloss on Proust, 'There is no escape from yesterday because yesterday has deformed us, or has been deformed by us.'[24]

Like Alice in her Wonderland, a persistent subtext in the memoir, Small shrinks, grows, changes, tumbles into the hole of his subconscious and needs to find his way out. The literalization of metaphor in the image of the tiny figure whirling through a vortex is a repeated motif through which Small suggests the disorienting, perspective-shattering experience of illness - something close to what Scarry describes as the 'world destroying quality of pain'[25] (Figure 6).

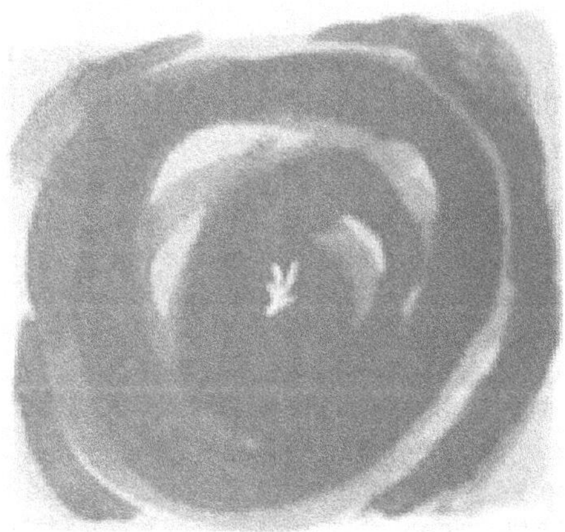

Fig. 6. Small, *Stitches* 165 (excerpt) © David Small. © Used with the permission of Pippin Properties, Inc.

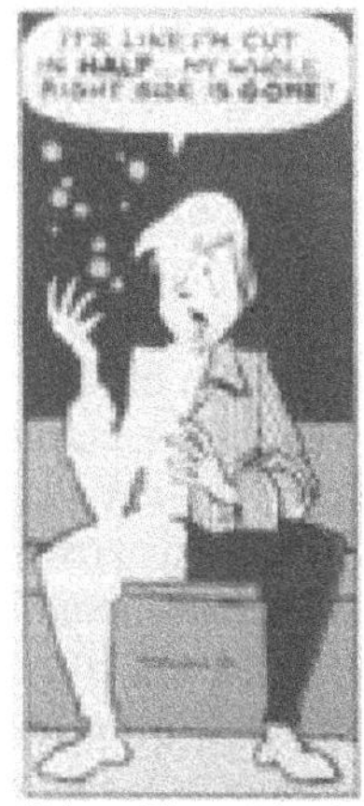

Fig. 7. Brian Fies, *Mom's Cancer* (excerpt) © Brian Fies. Used with the author's permission

Literalisation of metaphor is one of the simplest ways of representing pain in Comics - to take a different example, Brian Fies's memoir of his mother's cancer frequently renders the metaphors of illness material: he draws her with her left side blanked out when she has a stroke that freezes half of her body (Figure 7), and when she is balancing medicines with paradoxical and complicating side effects he depicts her walking a vanishing tightrope over a pit of dangers. This 'amplification through simplification'[26] responds to the frustrating 'nothing to show' of pain with visual translation of its metaphors and similes, and provides an objective correlative for this elusive and overwhelming encounter. Small frequently employs the representational shorthand of literalisation, though most often through dream sequences so that his use of symbols will not challenge the truth value of the story: because the representation of the real and imaginary through the comics medium is so fungible, it is easy to represent a literally splitting headache, or to draw a stabbing pain as a knife to the side. The metaphoric props of pain language are assembled seamlessly and rendered concretely.

Small is also often expressionistic. He uses abstraction and the blurring of boundaries between the inner self and the outer world in order to convey the disorienting, boundary shattering quality of pain and the way it permeates the subject's perception of the world. One of the most dazzling of these sequences comes after the operation. Small has gone into the hospital for what he has been told was the removal of a cyst: he has woken up with a wound stretching from his ear to his clavicle and with literally no voice, since during the operation one of his vocal chords was removed (Figure 8). In this scene, he is still unaware of the extent of the scar and that the operation removed a cancerous tumor, not a harmless cyst. He gets up to change his bandage, and in a mirror sees the evidence of the scar for the first time. The vision is presented to us in fragments and is doubly framed, first through the borders of the panel and then by the mirror of the bathroom cabinet. The mirror cuts off part of his head and his body beneath the shoulders: it shows him a reflection of himself, and that reflection is in parts. Earlier we examined aspect-to-aspect transition as a way to slow narration and create mood, but in this case it also shows the body broken into pieces. The image zooms in on the scar, as he and we vanish into the wound, which Small describes as a 'crusted black track of stitches; my smooth young throat slashed and laced back up like a bloody boot.' The scar is presented first horizontally, and then vertically, in a double exposure: in its horizontal aspect it resembles a mouth sewn into silence. And the wound seems to speak, or *something* speaks. Above the two vertical images of the scar is an unattributed fragment of dialogue: 'Surely this is not me.' 'No, friend. It surely is.' This scene mimics the dual movement of alienation and identification, the mirror that reflects Small back to himself as changed. On the next page the scar has faded to a patterns of lines and shadows; the facing panel transforms those lines into the stairs of the narrator's house, as his feet on the stairs ascend back to his room.

One of the striking elements of this sequence is the way it stutters between images, using the blanks around the pictures to heighten the emotional effect of the sequence and to deepen reader involvement as one puzzles through the connections between these different pieces. McCloud argues that comics can act as an 'art of the invisible' since the gutters or spaces between and around the panel boxes provide space for imagination, 'between the panels, none of our sense are required at all. Which is why all of our senses are engaged.'[27] Gutter language allows for the expression of the invisible, the unsayable; it also makes the reader a participant in the creation of the narrative. McCloud jokes that through gutter language the reader is made a partner in crime,[28] but we might call the reader instead a partner in witnessing. The suggestive gaps between the panels facilitate not simply proximity, but responsibility for co-crafting the narrative. This sequence exceeds language: much is implied here, but little is said. We need to navigate the space between the panels, to imagine or project Small's response, to imagine ourselves in his place. The scar speaks to us as well as to him: the dual movement of alienation and identification is also our own.

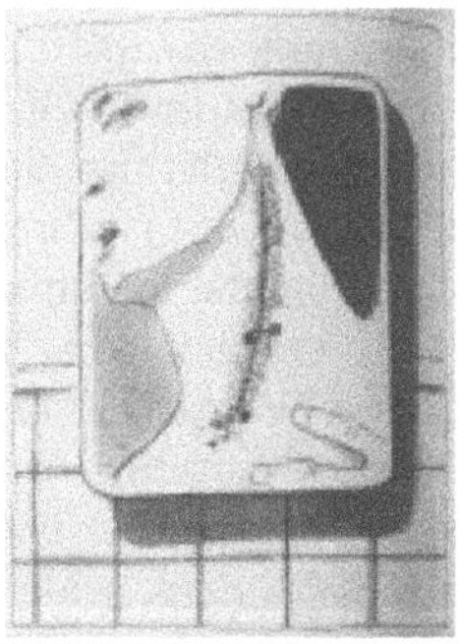

Fig. 8. Small, *Stitches* 190 (excerpt) © David Small

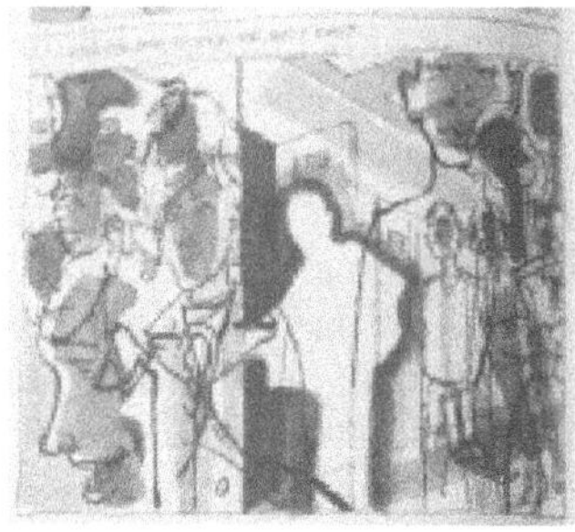

Fig. 9. *Stitches* 212 (excerpt). © David Small

Small's method of drawing figures frequently incorporates a literal and metaphoric core of shadow, a thick abstract wash that runs through the middle of his characters. Both Small's illness and family history form his black centre, and they threaten to swamp him in darkness and silence. 'When you have no voice you don't exist,' Small writes. 'Even among my old friends I felt invisible, a shadow flickering around the edges of every event.'[29] The party scene that Small draws reverses some of the conventions of figure drawing that he has established: in this picture, all the other figures are a mix of light and shadow while he is drawn as a thick outline framing nothing at all, a field of white (Figure 9). This negative definition mimics the reversal of black and white, of inside and outside, and of subject and field that is characteristic of an x-ray. The body is erased by darkness, while the bones show up, glowing white: but here the character is not even a skeleton, he is nothing at all. This vanished image replicates the vanishing of self, imposed by the disease and loss of voice. The disruption of convention lends itself to the representation of the intensity and disruptiveness of the encounter with pain. Small's experience of pain and isolation and his voicelessness threaten to obliterate his sense of self. He has recurrent dreams of disappearing into the cavern of his own mouth, or crawling into a building that, like the entrance to Wonderland, has a tiny door, and 'emerging each time, with the same sense of disbelief and despair, into that temple whose guts had been bombed.'[30] The word 'guts' makes the analogy visceral: Small is trapped in his own desecrated body and is unable to find his way out.

The destruction of language in Small's case is both figurative and literal, and the memoir dramatises the process of his return to speech and to self. The inability to speak the truth is part of his family's disease: their silence about his cancer is prefigured by their inability to speak of his grandmother's madness, his mother's lesbianism, and even the story of a great-grandfather who tried to commit suicide by drinking Drano and lived but never spoke another word since 'the poison had eaten away his vocal chords' (73). Two things give him back his voice. The first is a therapist who is not named in the book and appears in the comical, comforting guise of the white rabbit from *Alice in Wonderland*: his guide into the wonderland topsy-turvy reversals of his childhood experiences. The second thing that returns Small to language is art, and the book serves as a document of the power of art in testifying to illness and pain and constructing a language of recovery. The very first image of him in the book shows him drawing; in a later scene, he runs from a group of bullies, retreats into his room, begins to draw a picture and vanishes through the paper down a tunnel and into a cave where familiar cartoon characters greet him with open arms. Cartoons begin as his escape and turn out to be his cure. One of the most hopeful panels in the book depicts Small at his easel, surrounded by girls. The style of drawing is playful, the background is light and almost entirely lacks shadow. The text says, 'Art became my home. Not only did it give me back my voice, but art has given me everything I wanted or needed since.'[31] Art in the shape of comics is the dialectical response to the muteness of Small's childhood: it provides the language he needs to respond to his pain, and to make it into a thing of beauty.

Notes

[1] Ludwig Wittgenstein, *Philosophical Investigations*, trans. Elizabeth Anscombe (Oxford: Wiley-Blackwell, 2001), 384.
[2] Art Spiegelman, "Barefoot Gen: Comics after the Bomb," in *Barefoot Gen, Vol. 1: A Cartoon Story of Hiroshima* (San Francisco: Last Gasp, 2004), i.
[3] In 2011 a conference on Comics and Medicine at the Institute of English Studies, University of London, brought together critics, artists and medical practitioners in order to discuss both the representational possibility of medical comics and their potential contribution to medical and patient education. A growing body of interdisciplinary critical work has explored the contribution of comics in representing historic and collective trauma, psychic and physical illness, and in acting as both first-hand and second-hand witness to painful and traumatic experiences. Most of the work on trauma and comics has centered on *Maus*, and there is also a growing body of work on *Persepolis*. There is as yet no general study of trauma and comics, and many important works remain unexamined.
[4] Art Spiegelman, *In the Shadow of No Towers* (New York: Pantheon, 2004), iv.
[5] Susan Sontag , *On Photography* (New York: Picador, 2001), 20.
[6] Elaine Scarry, *The Body in Pain: The Making and Unmaking of the World* (Oxford: Oxford University Press, 1985), 20.

[7] Vladmir Nabokov, *Lectures on Don Quixote*, ed. Fredson Bowers (New York: Harcourt Brace, 1983), 56.
[8] Henri Bergson, *Laughter: An Essay on the Meaning of the Comic*, trans. Cloudesley Brereton (Los Angeles: Green Integer, 1998), 3.
[9] Ibid., 18.
[10] Ibid., 25.
[11] Comedic and fantasy violence continues alongside the development of sublimed violence in horror and superhero comics: the first belongs primarily to newspaper strips, while the second unfolds in comic books.
[12] Nonetheless, these pain cries were targeted by comics critics in the early seventies. In a 1971 *Times Education Supplement* editorial titled 'Violent and Deformed – the Prosecution Case' George Gale wrote, 'While violence is the main feature of these children's comics, the systematic destruction of the English language runs it a close second. The blows, falls, shrieks, crunches etc. are accompanied by a proliferation of non-words' (quoted in Martin Barker, *Comics: Ideology, Power and the Critics* [Manchester: University Press, 1989], 92).
[13] In *In the Shadow of No Towers* Spiegelman turns his back on the conventions of trauma comics that he helped establish in *Maus*: he abandons black and white for color, originality for pastiche, narrative for bricolage. The result is a complicated, layered, but far less emotionally engaging story. This is consistent with Spiegelman's critique: *In the Shadow of No Towers* rejects the easy seductions of narrative, in view of the way in which 9/11 had become a story used to mobilise a nation towards armed conflict.
[14] Justin Green, *Binky Brown Sampler* (San Francisco: Last Gasp, 1995), 10.
[15] Jared Gardner, 'Autography's Biography, 1972–2007,'*Biography* 31 (2008): 23.
[16] Green, *Binky Brown Sampler*, 4.
[17] The Wong-Baker pain scale, used in hospitals with children or people unable to comfortably use numbers or language to measure their pain, exploits this mode of identification with simplified, cartoon faces. You point to the face that is closest to the expression of your interior state: the cartoon face helps you measure and identify your own pain.
[18] Joe Sacco also uses typification as a tool for readerly identification. He draws in a mode of realist grotesque, but though his own face has a few identifying features - dark hair, thick lips, and a big nose - his eyes are obscured by thick, goggle-like glasses. These glasses serve to mask his face, and to remind us that in relation to the events he transcribes, he is our eyes. His role is as a set of eyes and ears, a mediator for the testimony of other people. We *see* the events he describes through him, but we never see him full-face.

[19] Mort Walker, *The Lexicon of Comicana* (Bloomington: iUniverse: 2000), 8. Walker's lexicon playfully responds to the need for a specific language for the emblems of cartooning. While some have quarreled with elements of Walker's nomenclature, many of his terms - plewds for sweat drops, hites for speed lines, and grawlixes, for curses - have entered into common usage both among critics and artists. See Dash Shaw, "Cartooning Symbolia," <http://www.dashshaw.com/ symbolia.html>, viewed March 18, 2012.
[20] Keiji Nakazawa, *Barefoot Gen* Vol. I: *A Cartoon History of Hiroshima* (San Francisco: Last Gasp, 2004), 237.
[21] David Small, Interview with Rebecca Touger, October 6, 2009 <http://www.smithmag.net/memoirville/2009/10/06/interview-david-small-author-of-stitches/>, viewed on October 15, 2010.
[22] McCloud, *Understanding Comics: The Invisible Art* (New York: HarperCollins, 1994), 74.
[23] Ibid., 103.
[24] Samuel Beckett, *Proust and Three Dialogues with Georges Duthuit* (Richmond: Calder, 1989), 13.
[25] Scarry, *Body in Pain*, 4.
[26] McCloud, *Understanding Comics*, 30.
[27] Ibid., 89.
[28] Ibid., 68.
[29] David Small, *Stitches: A Memoir* (New York: Norton, 2009), 213.
[30] Ibid., 242.
[31] Ibid., 30.

Bibliography

Acocella Marchetto, Marisa. *Cancer Vixen: A True Story*. Toronto: Knopf, 2006.

B. David. *Epileptic I*. Paris: L'Association, 2002.

Barker, Martin. *Comics: Ideology, Power and the Critics*. Manchester: University Press, 1989.

Barry, Lynda. *One! Hundred! Demons!* Seattle: Sasquatch Books, 2002.

Bechdel, Alison. *Fun Home: A Family Tragicomic*. Boston: Houghton Mifflin, 2006.

Beckett, Samuel. *Proust and Three Dialogues with Georges Duthuit.* Richmond: Calder, 1989.

Bergson, Henri. *Laughter: An Essay on the Meaning of the Comic*. Translated by Cloudesley Brereton. Los Angeles: Green Integer, 1998.

Fies, Brian. *Mom's Cancer*. New York: Abrams Image, 2006.

Gardner, Jared. 'Autography's Biography, 1972–2007.'*Biography* 31 (2008): 1-26.

Green, Justin. *Binky Brown Sampler*. San Francisco: Last Gasp, 1995.

Guibert, Emmanuel, Didier Lefèvre and Frédéric Lemercier. *The Photographer: Into War-Torn Afghanistan with Doctors without Borders*. Translated by Alexis Siegel. New York: First Second Books, 2009.

Herriman, George. *Krazy & Ignatz 1925-1926: There is a Heppy Lend Fur Fur A-waay*. Seattle: Fantagraphics, 2000.

Groensteen, Thierry. *The System of Comics.* Translated by Bart Beatty and Nick Nguyen. Jackson: University Press of Mississippi, 2007.

McCloud, Scott. *Understanding Comics: The Invisible Art.* New York: HarperCollins, 1994.

Nabokov, Vladimir. *Lectures on Don Quixote*. Edited by Fredson Bowers. New York: Harcourt Brace, 1983.

Nakazawa, Keiji. *Barefoot Gen*. Vol. 1*: A Cartoon History of Hiroshima*. San Francisco: Last Gasp, 2004.

Peeters, Frederik. *Blue Pills: A Positive Love Story*. New York: Houghton Mifflin Harcourt, 2008.

Pekar, Harvey, Joyce Brabner, and Frank Stack. *Our Cancer Year*. Philadelphia: Running Press, 1994.

Sacco, Joe. *Safe Area Gorazde: The War in Eastern Bosnia 1992-1995*. Seattle: Fantagraphics, 2002.

Satrapi, Marjane. *Persepolis: The Story of a Childhood.* New York: Pantheon, 2003.

Scarry, Elaine. *The Body in Pain: The Making and Unmaking of the World.* Oxford: Oxford University Press, 1985.

Seagle, Steven T. and Teddy Kristiansen. *It's a Bird.* New York: Vertigo, 2005.

Shaw, Dash. "Cartooning Symbolia." <http://www.dashshaw.com/symbolia.html>. Viewed March 18, 2012.

Small, David. *Stitches: A Memoir*. New York: Norton, 2009.

———. Interview with Rebecca Touger. October 6, 2009. <http://www.smithmag.net/memoirville/2009/10/06/interview-david-small-author-of-stitches/>. Viewed on October 15, 2010.

Sontag , Susan. *On Photography.* New York: Picador, 2001.

Spiegelman, Art. 'Barefoot Gen: Comics after the Bomb.' In Keiji Nakazawa, *Barefoot Gen*, vol. 1: *A Cartoon History of Hiroshima.* San Francisco: Last Gasp, 2004.

———. *In the Shadow of No Towers*. New York: Pantheon, 2004.

———. *Maus I: A Survivor's Tale: My Father Bleeds History*. New York: Pantheon, 1986.

———. *Maus II: A Survivor's Tale: And Here My Troubles Began.* New York: Pantheon, 1992.

Walker, Mort. *The Lexicon of Comicana.* Bloomington: iUniverse: 2000.

Williams, Ian. <http://www.graphicmedicine.org>. Viewed on July 19, 2011.

Wittgenstein, Ludwig. *Philosophical Investigations*. Translated by Elizabeth Anscombe. Oxford: Wiley-Blackwell, 2001.

Abbreviations

APA	American Psychiatric Association
ASD	Accouchement sans douleur [Painless Childbirth]
ASPO	American Society for Psychoprophylaxis in Obstetrics
BACE	Boston Association for Childbirth Education
CCCM	Corpus Christianorum Continuatio Mediaeualis
CGT	Confédération générale du travail [General Confederation of Labor]
DSM	Diagnostic and Statistical Manual of Mental Disorders
IASP	International Association for the Study of Pain
JAMA	Journal of the American Medical Association
JEGP	Journal of English and Germanic Philology
MCA	Maternity Center Association
PL	Patrologiae cursus completus: Series Latina. Edited by J.-P. Migne. 221 vols. Paris, 1857–1864.
PSSP	*Polnoe Sobranie Sochinenii i Pisem* [*Complete Works* (of Anton Chekhov)] in 30 vols. Moscow: Nauka, 1973-1988.
RSFSR	Rossiiskaia sovetskaia federativnaia sotsialisticheskaia respublika [Russian Soviet Federated Socialist Republic]
SSR	Sovetskaia sotsialisticheskaia respublika [Soviet Socialist Republic]

Notes on Contributors

Rebecca A. Adelman is an Assistant Professor of Media & Communication Studies at the University of Maryland, Baltimore County (UMBC), where her research and teaching interests include visual culture, citizenship and cultural studies of terrorism and war. Some of her work on these subjects appears in *The Journal of Men & Masculinities, Jura Gentium Cinema* and *Continuum: Journal of Media & Cultural Studies.*

Michal Altbauer-Rudnik is a fellow at the Israel Institute for Advanced Studies and Hanadiv post-doctoral fellow at the Department of History, The Hebrew University of Jerusalem. She teaches at The Hebrew University of Jerusalem and at Sapir College. Her research focuses on the social context of early modern lovesickness. She has published several works on this topic, such as 'Prescribing Love: Italian Jewish Physicians Writing on Lovesickness in the Sixteenth and Seventeenth Centuries' (2009) and 'Love, Madness and Social Order: Love Melancholy in France and England in the Late Sixteenth and the Early Seventeenth Centuries,' *Gesnerus* (2006). Her research interests include social history of medicine, cultural psychiatry and history of emotions.

Rebecca Anna Bitenc is currently working on a doctoral thesis in English Literature at Durham University, UK, after completing her M.A. in English, French and Psychology at the Albert-Ludwigs-Universität Freiburg, Germany. Her thesis on dementia in contemporary literature explores how the alleged loss of self in dementia is expressed across different genres - with a particular focus on the ethics of literary form. Her PhD project is funded by an Arts and Humanities Research Council Doctoral Scholarship.

Michèle Bokobza Kahan is Associate Professor in French Culture and Literature at the Department of French in Tel-Aviv University. She is the author of *Libertinage et folie dans le roman du 18ᵉ siècle* (2000) and *Dulaurens et son œuvre: Un auteur marginal, déviances discursives et bigarrures philosophiques* (2010). She has published articles on religious testimonial discourses about miracles and convulsions that occurred in early eighteenth-century Paris. Recently she published 'Ethos in Testimony,' *Eighteenth-Century Studies* 43 (2010), and 'Die Aufklärung im Dienst der Wunder,' in *Politik der Zeugenschaft*, ed. Sibylle Schmidt, Sybille Krämer and Ramon Voges (Bielefeld: Transcript, 2011).

Esther Cohen is Professor of Medieval History at the Department of History, The Hebrew University of Jerusalem. She has published on popular culture as well as on law and crime in the middle ages. During the past decade she has been working on pain in the middle ages. Her most important publications are *The Crossroads of Justice: Law and Society in Late Medieval France* (1993), *Peaceable Domain, Certain Justice: Crime and Society in Fifteenth-Century Paris* (1996) and *The Modulated Scream: Pain in Late Medieval Culture* (2010).

Na'ama Cohen-Hanegbi is a lecturer in medieval history at the department of History in Tel Aviv University and Hanadiv Post-Doctoral Fellow. She published articles in *Poetica* and in *Le sujet des émotions au Moyen Âge* on the conceptualisation and treatment of emotions in the Middle Ages. Her research field is the interactions between religion and medicine in the period.

Manuela Consonni is Senior Lecturer in Contemporary Jewish History and Head of the Italian Section in the Department of Romance and Latin American Studies, the Hebrew University of Jerusalem. She is the author of *Resistenza or Shoah: The Memory of the Deportation and Extermination in Italy, 1945-1985* (2010, Hebrew). Her articles appeared in *Partial Answers*, *Jewish History*, and *Quaderni Storici*. Her current research project is "'Bracketing Death': Philosophical and Anthropological Analysis of Death and the History of the Shoah."

Otniel E. Dror, MD, PhD (History) is Joel Wilbush Chair in Medical Anthropology and Head of the Section for the History of Medicine in the Medical Faculty of the Hebrew University of Jerusalem. His research focuses on the history of the study of emotions during the nineteenth and twentieth centuries. He is the author of *Blush, Adrenaline, Excitement: Modernity and the Study of Emotions, 1860-1940* (under revision for the University of Chicago Press). His articles have appeared in *Isis*, *Configurations*, *Science in Context*, and *Social Research*. His new book project is entitled: *The Adrenaline Century, 1900-2000*.

Sascha Benjamin Fink is a doctoral student at the Institute of Cognitive Science, University of Osnabrück, working on the role and status of introspection in neuroscientific research on consciousness and the problem of introspective disagreement. He is the author of 'Independence and Connections of Pain and Suffering' (*Journal of Consciousness Studies*, 2011) and a member of the Interdisciplinary Programme on Suffering and Pain at the Université de Luxembourg.

Ariela Freedman is Associate Professor at the Liberal Arts College, Concordia University. She works on First World War narratives, memory studies, literary modernism and comics. She is the author of Death, Men and Modernism (2003) and has recently published articles in a number of journals, including *Literature Compass*, *James Joyce Quarterly*, *Joyce Studies Annual* and *Journal of Modern Literature*. She is currently working on the German graphic artist Charlotte Salomon, and is developing a longer project on comics and pain.

Anna Leimumäki is working on a doctoral dissertation about illness narratives at the Department of Comparative Literature, University of Tampere (Finland). Her interests include interface between literary, social and health studies, meanings of illness, the process of narrativising experience and narrative devices. Having worked for several years in health-care projects, she is seeking new ways to develop more client-oriented practices in health care and to raise the consciousness of experience expertise.

Nourit Melcer-Padon completed her PhD thesis in English Literature at the Hebrew University in Jerusalem. Her thesis on the function of literary masks was awarded the Shlomniuk Prize for outstanding thesis in the humanities. She lectures in Italian and French literature at the Hebrew University of Jerusalem. Her fields of study range from literature and literary theory, to literary anthropology and cultural studies. She is currently engaged in research in the fields of witnessing and narrative techniques.

Paula A. Michaels is Associate Professor of History at the University of Iowa (USA), where she specialises in the social history of medicine and health in the former Soviet Union. She is the author of *Curative Powers: Medicine and Empire in Stalin's Central Asia* (2003), winner of the Association for Women in Slavic Studies Heldt Prize and a finalist for the PEN Center USA Literary Award. She is currently working on a transnational history of psychoprophylaxis, also known as the Lamaze method of childbirth.

Natalia Pervukhina-Kamyshnikova is Professor of Russian at the University of Tennessee, USA. She is the author of *Anton Chekhov: The Sense and the Nonsense* (1993) and *V. S. Pecherin: Emigrant na vse vremena* [*V. S. Pecherin: An Emigrant for All Seasons*] (2006). Her articles on Chekhov, Solzhenitsyn, S. Zayaitsky, Bulgakov, Herzen, and Pecherin have been published in USA, Canada, Poland, Israel and Russia. Her field of research includes Russian intellectual history, political and literary emigration and the historical representation of Russia in American scholarship and media.

Shlomith Rimmon-Kenan is Emeritus Professor of English and Comparative Literature at the Hebrew University of Jerusalem. She is the author of *The Concept of Ambiguity: The Example of James* (1977), *Narrative Fiction: Contemporary Poetics* (1983), and *A Glance Beyond Doubt: Narration, Representation, Subjectivity* (1996). She is the editor of *Discourse in Literature and Psychoanalysis* (1987). Her current fields of research are illness narratives and theory of interdisciplinarity.

Leona Toker is Professor in the English Department, the Hebrew University of Jerusalem. She is the author of *Nabokov: The Mystery of Literary Structures* (1989), *Eloquent Reticence: Withholding Information in Fictional Narrative* (1993), *Return from the Archipelago: Narratives of Gulag Survivors* (2000), *Towards the Ethics of Form in Fiction: Narratives of Cultural Remission* (2010), and articles on English, American and Russian literature. She is the editor of *Commitment in Reflection: Essays in Literature and Moral Philosophy* (1994). She has founded and is editing *Partial Answers: A Journal of Literature and the History of Ideas*.

Nathaniel Wolloch is an independent Israeli scholar. He received his PhD from the Hebrew University of Jerusalem. His fields of research include early modern cultural and intellectual history, the history of attitudes toward nature and animals, the Enlightenment, and the history of historiography. He is the author of *Subjugated Animals: Animals and Anthropocentrism in Early Modern European Culture* (2006) and *History and Nature in the Enlightenment: Praise of the Mastery of Nature in Eighteenth-Century Historical Literature* (2011).

R. F. Yeager is Professor and Chair, Department of English and Modern Languages, University of West Florida. His field of research is Medieval Literatures and Languages, especially Old and Middle English, He is the author of *John Gower's Poetic: The Search for a New Arion* (1990); a co-author of *Who Murdered Chaucer? A Medieval Mystery* (2003); editor of *On John Gower: Essays at the Millennium* (2007), editor and translator of *John Gower: The French Balades* (2011).

www.ingramcontent.com/pod-product-compliance
Lightning Source LLC
LaVergne TN
LVHW020650300926
849161LV00004B/880